Multilevel
Analysis *of*
Individuals
and Cultures

Multilevel Analysis *of* Individuals *and* Cultures

Edited by

Fons J. R. van de Vijver

Dianne A. van Hemert

Ype H. Poortinga

LEA Lawrence Erlbaum Associates
Taylor & Francis Group

New York   London

For more information about this and related titles, please visit www.researchmethodsarena.com.

Lawrence Erlbaum Associates
Taylor & Francis Group
270 Madison Avenue
New York, NY 10016

Lawrence Erlbaum Associates
Taylor & Francis Group
27 Church Road
Hove, East Sussex BN3 2FA

Printed in the United States of America on acid-free paper
10 9 8 7 6 5 4 3 2 1

International Standard Book Number-13: 978-0-8058-5892-1 (Softcover) 978-0-8058-5891-4 (Hardcover)

Library of Congress Cataloging-in-Publication Data

Multilevel analysis of individuals and cultures / author/editor(s), Fons J.R. van de
Vijver, Dianne A. van Hemert, and Ype H. Poortinga.
p. cm.
Includes bibliographical references and index.
ISBN 978-0-8058-5892-1 -- ISBN 978-0-8058-5891-4 1.
Sociology--Research--Methodology. 2. Multilevel models (Statistics) 3.
Cross-cultural studies. I. Vijver, Fons J. R. van de. II. Hemert, Dianne A. van. III.
Poortinga, Ype H., 1939-

HM571.M85 2008
300.7'2--dc22   2007033258

Visit the Taylor & Francis Web site at
http://www.taylorandfrancis.com

and the LEA and Psychology Press Web site at
http://www.psypress.com

Contents

Preface

The present volume provides an overview of issues in multilevel analysis and interpretation of data at the levels of individuals and cultures. This book is relevant and, we hope, of interest for researchers who study the relationship between behavior and culture. These include cross-cultural psychologists examining differences between countries in, for example, values, personality, and variables related to organizational behavior, as well as researchers in other fields who extend their datasets across cultural populations. The book is intended to be a source of information for the growing numbers of researchers in the social sciences who work with data at different levels, such as psychologists, economists, sociologists, cultural anthropologists, and political scientists.

AGGREGATION AND DISAGGREGATION

Conventional models in cross-cultural research simply combine individual and supraindividual factors and often assume uniformity of context, such as ecological conditions or cultural norms, for all individuals. More recent models increasingly address variables at different levels, such as individual scores that are aggregated at country level. The use of information at a higher level in the hierarchy of nested observations (aggregation) or at a lower level (disaggregation) leads to various interesting and often complex conceptual and methodological questions. This book explores central issues in the transfer of information across levels in the hierarchy: Under what conditions can information obtained at one level be validly applied at another level? Which procedures can be applied to determine cross-level applicability? What can be done in cases of incomplete applicability?

THEORETICAL, METHODOLOGICAL, AND EMPIRICAL DEVELOPMENTS

Theoretically, multilevel comparisons in cross-cultural research have their roots in various research traditions. One of these is the culture-and-personality school, which was an early attempt to employ psychological concepts derived from Freudian theory in order to describe entire cultural groups. Another approach in which the exchange between individual and societal level factors is clearly bidirectional can be found in cultural psychology; here individual and culture are seen as inherently linked. In a third approach, culture-comparative research, psychological data are collected on samples of participants from different cultures, and differences between samples tend to be explained in psychological terms.

For cross-cultural psychological research, two types of multilevel modeling are important. The first addresses the question whether there is comparability (or equivalence) of the meaning of data across cultures. The second kind of multilevel analysis comes under names such as *hierarchical linear models* (HLM) or *multilevel models*. A particular construct is seen as being influenced by factors at different levels of aggregation. Statistical techniques have been developed to incorporate all levels of aggregation in a single analysis so as to compare the relative influence of the predictors at the various levels.

Empirically there has been a steady increase in the availability of large datasets, in which individual-level variables are available for a wide number of countries. By now, a number of datasets with individual scores on psychological variables, such as values and personality dimensions, have been gathered in a substantial number of countries. Some of these data are available in the public domain either for free or for a small fee, such as the International Social Survey Program (http://www.issp.org), the World Values Survey (http://www.worldvaluessurvey.org), and the European Social Survey (http://www.europeansocialsurvey.org). It is realistic to assume that the number of such datasets will increase.

In summary, there are important developments in the three areas of theory, methodology, and empirical findings, which can be expected to give impetus to the further extension and application of multilevel models. The main aim of the present book is to advance these developments by presenting the work of various specialists who work in one or more of the three areas. Together, the chapters provide insight in characteristics of multilevel models as studied in various domains of cross-cultural psychology. The chapters also point to areas in which further work is needed.

OVERVIEW OF THE BOOK

The book is divided into four parts: the first part provides the conceptual background of multilevel analyses; the second part provides a methodological overview of multilevel approaches; the third, more empirical, section of the book describes models and applications of the multilevel issue in specific research domains; and the fourth part is meant to integrate the previous chapters.

In part I, two chapters set the stage by presenting theoretical and conceptual underpinnings. The Editors begin by outlining the basic conceptual issues in multilevel research involving individuals and cultures. They present a taxonomy of multilevel models based on the distinction between disaggregation and aggregation and on different degrees of interaction between levels. They also give an overview of different types of fallacies in multilevel research. Adamopoulos provides an overview of current models and past approaches to linking individual- and culture-level variables. He discusses definitions of level and culture, arguments for isomorphism and nonisomorphism between cultural and individual characteristics, and methodological issues in cross-level analyses (e.g., the ecological fallacy).

The two chapters in part II describe methodological aspects of multilevel research. Fontaine's contribution addresses the meaning of constructs at different levels of aggregation and discusses different approaches to multilevel equivalence, focusing on observed variables. He presents data-analytic techniques to deal with bias and equivalence across levels. Selig, Card, and Little describe the use of structural equation modeling in dealing with multilevel issues, focusing on latent variables. They distinguish multiple group mean and covariance structures (MACS) modeling for a small number of cultures and multilevel structural equation (MLSEM) modeling for dealing with a larger number of cultures.

Part III deals with multilevel applications and models in various promising research areas of psychology, including control, values, organizational behavior, social beliefs, well-being, personality, response styles, school performance, family, and acculturation. The earlier chapters of this part emphasize conceptual issues, while the later chapters are more empirically oriented and deal more with validity issues in aggregation models. Yamaguchi, Okumura, Chua, Morio, and Yates describe how cross-cultural insights are important for understanding the concept of control at both country and individual level. They present a conceptual analysis of control and the interactions between individual and cultural or contextual factors. Oyserman and Uskul deal with one of the most popular topics in cross-cultural research: the individualism-collectivism dimension. Their chapter explores this dimension at individual and country level and suggests ways in which the constructs can be conceptualized at both levels. Fischer's chapter deals with behavior of individuals within organizations as a function of three levels of factors: individual, organizational, and cultural. The potential for models that link these three levels is discussed, drawing from the relatively rich literature on organizational research.

The first of the more empirically oriented chapters is by Leung and Bond. They explore the issue of the similarity of meaning at individual and country level for social axioms or beliefs, presenting findings at the two levels of analysis. Correlates of social axioms at the individual and the country level are described. An overview of individual-level and country-level research on the correlates of happiness is given by Lucas and Diener. In addition, they present results of a multilevel factor analysis of well-being measures, establishing the comparability of the well-being construct at different levels of analysis. McCrae and Terracciano summarize research on the Five-Factor Model at the individual level and at the culture level. They also report new data on the culture-level correlates of personality factors. Smith and Fischer present a series of multilevel analyses on response styles, more specifically acquiescence and extreme response style, demonstrating interactions in response style effects between individuals' predispositions and their cultural context. Stanat and Lüdtke describe measures taken to ensure the equivalence of international assessments of student performance. They also review large-scale educational achievement projects and evaluate the contribution to our understanding of multilevel models in the domain of student performance.

Finally, chapters 13 and 14 describe research from another starting point: they begin with group (supraindividual) concepts and extrapolate to the level of the individual. Mylonas, Pavlopoulos, and Georgas describe different aspects of the family at the individual and country level of aggregation. Multilevel results are presented that are based on the large cross-cultural family project initiated by the third author. Nauck's contribution provides an overview of models of acculturation, in which variables at the levels of the individual and the ethnic group are studied jointly. In addition, empirical studies in the acculturation domain are interpreted from a multilevel perspective.

In part IV the Editors summarize basic problems and solutions offered in the various chapters. They provide an overview of the kinds of questions addressed in multilevel models, describe which problems have been solved, which theoretical and methodological issues are still open, and which areas look promising for the application of the various approaches and models.

Fons van de Vijver
Dianne van Hemert
Ype Poortinga

Author Note

The editors thank Rinus Verkooijen for his editorial assistance. We would also like to thank our reviewers, Todd D. Little, Kansas University and Ramaswami Mahalingam, University of Michigan. Finally, we would like to thank the team of Taylor and Francis (Debra Riegert, Rebecca Larsen, and Glenon Butler) for their skilful support.

Contributors

Editors

Fons van de Vijver
Tilburg University
Tilburg, The Netherlands

Dianne A. van Hemert
University of Amsterdam
Amsterdam, The Netherlands

Ype H. Poortinga
Tilburg University
Tilburg, The Netherlands

Authors

John Adamopoulos
Grand Valley State University
Allendale, Michigan, USA

Michael H. Bond
Chinese University of Hong Kong
Hong Kong, SAR

Noel A. Card
University of Illinois at Urbana
Champaign
Champaign, Illinois, USA

Hannah Faye Chua
University of Michigan
Ann Arbor, Michigan, USA

Ed Diener
University of Illinois
Champaign, Illinois, USA

Ronald Fischer
Victoria University of Wellington
Wellington, New Zealand

Johnny R. J. Fontaine
Ghent University
Ghent, Belgium

James Georgas
University of Athens
Athens, Greece

Kwok Leung
City University of Hong Kong
Hong Kong, SAR

Todd D. Little
University of Kansas
Lawrence, Kansas, USA

Richard E. Lucas
Michigan State University
East Lansing, Michigan, USA

Oliver Lüdtke
Max Planck Institute for Human
Development
Berlin, Germany

Robert R. McCrae
National Institute on Aging
Baltimore, Maryland, USA

Hiroaki Morio
University of Tokyo
Tokyo, Japan

Kostas Mylonas
University of Athens
Athens, Greece

Bernhard Nauck
University of Chemnitz
Chemnitz, Germany

Taichi Okumura
University of Tokyo
Tokyo, Japan

Daphna Oyserman
University of Michigan
Ann Arbor, Michigan, USA

Vassilis Pavlopoulos
University of Athens
Athens, Greece

James P. Selig
University of Kansas
Lawrence, Kansas, USA

Peter B. Smith
University of Sussex
Brighton, United Kingdom

Petra Stanat
Freie Universität Berlin
Berlin, Germany

Antonio Terracciano
National Institute on Aging
Baltimore, Maryland, USA

Ayse Uskul
University of Michigan
Ann Arbor, Michigan, USA

Susumu Yamaguchi
University of Tokyo
Tokyo, Japan

J. Frank Yates
University of Michigan
Ann Arbor, Michigan, USA

Part I

Conceptual Issues

1

Conceptual Issues in Multilevel Models

Fons J. R. van de Vijver, Dianne A. van Hemert, Ype H. Poortinga

Multilevel models are popular these days. Software engineering, semantics, organization studies, education, sociology, and psychology are among the branches of science with a keen interest in these models. Let us give an example. In the course of development children acquire common words for colors available in their language. At a young age children sharing the same language do not all know the same number of color words; there are individual differences. There are also cultural (linguistic) differences in the number of words known to young children. Each language has basic color terms, but the cross-language variability is considerable. Some languages have more terms than others; a given term may refer to a part of the visible spectrum for which there is more than one term in some other language. For example, many languages have a single word for the colors designated with blue and green in English (Berlin & Kay, 1969). It follows that the number of color words known by a child has an individual component and a language component. Differences between children within a language group will have to do with age and cognitive competence. Differences between children not speaking the same language are likely to be a function of the number of color words available in their respective languages. Thus, a cross-cultural study of children's color vocabulary requires different explanations for individual and cultural differences. Individual differences may be related to age, intelligence, and socioeconomic status, while the explanation of cultural differences would require a model of the emergence of color terms in various languages. As a consequence, differences between individuals within cultures should not be interpreted in the same way as differences between children with different mother tongues: The analysis of individual and cultural variance in the number of used color terms requires a multilevel model.

The present chapter gives an overview of current conceptualizations and models in the field of multilevel models. In the next section we introduce the most important basic distinctions in multilevel models and briefly review conceptualizations of cross-level transfer as proposed in the literature. The third section deals with interpretation issues in aggregation and disaggregation; the (dis)similarity of meaning of concepts and measures is discussed. The fourth section reviews methodological issues in multilevel analysis in cross-cultural research. The fifth section briefly discusses advances in statistical modeling which enable a more sophisticated treatment of multilevel data structures. More specifically, we describe cross-level equivalence models and hierarchical linear models. We draw conclusions in the final section.

WHAT ARE MULTILEVEL MODELS?

Three defining characteristics of multilevel models in cross-cultural psychology research require further explanation. First, in their minimal form such models include phenomena at two levels, such as the cultural level and the individual level. There should be a relationship between the two levels, which usually means that either there is a line of causation from cultural to individual factors with individual behavior being influenced by cultural context, or individual and cultural factors coconstitute or define each other. However, more advanced multilevel models often include at least three levels with feedback loops.

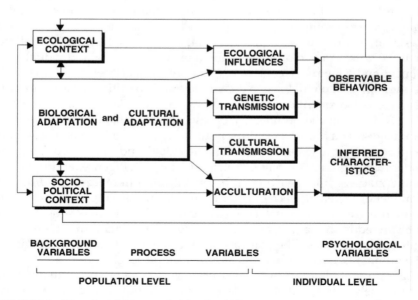

FIGURE 1.1   Ecocultural framework (after Berry, Poortinga, Segall, & Dasen, 2002).

For example, the ecocultural framework attempts to link cultural and ecological factors to psychological characteristics (see Figure 1.1; Berry, 1976; Berry, Poortinga, Segall, & Dasen, 2002). The antecedent variables of the framework are population-level characteristics, such as the eco-logical and the sociopolitical context. The outcome variables are observable behaviors (e.g., mother–child interactions), and individuals' inferred psychological characteristics (e.g., personality traits and cognitive styles). Through intervening process variables such as cultural transmission, population-level characteristics are assumed to influence individual-level characteristics. At the same time the outcome variables provide input for antecedent variables at the population-level, thereby defining dynamic and causal links. A second example of an elaborate multilevel model comes from acculturation research. Acculturation conditions such as the size of the ethnic group and immigration policy of the country of settle-ment are examples of relevant antecedent variables (Arends-Tóth & Van de Vijver, 2006; see Figure 1.2). Intervening variables are attitudes toward host and ethnic culture (acculturation orientations) and coping styles. Out-put variables are psychological adjustment (feelings of distress and well-being) and sociocultural competence in the host culture (e.g., knowledge of the mainstream language) and in the culture of origin (e.g., knowledge

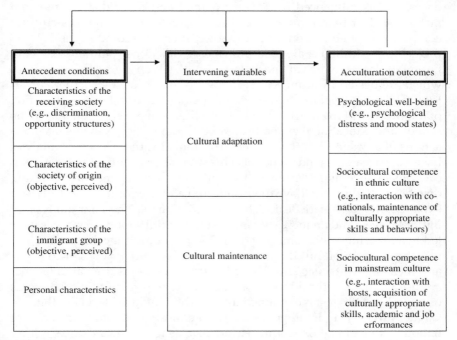

FIGURE 1.2 A conceptual framework for the study of acculturation (after Arends-Tóth & Van de Vijver, 2006).

of ethnic language). These three levels are linked in feedback loops (see also Nauck, this volume).

Other well-known examples come from developmental psychology, such as the developmental niche model (Super & Harkness, 1986, 1997), which holds that cultures structure the daily environments of infants. The niche has three interrelated subsystems: (1) the physical and social settings of the child; (2) the culturally regulated customs of childcare and child rearing; and (3) the parental ethnotheories of the caregivers. Another example from developmental psychology is Bronfenbrenner (1977, 1979), who viewed the individual's experience "as a set of nested structures, each inside the next, like a set of Russian dolls" (Bronfenbrenner, 1979, p. 22). Bronfenbrnner postulated four interrelated systems that together shape individual development: (1) the microsystem is defined by the attitudes and behaviors of persons in the immediate environment, such as peers, siblings, and parents; (2) the mesosystem includes settings such as the home, day-care center, and school; (3) the exosystem is made up of more distant settings, such as school boards and health care; while (4) the macrosystem identifies the broad cultural ecology of human development.

The second defining characteristic of multilevel models in cross-cultural psychology concerns the hierarchical structure (Smith, 2002). Multilevel studies start from hierarchical models in which individual behavior influences, and is influenced by, more proximal and more distal contextual factors. A clear hierarchy of nested structures is found in cross-cultural comparisons of educational performance, such as studied in the TIMMS project (e.g., Mullins et al., 2000; Stanat & Lüdtke, this volume). Pupils are nested in classes, which are nested in schools, which are nested in regions, which are nested in countries. Each level of this nested structure constitutes a distinct level of analysis. Mathematics performance is a function of intelligence of the individual student, climate of the class, quality of the school, and educational expenditure of the country level, as well as interactions of any subset of these levels. Traditionally, these levels of analysis have been treated as independent. This was mainly motivated by statistical convenience and reinforced by a history of independently working disciplines that tend to have their preferred and unique level of study and explanation. New statistical techniques that enable the joint analysis of multiple levels and an increased interest in multidisciplinary studies have led to a growing appreciation of the relevance of multilevel models.

A third aspect of multilevel models is the use of two types of concepts and measures: intrinsic and derived. *Intrinsic* concepts are variables that are used at their natural level. For example, variance in individual scores on a mathematics test is explained in terms of individual-level intelligence (as measured by an intelligence test) and educational quality in terms of national educational expenditure. Intrinsic usage implies that each level in the conceptual model or statistical analysis will have its own set of unique concepts and variables. The ecocultural model (Berry et al., 2002), the developmental niche model (Super & Harkness, 1986), and the experimental ecology model (Bronfenbrenner, 1979) are examples of models in which different variables are studied at individual and cultural level.

There is *derived* usage of concepts and measures when data are collected at one level and used at another level. Derived characteristics can either be aggregated or disaggregated. There is aggregation when data collected at a lower level are used as indices about a higher level. The use of derived characteristics is common in studies of country-level differences in psychological (individual-level) scores. In such studies some score statistic of a country sample of individuals, such as the mean or standard deviation, is used as a country-level indicator. For example, aggregated personality data are used to explain variance in social indicators, such as criminality rates.

There is disaggregation when data collected at a higher level are used at a lower level. In this case the available data pertain to social institutions, while expectations are derived about individuals. Society-level data that have been used in cross-cultural psychology include features such as human rights observance, enrolment ratios in formal education, age distribution, the country's status of individualism-collectivism, and gross national product per capita (GNP).

A study employs a multilevel design if data are based on a hierarchical structure and this multiple structure is considered in the data analysis. In general, we can distinguish between monolevel and multilevel studies on the one hand and between studies that use or do not use (dis)aggregated data on the other hand. These two dimensions are conceptually independent; their combination leads to the four cells of Table 1.1. The most common kinds of studies in the context of the current book are the multilevel models of the right column. However, monolevel studies that use (dis)aggregated data are also relevant here because they bring about various issues that are described in the present chapter and book (such as multilevel fallacies and possible meaning shifts after (dis)aggregation).

TABLE 1.1

Number of Levels in a Study and (Dis)aggregation

Use of (dis)aggregated data	Number of levels	
	One (Monolevel)	Two or more (Multilevel)
Yes	Monolevel studies using (dis)aggregated data	Multilevel studies using (dis)aggregated data
No	Monolevel studies using intrinsic data	Studies with intrinsic data at each level

A few examples may help to illustrate the distinction we introduce here. A study of the relationship between average intelligence scores in a country and educational expenditure is not a multilevel study. Rather, it is a monolevel study that applies aggregated individual-level intelligence data as country-level indicators. The research question and statistical analysis do not involve multiple levels because the analysis deals exclusively with country-level variables. As a further illustration, let us take a researcher who is interested in the relationship of gender and reading achievement. Gender is a dichotomous variable at individual level but a continuous variable at country level, as the "average" gender score refers to the proportion of males and females in a sample. An individual-level analysis would address male–female differences in reading achievement, while a monolevel analysis at class level would deal with the relationship between gender composition and reading achievement based on data aggregated at class level (e.g., do classes with more girls perform better on reading achievement tests?). An analysis of whether boys perform better in classes with more girls would require a multilevel approach; here individual- and cross-level data are to be considered simultaneously.

AGGREGATION/DISAGGREGATION AND INTERACTION IN MULTILEVEL MODELS

The basic issues of addressing phenomena at two or more hierarchically nested levels and studying relations between levels can be represented in various ways. Existing models can be said to differ in two dimensions. The first refers to the use of *intrinsic or derived (either aggregated or disaggregated) variables,* as described above. The use and interpretation of intrinsic variables in multilevel models is usually straightforward. However, more conceptual issues arise in the use and interpretation of derived variables. The second dimension involves the *nature of the relation (interaction)* between the dimensions. For example, in some models higher levels influence lower levels, like educational expenditure influences reading achievement at individual level. In other models variables at different levels can jointly produce an outcome, like reading performance of male and female pupils (at individual level) and gender composition of the class (at class level). We will describe these two dimensions in more detail.

Derived Models: Isomorphism and Nonisomorphism

How can individual-level and nation-level constructs be linked? We distinguish two kinds of relationships: isomorphic and nonisomorphic relationships. Phenomena at two different levels show an *isomorphic* relationship if there is a monotonic function describing the relationship between them. Such a relationship amounts to identity of concepts at different levels; individual and cross-cultural differences have the same meaning. Isomorphism is a layered, hierarchical concept; various kinds of isomorphism can be distinguished, ranging from identity of functions (see also Adamopoulos, this volume) to identity of scores across levels. The second kind of relationship to link individual- and culture-level phenomena can be called nonisomorphic, which is a generic term for all kinds of models in which individual and cultural aspects do not have the same structure.

Isomorphic Models

The various isomorphic models that have been proposed in the cross-cultural literature can be reduced to two kinds, depending on whether the emphasis is on individual characteristics as determined by cultural features or vice versa. The latter kind is illustrated by anthropological work on personality and culture, starting with the notion of "Volksseele" (soul of the people) that was common in the late 19th and early 20th century (Wundt, 1912). In the 20th century, culture-level psychological concepts were frequently formulated in the culture-and-personality school (Bock, 1999; Jahoda, 1982). Benedict (1934) viewed culture as "personality writ large"; she characterized an entire cultural population in terms of a unique personality configuration that supposedly applied to all its members. Later researchers relaxed this assumption of strict homogeneity, attributing the same basic character or modal character to all individuals within a culture (Kardiner & Linton, 1945). Still later this was further weakened to become "national character," a collection of characteristic traits present among the citizens of a particular nation (Peabody, 1967, 1985). The culture-and-personality school has shown a shift from a single overarching personality syndrome shared by virtually all members of a culture to sets of psychological traits which across cultures show partly overlapping distributions. All these approaches shared the view that culture can be seen psychologically as a kind of shared frame with a limited degree of intracultural variation; Hofstede (1991) refers to culture as collective programming of the mind. In short, these approaches tend to describe the main characteristics of a culture's modal personality by means of a small set of orientations or values.

The other kind of isomorphic models emphasizes the influence of culture on psychological features and views psychological phenomena as "culture writ small." Several of the wide range of models proposed in this line of thinking deal with the relationship between language and cognition. The Sapir-Whorf hypothesis is a good example (Whorf, 1956). The strong form of this hypothesis holds that our mental functioning is determined to an important extent by linguistic features and that it is difficult to transcend in our thinking the boundaries of our language.

Another example is constituted by social representations. These entail shared beliefs and attitudes within cultures about a wide variety of topics ranging from money to diseases (Moscovici, 1982; Wagner & Hayes, 2005). Social representations provide culturally accepted theories of these topics; they do not represent simply opinions or attitudes, but theories or branches of knowledge in their own right that lead to the discovery and organization of reality. Social representations contain a mixture of affective and cognitive components; they are about what culture "teaches" its members. A third example of top-down isomorphic models comes from cognitive anthropology. Lévy-Bruhl (1922; see also Segall, Dasen, Berry, & Poortinga, 1990) argued that "primitives" (we would now say "illiterates") have a prelogical way of thinking, with limited attention to laws of logic and causal relationships. An influential example of a top-down isomorphic model has been formulated by Vygotsky (1978) who argued that higher mental functions can only develop in the individual if they are already present in the society.

Nonisomorphic Models

Individualism-collectivism is probably the best example in cross-cultural psychology of a concept for which nonisomorphism has been postulated at the individual and cultural level (e.g., Oyserman & Uskul, this volume; but see Adamopoulos, this volume). The lack of isomorphism was not based on a theoretical claim but is a consequence of empirical findings failing to support complete isomorphism. Triandis (2001) argues that individualism and collectivism are opposite poles of a single dimension at country level, whereas analyses at individual level frequently show two factors, sometimes related but at other times even orthogonal. Such a pattern indicates that the psychological meaning at individual and country level cannot be identical. Triandis, Leung, Villareal, and Clack (1985) proposed the terms *individualism* and *collectivism* to refer to the country-level dimension and the terms *idiocentrism* and *allocentrism* to refer to the related concepts at individual level. Triandis argues that the distinction between the two levels allows us to describe the behavior of allocentrics in individualist societies and of idiocentrics in collectivist societies. The latter should find "their culture stifling and try to escape it," whereas the former "join groups, gangs, unions, and other collectives" (2001, p. 910). Still, Triandis assumes a fair deal of correspondence between cultural customs and individual habits.

Isomorphism versus Nonisomorphism

It is probably fair to state that isomorphism is the (implicit) rule in cross-cultural psychology and that nonisomorphism is the exception. To the best of our knowledge, no theories have been developed in cross-cultural psychology that specify complete nonisomorphism between individuals and their cultural context. There are good reasons for this preference. Isomorphic concepts are easier to understand, as theory and data from one level can be applied directly at another level, and hypotheses and theories are easier to formulate for isomorphic concepts than for (partially) nonisomorphic concepts. In addition, it is plausible that there should be overlap between concepts at two levels even if that overlap is incomplete. For example, twin research clearly shows that individual differences in intelligence have an important genetic component, whereas country differences are more strongly related to educational expenditure per capita (e.g., Georgas, Weiss, Van de Vijver, & Saklofske, 2003; Van de Vijver, 1997). These findings suggest that intelligence does not show complete isomorphism at individual and country level and that we need partly or entirely dissimilar models to account for individual and country differences in intelligence scores. If the meaning of intelligence scores, or any other measure, is not the same at both levels, the question should be addressed whether a single concept can be used at both levels. The proposal by Triandis et al. (1985) to employ different terms at individual and country level to refer to the related though distinct concepts of individualism and collectivism is in line with this reasoning; it avoids the inevitable interpretation problems which arise when a single concept is used that has a different meaning at individual and country level.

Interaction Models: No Interaction, Static, and Dynamic Interaction

Interactions addressing processes between levels have received scant attention in the multilevel literature (but see Blakely & Woodward, 2000). Three different kinds of interactions between levels can be envisaged. The first possibility is that there is *no interaction* between levels. This outcome is found when the two levels are either entirely independent (complete absence of isomorphism) or entirely dependent (fully isomorphic). Full independence in aggregation models implies that there is no structural relationship between levels; structural relationships between variables defining a construct at one level have no correspondence with structural relationships at another level. The classical culture-and-personality school provides an example of complete dependence; individual personality is covered by the cultural personality.

The second type of interaction can be called *static* or *statistical*. It is observed in a study whenever the statistical interaction term linking individual- and culture-level data in a multilevel analysis reaches a significant value. Such an interaction would be found if high idiocentrics in individualist countries show a higher self-esteem than high idiocentrics in collectivist countries, whereas low idiocentrics in individualist countries show a lower self-esteem than low idiocentrics in collectivist countries. In this example, the interaction would lead to an amplification of individual and cross-cultural differences. Obviously, such an interaction could also point to attenuation of differences.

The third kind of interaction can be called *dynamic*. The emphasis here is on outcomes of dynamic feedback loops of phenomena at different levels. Many instances of dynamic interactions are found in evolution theory. The morphology of a species can be seen as the result of both the genetic input at individual level and environmental changes in and constraints by the environment. The exchange between the individual and environmental factors requires a dynamic multilevel model. It could be argued that all interaction models in cross-cultural psychology are dynamic in the sense that behavioral outcomes have evolved during a person's lifetime. However, many interactions may be stable after their initial period of development. For example, individuals who are extraverted and live in a culture that does not value extraversion may build up enough experience in childhood and adolescence to express or inhibit their extraversion in a socially accepted manner once they have become adults. Therefore, we think that it makes sense not to call all interactions dynamic.

Combining (Dis)aggregation and Interaction: A Taxonomy of Multilevel Models

In Table 1.2, the three types of interaction (no, static, and dynamic) are combined with intrinsic and derived use of variables and concepts. Among the latter, a distinction is made between isomorphic and nonisomorphic structures, leading to nine cells. We can illustrate these nine cases using the concepts of individualism and collectivism. Suppose a questionnaire is administered to samples of individual respondents in various countries and we are interested in the question of whether the two factors (individualism and collectivism) show up at individual and country level.

The first column of Table 1.2 refers to studies in which different constructs and variables are measured at individual and country level. For example, individualism at country level would be measured by indicators such as the average number of persons per household and number

TABLE 1.2

Taxonomy of Multilevel Models: (Dis)aggregegation and Interaction

Type of interaction	Intrinsic concepts and variables	Derived (disaggregated/aggregated) concepts and variables	
		Nonisomorphic relations between levels	Isomorphic relations between levels
No interaction	Case 1	Case 4	Case 7
Static	Case 2	Case 5	Case 8
Dynamic	Case 3	Case 6	Case 9

or proportion of national laws that protect individual freedom (Triandis, 1995). Measurements at individual level could be questionnaire items that focus on individual autonomy and independence. In case 1, the country-level and individual-level measures are unrelated to each other; for example, proportions of laws on individual rights in various countries are not related to the mean score on the questionnaire. There would be a static interaction of individual- and country-level individualism (case 2) if country-level individualism would reinforce (or attenuate) individual-level individualism. Finally, case 3 occurs if there are feedback loops between individualism at individual and country level. For example, country-level individualism leads to higher levels of individual-level individualism (persons feel stimulated in their individualist tendencies by their environment), which then leads to changes at culture level (e.g., more legislation in which individual rights are protected).

The last two columns in Table 1.2 presume that aggregated or disaggregated data are used. Case 4 (no interaction, nonisomorphic structure) occurs if the idiocentrism scores of individuals are different in meaning from and are not affected by their countries' standing on individualism. The absence of any interaction indicates that the individual- and country-level constructs are entirely unrelated. Case 4 is the most extreme case of lack of cross-level influence. By aggregating individual-level scores at country level, an entirely new concept emerges that has its own meaning. For example, individualism-collectivism has been said to refer to a combination of relatedness (need for having strong relational ties) and autonomy, as in Kagitcibasi's (2005) model. It is easy to see how these two concepts can be unrelated at individual level (as argued by Kagitcibasi); autonomous persons may feel either a weak or a strong need to affiliate with other persons. However, the two concepts are polar opposites at country level; countries in which autonomy is emphasized show less cohesive families and communities.

There would be a static interaction (case 5) if individualism and collectivism (or idiocentrism and allocentrism) do not have the same structure at the two levels, but some individual-level components can be predicted from a country's standing on the concept. For example, one can imagine that filial piety (Ho, 1996) is influenced by both country-level individualism-collectivism and individual-level idiocentrism-allocentrism. There would be a static interaction if, say, allocentrics in a collectivist society would show more filial piety than could be expected on the basis of their allocentrism score level. There would be a dynamic interaction (case 6) if, say, the idiocentrism of individuals and individualism of countries are connected in positive or negative feedback loops. For example, the focus on idiocentrism of individuals provides the impetus for an individualist political movement to develop institutions that facilitate this autonomy (e.g., facilities for handicapped people).

Another set of interactions arises when there is identity of structures at individual and country level (isomorphism; third column of Table 1.2). The three examples just given can also serve here, with one essential distinction: concepts now have the same meaning at individual and country level. A single pair of concepts would be sufficient to describe both individual and country differences. Case 7 (isomorphic structure, no interaction) is the simplest case; the concepts are identical at both levels, and they are completely dependent and exchangeable. Cases 8 (static interaction) and 9 (dynamic interaction) show some cross-level influence. For example, collectivism at individual level may be encouraged in a collectivist country and discouraged in an individualist country. Longitudinal studies would be needed to examine how changes at individual and country level can affect each other.

METHODOLOGICAL ISSUES IN AGGREGATION AND DISAGGREGATION

The main methodological issues in aggregation and disaggregation are validity concerns in cross-level inferences, identifying structure in cross-cultural datasets, and developing a taxonomy of multilevel fallacies.

Validity Concerns in Cross-Level Inferences

The use of intrinsically individual and cultural variables as a rule does not raise validity concerns. However, derived variables can be open to multiple interpretations and disputable inferences. Two validity issues jeopardize aggregated and disaggregated scores: the applicability of scores at other levels of (dis)aggregation and shifts of meaning after (dis)aggregation. Applying scores from one level to another level can easily result in invalid interpretations. For example, Hofstede (2001) defines individualism-collectivism as "the relationship between the individual and the collectivity that prevails in a given society" (p. 209). In his work, individualism-collectivism is an interval-level country characteristic (see also Oyserman & Uskul, this volume). However, much cross-cultural literature transforms individualism, often implicitly, to a psychological characteristic by attributing this country characteristic to all individuals living in the country. The reasoning goes as follows: Japan is a collectivist country; therefore, any Japanese is a collectivist. This simplified reasoning can be easily refuted. It is clear that it neglects individual differences within a country and can only be valid for phenomena that do not show any intracultural variation, which is very uncommon in psychological data.

The second problem with (dis)aggregation of data is possible shifts in meaning. Well-known is the question of how group differences on IQ tests should be interpreted. Several authors (e.g., Furby, 1973; Scarr, 1985) have referred to some analogue like the following. When maize is grown on two plots with different soil structure and nutrients, the maize plants will show intra- and interplot differences in stem length. Intraplot differences are mostly due to individual (genetic) differences between the maize plants, whereas interplot differences are mainly caused by environmental differences. Although the cause for differences at one level is not the same as at another level, the length of the stem of any single maize plant is influenced by both causes; depending on the frame of reference, one or the other cause should be emphasized. Sonke, Poortinga, and De Kuijer (1999) were interested in the reaction times of Dutch and Iranian students to Arabic letters and simple figurative stimuli. The Iranian students had a better performance on the Arabic letters task and a lower performance on figurative stimuli as compared to the Dutch students. If both tasks would be seen as measures of speed of responding to visual stimuli, the lack of consistency in the cross-cultural score differences would be hard to interpret. The authors argued that differences in stimulus familiarity can explain the cross-cultural score differences. Thus, differences in mean reaction time between two cultural samples turned out to be a measure of stimulus familiarity rather than speed of responding, shifting the meaning of the reaction time tasks. Individual differences in familiarity with the stimulus sets presumably were small within each of the student samples and unlikely to explain much of the variation in the intracultural score differences. However, cross-cultural differences in familiarity were relatively large and it is likely that familiarity explains the cross-cultural differences in reaction time. Again, differences in scores of individuals from the same country need not have the same meaning as differences in scores of those from different countries.

Identifying Structure in Cross-Cultural Datasets

An important issue in many multilevel studies is the identification of the structure underlying an instrument to identify its meaning. This problem is usually solved in monolevel studies by conducting some multivariate analysis that addresses the dimensionality of the elements of the instruments, such as an exploratory factor analysis of the interitem correlation matrix. How can the problem of structure be solved in multilevel studies? Suppose we have administered a coping questionnaire, measuring problem- and emotion-focused coping in two countries, and that we are interested in the question of whether the two countries show differences in coping styles. It is relatively common in such a situation to combine the raw scores of both countries in a single data matrix and to conduct a factor analysis on this matrix to examine the dimensionality of the coping questionnaire. The problem with this data analysis is the confounding of individual and country differences; as a consequence, the observed factors are hard to interpret.

A fairly common solution is to standardize the data per culture prior to the factor analysis in order to remove country differences from the data matrix. Standardization is also often used to avoid confounding of cross-cultural differences in the target construct with cross-cultural differences in response styles. However, the disadvantages of standardization should not be underestimated (Fischer, 2004). First, standardization leads to loss of information about the absolute positions of individuals on response scales and of cultures. Statistical techniques that make use of score level and metric, such as analysis of variance and structural equation modeling, can no longer be used in a simple manner after double standardization. A second disadvantage involves effects of standardization on the outcomes of statistical techniques, such as exploratory factor analysis. For example, the ipsatization of scores (i.e., total scores are the same for all individuals) that is implied in standardization results in negative average interitem correlations, which affects the factorial structure (e.g., Ten Berge, 1999).

Leung and Bond (1989) distinguished four types of analyses to identify factors or dimensions in a cross-cultural dataset with questionnaire items. It is interesting to link these to current thinking on multilevel models.

A *pancultural analysis* is conducted of the scores of an entire set of respondents, regardless of cultural background. This analysis, which is usually carried out on the basis of nonstandardized data, produces factors or dimensions that combine individual and cultural factors. As indicated above, factors may be difficult to interpret. If many items show substantial cross-cultural differences, a global factor may emerge or may be boosted by the cross-cultural differences. An *intracultural analysis* takes the data of a single cultural sample. The use of mean scores of countries (also called "citizen scores"; Smith, Bond, & Kagitcibasi, 2006) to examine relationships at country level is called a *cultural* or *ecological analysis*—after Robinson's (1950) ecological correlations. Such an analysis usually has a small number of observations, because each country constitutes one case. A sample size of several countries is needed even though common criteria for sample sizes do not necessarily apply at country level (relatively high internal consistencies of data tend to be found at country level, since the aggregation of individual data in ecological analyses reduces random fluctuation). The fourth type of analysis is called *individual analysis*; individual dimensions are derived from an analysis on all individuals in the entire dataset, but only after a double standardization, first per individual and then per item within each sample.

Building on the classification by Leung and Bond (1989), it can be argued that the examination of structure in multilevel models including individual-level data requires at most three types of data organization. The first is the *ecological dataset*, which contains country-level scores, based on aggregated individual-level data. This matrix provides information about the nature of country-level structure. It is an empirical question whether or not the structure at country and individual level is identical (cf. chapters by Fontaine and by Selig et al., this volume). The second type of data organization is composed of the *individual-level datasets per culture*. These datasets provide information about similarities and differences of individual-level data across the cultures included in a study. Data analyses have to determine to what extent the individual-level datasets are comparable or equivalent across countries. In particular when the number of cultures in a study is large, individual-level matrices are often combined in a single *pooled within-group covariance matrix,* based on the pooled individual-level dataset. This usually takes the form of a covariance matrix in which data of all cultures are combined. The matrix is the average covariance matrix per culture, weighted for sample size. An analysis of this matrix provides insight in the global structure of an instrument. Starting with the working assumption of identity of factors or dimensions across cultures, the analysis of the pooled data matrix gives us the best approximation of the global structure.

There are two limitations on the use of pooled within-group covariance matrices. First, working with this matrix assumes that all cultures show the same underlying structure. If an instrument would yield different factor solutions in different groups, pooling the covariance matrices may actually be counterproductive, as any pooling of the data will hide salient cross-cultural differences. This can be examined by comparing the factor solution in each culture with the structure found in the pooled solution (Van de Vijver & Poortinga, 2002). Second, pooling requires a large number of countries in a study (Selig et al., this volume).

A Taxonomy of Multilevel Fallacies

Multilevel fallacies can take different forms (see also Blakely & Woodward, 2000). We distinguish four types of errors, which are based on two dichotomous underlying classifications (see Table 1.3). The first refers to

TABLE 1.3

Four Types of Fallacies in Multilevel Research

	Direction of cross-level inference	
What is (dis)aggregated?	Aggregation	Disaggregation
Construct or relationship of constructs	*Type A*	*Type B*
Score levels	*Type C*	*Type D*

Source: after Van de Vijver & Poortinga, 2002.

the distinction between construct- and level-application errors. A construct-application or "structural" error refers to the use of concepts (or relationships between concepts) at levels to which they do not apply (e.g., idiocentrism applies to individuals and not to countries, while the opposite holds for individualism). Level-application errors or "quantitative" errors involve the use of score levels (quantities) at a level where they are not valid; for example, a low GNP of a country does not mean that all its inhabitants have a low income. The second dichotomy in Table 1.3 draws a distinction between errors due to aggregation and errors due to disaggregation.

Type A in Table 1.3 involves construct-aggregation fallacies; constructs (or relations of constructs) of lower-order units are incorrectly applied to higher order units. Schwartz (1992, 1994) argues that values at individual level and culture level (the latter are based on individual-level scores aggregated per country) do not have the same structure; the country-level structure is simpler than and only partially overlaps with the individual-level structure. Consequently, it would be incorrect to apply the same constructs to refer to individual-and culture-level values. To determine whether construct fallacies have been committed, the question has to be answered as to what extent variables measure the same constructs at an individual and cultural level (see Fontaine; Selig, Card, & Little, this volume; Muthén, 1991; Van de Vijver & Poortinga, 2002). Statistical techniques to analyze cross-level equivalence examine to what extent factors or dimensions that are identified at one level can also be found at a lower or higher level of aggregation. For example, Van de Vijver and Poortinga (2002) found that postmodernity in the World Values Survey showed the same, unidimensional factor at individual and country level. This finding was interpreted as evidence for the similarity of meaning at individual and country level. McCrae, Terracciano et al. (2005) found good similarity for the five-factorial structure of the Revised NEO Personality Inventory at individual and country level. Cheung, Leung, and Au (2006) did not find support for the multilevel equivalence of the entire five-factorial structure of social axioms at the two levels. One of the factors, social cynicism, showed good equivalence; the other four factors showed strong correlations at country level while they were uncorrelated at individual level (see also Leung & Bond, this volume).

A type B error is committed when a higher level construct or relationship is incorrectly applied to a lower level of aggregation. At country level there is a negative relationship between GDP and fertility (as measured by the average number of children per head of population). Entwistle and Mason (1985) examined the relationship between socioeconomic status and fertility within countries. A negative relationship is usually found in more affluent countries, whereas a positive relationship between status and fertility tends to be found in less affluent countries. The between-country relationship does not hold at a lower level, illustrating the Type B cross-level error. Although variation in the relationship across aggregation levels excludes interpretation in common terms, this should not be seen as problematic. Rather it indicates the need for an explanation that makes the pattern of findings understandable. For example, it has been suggested that children can serve different functions across societies; namely, an economic function (in contributing to the care of the parents when they grow old) and a psychological function (adding to the quality of life of parents) (Kagitcibasi, 2005). Economic care is more salient with low affluence while the psychological function gains salience with high affluence.

In type C and type D fallacies, quantitative differences in score scales are incorrectly applied at a lower or higher level. These fallacies have been more extensively studied and documented than structure-oriented fallacies. Richards, Gottfredson, and Gottfredson (1990/1991) coined the term *individual differences fallacy* to describe situations in which aggregation of individual characteristics does not give an adequate picture of the aggregate-level characteristic (type C error). An example is the dissimilarity of within- and between-plot differences of maize, mentioned before. The (average) plot difference in stem length, which is based on individual maize plants, does not reflect genetic differences. The cross-cultural literature on intelligence provides another example. Although there is ample evidence that factor analyses of intelligence tasks yield similar structures across ethnic groups in a society (Irvine & Berry, 1988; Jensen, 1980; Van de Vijver, 1997), controversies on the interpretation of quantitative differences in scores are still continuing after decades.

The reverse error, the application of characteristics of countries to individuals (type D error), is commonly known as the *ecological fallacy* (Robinson, 1950; cf. also Hofstede, 1980, 2001). Robinson distinguished between individual correlations and ecological correlations:

> In an individual correlation the variables are descriptive properties of individuals, such as height, income, eye color, or race, and not descriptive statistical constants such as rates or means. In an *ecological correlation* the statistical object is a *group* of persons. (p. 351, italics in original)

Ecological correlations are used widely in quantitative sociological analyses, but according to Robinson their purpose is to gain information about the behavior of individuals: "Ecological correlations are used simply because the correlations between the properties of individuals are not available. In each instance, however, the substitution is made tacitly rather than explicitly" (p. 352). Robinson showed that ecological correlations tend to be higher than individual correlations. To illustrate the two levels, he referred to correlations between literacy and skin color in census data from the United States. Individual-level correlations, calculated separately for various U.S. states, were much lower than the ecological correlation computed on the rates (i.e., means) of the two variables for the same states (see also Stanat & Lüdtke, this volume). Another example of a type D error is the inapplicability of percentages of a population as a basis for scores of individuals (the rate of pregnant women in a group cannot serve as a score for any individual woman). The example may be misleadingly simple; it is easy to see that the percentage is a continuous variable that can only be dichotomous at individual level. However, with psychological data the error tends to be far less conspicuous.

We like to emphasize that the application of group-level characteristics to individuals is not always problematic; it can make good sense also in psychology to attribute a group characteristic to all its individual members. Language with its many ramifications is one example; other examples can be found in small traditional societies where everyone by and large shares the same religious beliefs and a more or less common set of practices. In general, disaggregation leads to misrepresentation when a trait is distributed unequally over individuals, but not when it is homogeneous in a population. For the study of homogeneously distributed traits, information can be gathered from a small number of individuals, who serve as informants for their cultural population. In research with informants it is assumed that the same results would be obtained if any, or all, of the informants would be exchanged for others. Exchangeability is supposed to be near perfect in the study of language where an analysis is often based on observation of only a few speakers. In psychology the exchangeability of respondents is usually low and in order to gain results that apply to a population as a whole it is necessary to have data from a sample of respondents that can be deemed representative for that population with all its individual and subgroup diversity.

RECENT STATISTICAL ADVANCES IN MULTILEVEL MODELING

Scientists working on the interface of individual and culture have a long-standing interest in conceptual issues of multilevel models. The statistical treatment of the data, however, has always been problematic. No statistical tools were available to link cultural factors to individual outcomes in a statistically adequate manner. More specifically, for a long time it has been impossible to assess whether individual and country differences in aggregated individual-level scores have the same psychological meaning.

Also, classical regression models could not combine individual- and culture-level predictors and dependent variables.

In the last few decades, statistical techniques have been developed in two directions. First, when identical underlying constructs of traits are not reflected by identical behavior manifestations across cultural populations, measures of such constructs cannot be compared at face value. This is referred to as the problem of equivalence or comparability of data across cultures (Van de Vijver & Leung, 1997; Fontaine, this volume). Thus, lack of equivalence or bias refers to shifts in meaning of score variables across cultural groups. Conceptually, there is a close relationship between equivalence across cultures and across levels. Scores of individuals in two cultures cannot be taken to be equivalent when an additional variable has to be introduced to account for differences at the culture level. In multilevel research it is accepted that the interpretation of data may have to vary across levels. Statistical tools are now available to test the identity of the structure shown by an instrument at different levels of aggregation (Hox, 2002; Muthén 1991, 1994; applications can be found in Cheung, Leung, & Au, 2006; Van de Vijver & Poortinga, 2002; Van de Vijver & Watkins, 2006).

The second development in statistical analysis concerns cross-level relationships of variables. In cross-cultural psychology we are not only interested in cross-level equivalence of constructs; identity of predictor–outcome relations is also often a major topic of study. For example, in educational research a difference has been found in the verbal ability of boys and girls, with girls on average gaining higher scores. Hence, an above average mean score for a school class is likely to reflect the presence of a high proportion of girls in that class, and a below average mean score a high proportion of boys. In this case there is a shift in the meaning of the test score variable across the two levels from cognitive ability to gender ratio. However, this shift in meaning is assumed to be equivalent across all school classes in a dataset. The cross-cultural psychologist would be interested in the question to what extent the gender difference in scores is invariant across cultural contexts and the gender ratio has the same influence on the verbal ability scores across these contexts. Country-specific features may challenge the equivalence of this relationship (Esping-Andersen & Przeworski, 2001). Recent statistical advances have made it possible to address the identity of relationships across different cultural contexts; these models have become known under various names such as hierarchical linear modeling and random components modeling (Hox, 2002; Raudenbusch & Bryk, 2002). Thus, it can be established whether or not the difference between boys and girls in verbal ability is the same in all cultures, and the influence of factors with a possible bearing on the relationship can be evaluated.

The two kinds of multilevel models we distinguish, the cross-level equivalence and the hierarchical linear models, are flexible tools. Both models can deal with any level of invariance across cultural groups. For example, modern statistical programs can deal with partial invariance of constructs and restrict the cross-level comparison to the invariant parts. This flexibility has important advantages for cross-cultural research. Multilevel models can help to bring about more nuances and help researchers to replace the equivalent versus nonequivalent dichotomy by more graded interpretations.

CONCLUSION

The current chapter provided various definitions and distinctions that are relevant in multilevel models. These models use nested structures in which lower-order units, such as individuals, are embedded in higher-order units, such as cultures. The relationships between lower and higher orders were addressed. Two kinds of relationships can describe most models and research. The first deals with cross-level equivalence, involving the extent to which constructs have the same structure at different levels of aggregation. For example, do individual and country differences in intelligence have the same meaning? Cross-level equivalence is an important and often neglected issue in cross-cultural studies. The second relevant type of models deals with relations between lower and higher orders and typically involves different variables at each level. For example, what is the relative contribution of differences in intelligence (at individual level) and educational expenditure (at country level) to individual differences in a cross-national assessment of reading achievement?

An important distinction in multilevel models is between intrinsic and derived characteristics. The former applies when each level in the hierarchy has its own variables; the example of reading achievement employs variables (intelligence and educational expenditure) at their natural level of observation. Derived characteristics are based on aggregated or disaggregated data; for example, gender is aggregated to class level in order to examine the influence of gender composition on educational achievement. Derived characteristics constitute more methodological challenges than intrinsic characteristics, due to possible shifts in meaning after (dis)aggregation. The issue of meaning shifts looms large when only a few countries are available in a study and an analysis of the country-level structure of the construct is not feasible.

Multilevel fallacies, such as the incorrect attribution of culture characteristics to individual members of the culture, constitute another methodological challenge. We presented a taxonomy of multilevel fallacies. Recent statistical advances in multilevel modeling have equipped us with good tools to address major issues in the conceptualization and analysis of multilevel structures.

We are now at a point in time where multilevel modeling has to make the transition from a psychometric innovation to a substantive contribution to the field. We are of the opinion that the conceptual relevance of the problems considered in multilevel models and the availability of relevant computer programs can contribute substantially to the growth of interest in these models. The litmus test of these models is their success in providing creative answers to old and new problems in the analysis of relationships between behavior and culture.

REFERENCES

Arends-Tóth, J., Van de Vijver, F. J. R., & Poortinga, Y. H. (2006). The influence of method factors on the relation between attitudes and self-reported behaviors in the assessment of acculturation. *European Journal of Psychological Assessment, 22,* 4–12.

Benedict, R. (1934). *Patterns of culture.* New York: Houghton Mifflin.

Berlin, B., & Kay, P. (1969). *Basic color terms: Their universality and evolution.* Berkeley: University of California Press.

Berry, J. W. (1976). *Human ecology and cognitive style: Comparative studies in cultural and psychological adaptation.* New York: Sage/Halsted.

Berry, J. W., Poortinga, Y. H., Segall, & M. H., Dasen, P. R. (2002). *Cross-cultural psychology: Research and applications* (2nd ed.). Cambridge: Cambridge University Press.

Blakely, T. A., & Woodward, A. J. (2000). Ecological effects in multi-level studies. *Journal of Epidemiological Community and Health, 54,* 367–374.

Bock, P. K. (1999). *Rethinking psychological anthropology* (2nd ed.). Prospect Heights, IL: Waveland Press.

Bronfenbrenner, U. (1977). Toward an experimental ecology of human development. *American Psychologist, 32,* 513–531.

Bronfenbrenner, U. (1979). *The ecology of human development: Experiments by nature and design.* Cambridge, MA: Harvard University Press.

Cheung, M. W., Leung, K., & Au, K. (2006). Evaluating multilevel models in cross-cultural research: An illustration with social axioms. *Journal of Cross-Cultural Psychology, 37,* 522–541.

Entwistle, B., & Mason, W. M. (1985). Multi-level effects of socioeconomic development and family planning in children never born. *American Journal of Sociology, 91,* 616–649.

Esping-Andersen, G., & Przeworski, A. (2001). Quantitative cross-national research methods. In N. J. Smelser & P. B. Baltes (Eds.), *International encyclopedia of the social and behavioral sciences* (pp. 12649–12655). New York: Elsevier Science.

Fischer, R. (2004). Standardization to account for cross-cultural response bias: A classification of score adjustment procedures and review of research in JCCP. *Journal of Cross-Cultural Psychology, 35,* 263–282.

Furby, L. (1973). Implications of within-group heritabilities for sources of between-group differences: IQ and racial differences. *Developmental Psychology, 9,* 28–37.

Georgas, J., Weiss, L., Van de Vijver, F. J. R., & Saklofske, D. H. (Eds.). (2003). *Cultures and children's intelligence: A cross-cultural analysis of the WISC-III.* New York: Academic Press.

Ho, D. Y. F. (1996). Filial piety and its psychological consequences. In M. H. Bond (Ed.), *Handbook of Chinese psychology* (pp. 155–165). Hong Kong: Oxford University Press

Hofstede, G. (1980). *Culture's consequences: International differences in work related values.* Beverly Hills, CA: Sage.

Hofstede, G. (1991). *Cultures and organizations: Software of the mind.* London: McGraw-Hill.

Hofstede, G. (2001). *Culture's consequences* (2nd ed.). Thousand Oaks, CA: Sage.

Hox, J. J. (2002). *Multilevel analysis: Techniques and applications.* Mahwah, NJ: Lawrence Erlbaum.

Irvine, S. H., & Berry, J. W. (1988). The abilities of mankind: A revaluation. In S. H. Irvine & J. W. Berry (Eds.), *Human abilities in cultural context* (pp. 3–59). Cambridge: Cambridge University Press.

Jahoda, G. (1982). *Psychology and anthropology: A psychological perspective.* London: Academic Press.

Jensen, A. R. (1980). *Bias in mental testing.* New York: Free Press.

Kagitcibasi, C. (2005). Autonomy and relatedness in cultural context: Implications for self and family. *Journal of Cross-Cultural Psychology, 36,* 403–422.

Kardiner, A., & Linton, R. (1945). *The individual and his society.* New York: Columbia University Press.

Leung, K., & Bond, M. H. (1989). On the empirical identification of dimensions for cross-cultural comparisons. *Journal of Cross-Cultural Psychology, 20,* 133–151.

Lévy-Bruhl, L. (1922). *Mentalité primitif.* Paris: Alcan.

Little, T. D. (1997). Mean and covariance structures (MACS) analyses of cross-cultural data: Practical and theoretical issues. *Multivariate Behavioral Research, 32,* 53–76.

McCrae, R. R., Terracciano, A., & 79 Members of the Personality Profiles of Cultures Project (2005). Personality profiles of cultures: Aggregate personality traits. *Journal of Personality and Social Psychology, 89,* 407–425.

Moscovici, S. (1982). The phenomenon of social representations. In R. M. Farr & S. Moscovici (Eds.), *Social representations* (pp. 3–70). Cambridge: Cambridge University Press.

Mullins, I. V. S., Martin, M. O., Gonzalez, E. J., Gregory, K. D., Garden, R. A., O'Connor, K. M. et al. (2000). *TIMSS 1999, International mathematics report.* Boston: IEA.

Muthén, B. O. (1991). Multilevel factor analysis of class and student achievement components. *Journal of Educational Measurement, 28,* 338–354.

Muthén, B. O. (1994). Multilevel covariance structure analysis. *Sociological Methods & Research, 22,* 376–398.

Peabody, D. (1967). Trait inferences: Evaluative and descriptive aspects. *Journal of Personality and Social Psychology Monographs, 7,*

Peabody, D. (1985). *National characteristics.* Cambridge: Cambridge University Press.

Poortinga, Y. H., & Van de Vijver, F. J. R. (1987). Explaining cross-cultural differences: Bias analysis and beyond. *Journal of Cross-Cultural Psychology, 18,* 259–282.

Raudenbush, S. W., & Bryk, A. S. (2002). *Hierarchical linear models* (2nd ed.). Newbury Park, CA: Sage.

Richards, J. M., Gottfredson, D. C., & Gottfredson, G. D. (1990/1991). Units of analysis and item statistics for environmental assessment scales. *Current Psychology: Research and Reviews, 9,* 407–413.

Robinson, W. S. (1950). Ecological correlations and the behavior of individuals. *American Sociological Review, 15,* 351–357.

Scarr, S. (1985). Constructing psychology: Making facts and fables for our times. *American Psychologist, 40,* 499–512.

Schwartz, S. H. (1992). The universal content and structure of values: Theoretical advances and empirical tests in 20 countries. *Advances in Experimental Social Psychology, 25,* 1–65.

Schwartz, S. H. (1994). Beyond individualism and collectivism: New cultural dimensions of values. In U. Kim, H. C. Triandis, C. Kagitcibasi, S. C. Choi, & G. Yoon (Eds.), *Individualism and collectivism: Theory, method and applications* (pp. 85–119). Thousand Oaks, CA: Sage.

Segall, M. H., Dasen, P. R., Berry, J. W., & Poortinga, Y. H. (1990). *Human behavior in global perspective: An introduction to cross-cultural psychology.* New York: Pergamon Press.

Smith, P. B. (2002). Levels of analysis in cross-cultural psychology. In W. J. Lonner, D. L. Dinnel, S. A. Hayes, & D. N. Sattler (Eds.), *Online readings in psychology and culture* (unit 2, chapter 7). Bellingham, WA: Center for Cross-Cultural Research, Western Washington University. Retrieved October 31, 2006 from http://www.wwu.edu/~culture.

Smith, P. B., Bond, M. H., & Kagitcibasi, C. (2006). *Understanding social psychology across cultures: Living and working in a changing world.* London: Sage.

Sonke, C. J., Poortinga, Y. H., & De Kuijer, J. H. J. (2002). Cross-cultural differences on cognitive task performance: The influence of stimulus familiarity. W. J. Lonner, D. L. Dinnel, D. K. Forgays, & S. A. Hayes (Eds.), *Merging past, present, and future in cross-cultural psychology: Selected papers from the Fourteenth International Congress of the International Association for Cross-Cultural Psychology* (pp. 146–158). Lisse, the Netherlands: Swets & Zeitlinger.

Super, C. M., & Harkness, S. (1986). The developmental niche: A conceptualization at the interface of child and culture. *International Journal of Behavioral Development, 9,* 545–569.

Super, C. M., & Harkness, S. (1997). The cultural structuring of child development. In J. W. Berry, P. Dasen, & T. S. Saraswathi (Eds.), *Handbook of cross-cultural psychology: Vol. 2. Basic processes and human development* (pp. 1–39). Boston: Allyn & Bacon.

Ten Berge, J. M. F. (1999). A legitimate case of component analysis of ipsative measures, and partialling the mean as an alternative to ipsatization. *Multivariate Behavioral Research, 34,* 89–102.

Triandis, H. C. (1995). *Individualism and collectivism.* Boulder, CO: Westview Press.

Triandis, H. C. (2001). Individualism-collectivism and personality. *Journal of Personality, 69,* 907–924.

Triandis, H. C., Leung, K. Villareal, M. V., & Clack, F. L. (1985). Allocentric versus idiocentric tendencies: Convergent and discriminant validation. *Journal of Research in Personality, 19,* 395–415.

Van de Vijver, F. J. R. (1997). Meta-analysis of cross-cultural comparisons of cognitive test performance. *Journal of Cross-Cultural Psychology, 28,* 678–709.

Van de Vijver, F. J. R., & Leung, K. (1997). *Methods and data analysis for cross-cultural research.* Newbury Park, CA: Sage.

Van de Vijver, F. J. R., & Poortinga, Y. H. (2002). Structural equivalence in multilevel research. *Journal of Cross-Cultural Psychology, 33,* 141–156.

Van de Vijver, F. J. R., & Watkins, D. (2006). Assessing similarity of meaning at individual and country level: An investigation of a measure of independent and interdependent self. *European Journal of Psychological Assessment, 22,* 69–77.

Vygotsky, L. S. (1978). *Mind in society: The development of higher psychological processes.* Cambridge, MA: Harvard University Press.

Wagner, W., & Hayes, N. (2005). *Everyday discourse and common sense: The theory of social representations.* Basingstoke, UK: Palgrave Macmillan.

Whorf, B. L. (1956). *Language, thought and reality: Selected writings of Benjamin Lee Whorf* (J. Carroll, Ed.). Cambridge, MA: MIT Press.

Wundt, W. (1912). *Elemente der Völkerpsychologie: Grundlinien einer psychologischen Entwicklungsgeschichte der Menschheit.* Leipzig, Germany: Kroener.

2

On the Entanglement of Culture and Individual Behavior

John Adamopoulos

Nature loves hierarchies (Simon, 1973, p. 5)

Nature loves to hide (Heraclitus, ca. 500 BCE/1960, fr. 123)

The main thesis of this chapter is that these two statements are of great significance in the analysis of psychological phenomena. The universe that psychologists explore is organized in levels of abstraction or generality that may or may not be closely connected to each other and easy to identify. One of the main tasks of psychological research is to discern the components of this structure and to describe processes within and, possibly, across levels.

Psychology has had a long history of struggle with the problem of bringing together and integrating conceptual developments that occur at different levels of generality. The levels involved most frequently in this struggle reflected biological and organismic (experiential) explanations of behavior (e.g., Goodson & Morgan, 1976). In the past, each of these levels was usually considered irrelevant to the other's explanatory capabilities. For example, Silverstein (1976) proposed that even though psychologists assume that there is a neurophysiological event underlying every experience, there is no need to seek explanations for experiences or behavior that are grounded in human neurophysiology because such explanations will necessarily be different from those obtained at the organismic level. Drawing from his split-brain research, Sperry (1982) has made a similar argument regarding the relative independence of mental constructs from underlying physiological processes.

The complexity of the problem of explanation at different levels is even more evident in recent theoretical disagreements. In cognitive psychology, for instance, there have been calls to investigate memory independently as a network of concepts and relations and as a neurophysiological system (e.g., Anderson, 1990). Other theorists, however, have assumed a greater correspondence between brain and cognitive activity, as in the case of parallel distributed processing models of memory (e.g., Rumelhart & McClelland, 1986). Similarly, while arguing for a much more integrative approach, Cacioppo, Berntson, Sheridan, and McClintock (2000) have pointed to the tension between biological and social approaches in the study of behavior:

> The differences in levels of analysis have resulted in distinct histories, research traditions, and technical demands, leaving what some regard both as an impassable abyss between social and biological approaches and as evidence of the impending demise of psychology as a discipline. (p. 829)

In recent years the problem of levels of analysis has been extended to the contrast of theoretical explanations of individual behavior and cultural practice. "Culture" (frequently used as a referent to a particular population) and "behavior" (as a referent to a particular individual) are typically conceptualized in cross-cultural research as belonging to different, albeit contiguous, levels. For example, the ecocultural framework explicitly attempts to draw connections between population-level and individual-level variables via a variety of biological and sociocultural adaptations and transmission processes (Segall, Dasen, Berry, & Poortinga, 1999). The clear assumption of this widely used approach to the explanation of cross-cultural differences is that adaptations directly link variables at a population level (e.g., subsistence economy) to individual psychology (e.g., parental practices) with no intermediate level necessary.

The statements about nature's possible predilections that open this chapter have two important implications for any theoretical analysis in cultural research. First, paraphrasing Simon, we may argue that the problem of the levels of analysis in cross-cultural psychology is real and important because nature is organized hierarchically. Second, drawing from Heraclitus, we may suspect that such organization is not as simple or easy to understand as it might seem at first glance. In fact, even the use of the word *entanglement* in the title of this chapter is meant to reflect some of these issues. On the one hand it points to the inextricable connection between culture and behavior. On the other, it alerts us to the slightly unsavory character of this problem, the complicated mess that awaits explanation.

This chapter considers the problem of levels of analysis in cross-cultural psychology by focusing on questions about its significance. The core theme is the question of whether or not phenomena at the individual and cultural levels should be expected to have similar theoretical structures (i.e., be isomorphic). It also examines potential troubles with inference at the two levels of culture and individual behavior.

The chapter begins with a general statement of the problem of levels in cross-cultural research and introduces the notion of isomorphism between levels. It then focuses on the analysis of different assumptions about the direction of causality in individual-culture relationships, always working from the perspective that the exploration of the problem of levels will inevitably lead to a better understanding of human behavior. Specifically, this chapter considers approaches that are more-or-less *unidirectional* in that they emphasize the primacy of either the culture or intrapsychic processes in determining individual behavior, and contrasts them to approaches that assume a *reciprocal* relationship between the culture and the individual human being. Problems associated with mixing levels of measurement of variables and levels of inference about phenomena are briefly summarized. As a final word of caution about making inferences at the cultural level, the idea of individualistic biases in the conceptualization of individual-culture relationships is reviewed in this section.

The central part of the chapter examines two theoretical orientations to the problem of levels that are in many ways antithetical to each other. The first is based on the assumption that there is no *necessary* reason to expect any isomorphism in the structure of phenomena investigated at the individual and cultural levels. The second orientation is based on the assumption that there are continuities across levels, such that structurally similar explanatory propositions can be used for phenomena studied at different levels. The reasoning behind each of these two approaches is outlined and is supported by examples of the absence or presence of isomorphism, respectively.

In reading this section it is important to keep in mind that the recent interest in the problem of levels of analysis in psychology—and in cross-cultural psychology in particular—does not mean that this is a new idea. As I have already suggested, scientists and philosophers of science have long been fascinated by this issue. Consequently, many of the relevant arguments were developed years ago. One of goals of this section is to bring much of that early discussion forward and to integrate it with more recent analyses of the problem.

The final section of the paper revisits individual-culture relationships by examining and summarizing many remaining problems that await solution. For example, the definition of a "level" is taken up, along with various issues regarding the selection of appropriate "levels" in theoretical systems that involve both individuals and cultural communities and the aggregation of individual members of a culture. An outline of the basic elements necessary for a solution to some of these problems is presented, though a complete treatment of these issues is still not available. The discussion centers primarily on theoretical and secondarily on methodological issues; statistical matters form a different component of the problem.

LEVELS, ISOMORPHISM, AND CROSS-CULTURAL RESEARCH

Comparisons across levels of a system, whether they refer to individual and culture, to species and genera, or, more playfully, to human and extra-terrestrial life forms in philosophical discourse—ultimately introduce the concept of *isomorphism*. This widely used term does not have the same precise definition across disciplines, though it is typically used in comparative contexts where some form of parallelism in structure or function across levels is sought or described. For example, in mathematical set theory isomorphism refers strictly to a one-to-one correspondence between two sets such that all properties in one set must be found in the other. When such correspondence is not present, a function that accounts for structural similarities is referred to as a homomorphism. Along similar lines, topologists distinguish one-to-one correspondence between objects ("homeomorphism") from the mere possibility of deforming one object into another ("isotopy") (Prasolov, 1995).

Evolutionary biology has a long history of significant argumentation over the terms and substance of cross-level comparisons. The term *homology* has been used to refer to isomorphic relations, but distinctions among types of isomorphisms have been recognized and have led to further terminological refinement. For example, "homology" refers to relationships due to common ancestry, whereas the term *homoplasy* refers to similarity not explicitly understood in terms of common ancestry. Gould's (2002) extensive analysis of the problem of structural similarity in the theory of evolution leads to the conclusion that such similarity exists in varying degrees and accounts for observed *parallelism* among related organisms and *convergence* among unrelated ones.

Systems theorists, whose focus has typically been on cross-level continuity, have frequently described isomorphism as appearing in varying degrees of similarity. James G. Miller (1978) uses the terms *isomorphism* and *homology* to refer to formal identities between different kinds of systems. "Formal identity" in this case is understood as similarity that is manifested in equivalent functions that relate sets of variables within each of the systems under consideration. In a relatively early statement on this issue, von Bertallanfy (1968) proposed that "a consequence of the existence of general system properties is the appearance of structural similarities or isomorphisms in different fields. There are correspondences that govern the behavior of entities that are, intrinsically, widely different" (p. 33). He advocated the search for unity in science by concluding that "the world… shows structural uniformities, manifesting themselves by isomorphic traces of order in the different levels or realms" (p. 49).

It seems that the term *isomorphism*, as used in the sciences, does not always imply identity, but more commonly involves degrees of similarity.

This broader conceptualization appears particularly well suited for cross-cultural psychology, where the debate about levels is relatively recent and some definitional flexibility is indicated. Therefore, I propose that *isomorphism* be used to denote significant parallelism between constructs but not necessarily complete identity or one-to-one correspondence. The term should be used to indicate that the structure of constructs or the functional relationship between two or more variables is similar in form (i.e., is equivalent) across different levels of a system, as in an individual and an aggregation of individuals within a community, or individuals *within* a culture and *across* cultures. A further distinction can be made between isomorphism as it applies to theoretical terms on the one hand and to empirical constructs and the meaning of obtained scores on various measures on the other. It can even be argued that different expectations for isomorphism are appropriate for these two domains, with one-to-one correspondence being a reasonable goal for the latter. The main focus of this chapter is on theoretical relationships and thus the more flexible definition of isomorphism is adopted.

Isomorphism in Cross-Cultural Research

A number of statements attest to the significance that the debate about levels has achieved in current thinking in cross-cultural psychology. In an early analysis of the problem, Shweder (1973) provided several empirical examples of the lack of what we might term intracultural and cross-cultural isomorphism. He documented such lack of isomorphism in a number of empirical cases, including the behavioral correlates of nurturance versus egoism at the *intra*cultural and *inter*cultural levels, and the categories used to code *intra*group versus *inter*group interaction. On the basis of his cogent analysis, Shweder (1973) concluded that "it is just possible that the psychological variables that will one day describe differences among cultural communities are not the same as those that will describe differences among individuals within any or all cultural communities, and vice versa" (p. 544).

By and large cross-cultural psychologists did not heed this warning during the following decade. I believe part of the reason was a growing suspicion that such an argument could ultimately be used to challenge the significance of the scientific contribution of cross-cultural psychology—a discipline with a strong universalist orientation that often relied on broad commonalities in *individual* experience to account for similarities across *cultures* (cf. Adamopoulos & Lonner, 1994). In fact, within a few years, Shweder (1986) challenged the disciplinary independence and ability of cross-cultural psychology to offer insights into psychocultural processes and described it as a mere extension—a poor relative, perhaps, or, better yet, a "frustrated gadfly" (Shweder, 1990, p. 12)—of general psychology. He advocated instead a much more relativist "cultural psychology" that emphasized the primacy of local explanations of behavior over those favoring pancultural psychological principles.

Early hesitation notwithstanding, cross-cultural psychologists have recognized fully the significance of this problem since the early 1980s. Hofstede (1980) was among the first to raise the problem of levels of analysis as a significant issue in cross-cultural psychology, describing potential methodological flaws in research that attempted in various ways to cross the individual–culture boundary. Since the 1990s, there has been a flurry of activity in this area as recognition of the problem of levels has become widespread in psychology (e.g., Nezlek, 2001). Cross-cultural psychologists have acknowledged the relevance of the problem to their particular interests (i.e., individual–culture relationships) and have set about to formulate responses to it (Smith, 2002, 2004). To a large extent, approaches to the problem in the social sciences have focused on analytical matters (e.g., Hox, 2000; Little, Schnabel, & Baumert, 2000; Selig, Card, & Little, this volume). However, there are abundant conceptual issues associated with this problem, as has already been implied, even if we confine our interests to individual–culture interactions. What is the nature of such interactions, and why are they theoretically important?

INDIVIDUAL–CULTURE RELATIONSHIPS

Theoretical Power

There appears to be a near consensus among cross-cultural psychologists that awareness of the problem of levels and associated fallacies necessarily will lead to more powerful explanations in psychology (e.g., Smith, 2002). Such fallacies frequently emerge from overreaching in attempts to draw connections between individuals, their behavior, and culture. Therefore, it is important to outline common types of individual–culture relationships in cross-cultural psychology and the kinds of explanations such presumed relationships entail.

A major distinction in understanding individual–culture relationships involves their unidirectional versus bidirectional or reciprocal character. It is perhaps a sign of the relative youth of the field that current research programs in cross-cultural psychology tend to focus on unidirectional relationships, based on the assumption that the relative impact of the culture on the individual is greater than the impact of the individual on the culture. Theories with elaborate reciprocal influences between individual and culture remain, for the most part, a chimera, though a reasonable argument can be made that reciprocity is a minor issue at this point and that cultural influences on individual behavior should be what cross-

TABLE 2.1

Examples of Cultural Research Approaches Involving Different Levels of
Variable Measurement and Inference

		Level of measurement	
		Individual	**Culture**
Level of Inference	**Individual**	*Example*: Development of culturally sensitive models of individual functioning (e.g., Triandis et al., 1984) *Possible problem*: Culturally uninformative	*Example*: Study of individual functioning based on characteristics of individual's culture (e.g., Individualism/Collectivism; Hofer et al., 2005) *Possible problem*: Ecological fallacy
	Culture	*Example*: Study of cultural values based on individual responses (e.g., Hofstede, 1980) *Possible problem*: Reverse ecological fallacy	*Example*: Hologeistic study of parenting styles (e.g., Rohner, 1975) *Possible problem*: Not applicable to individual behavior

cultural psychologists must emphasize in the current state of development of their discipline.

Unidirectional Relationships

Four perspectives on unidirectional relationships can be observed. Table 2.1 summarizes these perspectives, which are generated by the level (individual or culture) at which relevant variables are measured, and the level at which interpretations or conclusions are drawn. Two of the perspectives measure variables and reach conclusions at the same level (individual-individual or culture-culture) and present fewer conceptual challenges in this context. The remaining two perspectives involve cross-level interpretations and thus pose a greater challenge to researchers because they are subject to particular methodological difficulties (Hofstede, 2001).

Culture-oriented research in which variables are measured at and refer to the individual level of functioning can be powerful alternatives to mainstream psychological research that has, until recently, avoided dealing with potentially significant cultural influences on behavior (Adamopoulos & Lonner, 2001). An interesting and unusual application of such an approach is the modeling by Triandis et al. (1984) of perceptions of social behavior. The procedure involves the estimation of the likelihood of performing different behaviors in various social contexts by different actors with specific attributes (e.g., men, women, members of a particular culture or a socioeconomic class). Individual cognitive structures of the manner in which persons understand their world can be derived from such data. Variants of this approach were used by Adamopoulos (1982) to study the dimensionality of the social environment, and by Adamopoulos and Stogiannidou (1996) to develop a culturally sensitive approach to the understanding of social action.

The investigation generated personal psychological structures, but by varying the general context of the research procedure Triandis et al. (1984) were able to outline a procedure for cultural description as well. For example, they proposed selecting individuals from different socioeconomic and educational backgrounds, with differing family experiences, and employing targets of action who differed in religion, race, and other demographic and cultural factors. Such analyses would be expected to yield rich, if not comprehensive, descriptions of particular cultures, and, eventually, lead to models of social behavior that would be characteristic of specific cultures.

Naturally, such description is ultimately limited and may be of little relevance to the exploration of any possible individual–culture relationships. For example, it may be simply wishful thinking that cognitive structures obtained from individual members of a particular culture may yield significant clues about shared structures at the level of the cultural community, and thus this type of analysis may fail to reveal any theoretically interesting correspondence between the two levels.

A parallel argument can be developed for research in which variables are both measured at the level of culture and are used to draw conclusions at the same level. An example is Rohner's (1975) holocultural study of parenting styles with culture-level ratings derived from ethnographic records. Rohner (1975, 1986) reported significant relationships between social and economic conditions, parental acceptance or rejection, and psychological and behavioral outcomes for children. These outcomes may make sense to people raised in such a context, but it is impossible to state with any degree of certainty that a particular person's psychological makeup is directly affected by the variables featured in Rohner's culture-level model.

Cases in which the measurement of variables occurs at one level but their application occurs at another level are both more common and more problematic in cross-cultural psychology. Hofstede's (1980) work was an early attempt to use variables measured at the individual level in order to form culture-level indices regarding work values. He was among the first to recognize the possibility that any cultural indices constructed in this fashion may be meaningless unless theoretical relationships among variables are shown to hold at both the individual and cultural levels (see also Schwartz, 1992, for a similar argument). Along the same lines, Richards, Gottfredson, and Gottfredson (1990/1991) confirmed the possibility that variables measured at the individual level (students) may not always apply to the aggregate (classrooms)—a condition they termed the "individual differences fallacy."

Hofstede (2001) labeled this potential weakness of inference the "reverse ecological fallacy," in order to contrast it with the "ecological fallacy," which is the analysis of individual functioning based on the culture-level measurement of relevant variables or even on the *assumption* that certain theoretical relationships are valid among individuals simply because they can be found at the level of cultures. The ecological fallacy is an extremely common occurrence in cross-cultural psychology, is easily accepted among the practitioners of the field—as long as the particular theoretical relationships appear reasonable—and can be found even in methodologically sophisticated research. The most common assumption in recent years has been that individuals from cultures that are high on individualism or collectivism can be assumed to be individualists or collectivists, respectively. Thus, individual research participants are frequently not measured on these dimensions, even though constructs assumed to be influenced by culture are frequently modified by a wide variety of other factors. Klassen (2004), for example, in a meta-analysis of self-efficacy beliefs across cultures, found both that cultures differ in self-efficacy levels and that aggregate-level beliefs were affected by sociopolitical changes. Clearly, any attempt to make inferences at the individual level based on such aggregate-level data would be suspect.

It is only unusually thoughtful research that addresses this issue directly, and even in such cases a number of assumptions are made. For example, Hofer, Chasiotis, Friedlmeier, Busch, and Campos (2005) contrasted individual motives in several cultures using a TAT-type measure. They framed their expected differences in terms of individualism-collectivism, but the construct was not measured at the level of research participants. Instead, the investigators relied on culture-level indices provided by Hofstede (2001). In an additional step that mitigated the probability of the ecological fallacy, the researchers measured individual values, which are conceptually related to individualism-collectivism. However, this degree of caution is still relatively unusual, and it is often difficult to gauge the degree to which a particular investigation in this tradition is subject to the fallacy.

Reciprocal Relationships

Though it is likely that they are common in nature, bidirectional influences between culture and behavior are far less common in cross-cultural theory, probably because of their complexity. However, in theoretical discussions reciprocal relationships between culture and the individual are widely acknowledged. For example, the ecocultural framework explicitly assumes that while cultural adaptations may influence both the "inferred characteristics" and "observable behaviors" of the individual, the latter may in turn affect such variables as the ecology and the sociopolitical system at the population level (e.g., Berry, Poortinga, Segall, & Dasen, 2002).

Acknowledgment of reciprocity aside, most cases where the ecocultural framework has been used—explicitly or implicitly—concern cultural influences on individual behavior (cf., Lonner & Adamopoulos, 1997). In fact, it has often been assumed *explicitly* that such influences are far more powerful than the other way around (e.g., Smith, 2002). Other major frameworks used in cross-cultural comparisons also tend to make similar assumptions. Adamopoulos and Lonner (2001), for example, have pointed out that the self-construal approach developed by Markus and Kitayama (1991) implicitly but clearly explains the emergence of an independent or interdependent self as a function of the individual's culture. Thus, while an impressive number of intrapsychic processes—cognitive and motivational—are interpreted via the individual's *self-schema*, the latter is thought to be the product of a shared, and frequently not measured, abstraction at the population level (i.e., culture). Precisely what variables make up this abstraction is never clearly articulated, though presumably relevant individual- and culture-level processes are involved in reciprocal causal relationships.

The analysis of reciprocal relationships can be particularly useful in the development of culture-specific models of presumed pancultural structures. For example, the manifestation of cultural collectivism at the level of individual behavior can be studied in one of two ways:

1. One can simply go to different cultures and study a phenomenon (e.g., individual determinants of social behavior) independently. Naturally, this may yield little understanding or not even reveal the possibility that there are important underlying commonalities in the way the construct is conceptualized across cultures because of strong, albeit superficial, differences in its local manifestations. For example, in one culture individuals may weigh family obligations very heavily, whereas in another culture they may frame their behavior around work responsibilities. While seemingly different at the level of manifest behavior, these two may have a strong, though hidden, common theme of responsibility to the collective. The implicit assumption of unidirectional, culture-to-individual influences obscures this theme. In other words, studying a particular construct or phenomenon independently in different cultures and assuming a unidirectional influence—as is frequently the practice—makes it more likely to miss important underlying commonalities. On the other hand, assuming a reciprocal relationship in different cultures, studied together, makes it more likely to search for common denominators and build explanatory models with greater theoretical power. This idea is further explained below.
2. One can appreciate that collectivism may be a cultural characteristic that manifests itself differently across cultures. Starting from a testable assumption of universality, an investigator may identify cultural variants of the construct—for example, collectiv-

ism based primarily on social duty among Hindu Indians (e.g., Joan G. Miller, 1994) but on family connectedness in Greece (e.g., Georgas, 1993). A model of reciprocal influences will facilitate the identification of a universal construct as well as the description of its function as a determinant of individual behavior.

The "cultural psychology" tradition mentioned earlier in this chapter views reciprocal relationships between culture and the individual as the very definition of the discipline. In fact, both Shweder (1991, p. 2) and Joan G. Miller (1997), among many others, explicitly stated that individuals and cultures are constitutive components of each other—they "make each other up." Naturally, it is very difficult to distinguish between "levels" within this orientation. It seems to me that, to use Shweder's wonderful phrase, the "astonishment" of cultural psychology is that the independent self *is* (part of) the definition of individualism, the behavior of individuals *is* (part of) the very definition of culture—in other words, that the individual psyche *is* the cultural context. In this tradition the "problem of levels of analysis" becomes a pseudoproblem because variables that are usually considered to be at different levels blend into and become constitutive parts of each other. Thus, the "levels problem" defies precise description and poses no clear methodological concerns for the devotees of this orientation.

Researcher Bias in the Conceptualization of Individual–Culture Relationships

There exists among researchers a general expectation that explicit awareness of the problem of levels may mitigate the effects of cultural biases, and, in particular, of a Western, individualistic perspective in psychological explanation (e.g., Bond, 2002; Oyserman, Coon, & Kemmelmeier, 2002; Smith, 2002). For example, the golden methodological standard in cross-cultural research in the period from 1960 to 1980 was a procedure referred to as the "emic–etic" approach by Berry (1969, 1989), or its variant, the "locally inductive" approach (Malpass, 1977). Essentially, these approaches involve the use of theoretical abstractions developed within the confines of a particular culture (typically a Western one) to develop locally applicable construct definitions in other cultural contexts. This complex process necessarily involves as a first step moving from the individual level—where most monocultural psychological theories are developed—to a cultural abstraction (a cultural "emic" in the culture of origin). The next step is the assumption of a pancultural construction ("imposed etic"). This is followed by the development of culturally sensitive variants of the construct ("emics" in one or more other cultures) and their measurement—typically performed at the individual level. Finally, a cultural universal ("derived etic") is inferred.

This rather convoluted research paradigm is a stark reminder of the fact that inferences about individual behavior can easily be distorted if we lose sight of processes that occur or are more clearly observed at a higher level of abstraction (culture). Along the way, cross-cultural researchers must master diverse skills involving the study of intrapersonal, interpersonal, and cultural processes. The basic idea behind this set of methodological procedures is that awareness of culture-level processes that may affect individual behavior can help the investigator avoid a number of problems:

Theoretical Prestige Trumps Local Objections

Western psychology, by virtue of precedence, has generated much of the theoretical system currently in vogue. Established theories are generally more prestigious and can easily displace limited, local efforts at explaining various psychological phenomena in other geographical and cultural regions of the world. For example, there is no reason why Western scientists would question the universal relevance or validity of the "fundamental attribution error" (i.e., the overwhelming reliance by observers on internal explanations of the behavior of others), unless they were aware of culture-level differences like individualism and collectivism or similar constructs (e.g., Joan G. Miller, 1984). Polite objections by local scientists can be ignored in the face of a large number of prestigious publications attesting to the ubiquitousness of the process. Most scientists may not like to admit it, but this process is a variant of Kuhn's (1962) description of the manner in which scientific communities suppress anomalous research findings and theoretical ideas during periods of "normal science."

Western Rationality and Analytical Orientation Overwhelm Alternative Perspectives

Kuhn (1962) based his analysis of the process of scientific growth on the notion that "normal science" is predicated upon the scientific community's views and beliefs about the world. In light of his argument, we can extend the point made earlier regarding the dominant role of Western psychology to propose that non-Western perspectives have not received appropriate attention, despite calls for greater tolerance for divergent orientations (e.g., Shweder, 1986).

Recently, Nisbett, Peng, Choi, and Norenzayan (2001) made an important case for the reconsideration of the content–process distinction in cognition based on the argument that fundamentally different systems of thought are found in different parts of the world. Specifically, they proposed that Western philosophical systems are more analytic, whereas East Asian systems are more holistic. Though one can disagree with the particular way Nisbett et al. (2001) split the world—for example, they seem to ignore a strong contextualist undercurrent and a significant concern with individual responsibility toward the communal good in aspects of Ancient Greek thought—the distinction between holistic and analytical systems of thought can explain important directions in the history of modern psychology.

Individualistic Notions of Agency Cancel Culture-Based Explanations

Nisbett et al. (2001) related analytical thought to the development of notions of personal agency and holistic thought to the emergence of collective agency. This distinction offers an efficient account of the formation of modern theories of agency and intentionality in American psychology. Many of these theories celebrated the individual almost to the exclusion of any consideration that culture can play anything but a minor role in the formation of individual intentions. For example, the well-known theory of behavioral intentions by Fishbein and Ajzen (1975) explicitly assumed that all determinants of individual intentions are intrapsychic, and, further, that all "external" influences (cultural or otherwise) are filtered through these intrapsychic components. More recent extensions of the theory, while generally acknowledging the influence of sociocultural factors, do not deviate significantly from this basic assumption (Ajzen, 2001). The theory of planned behavior (e.g., Ajzen, 1991) still rests upon the notion that individual processes *mediate* the effects of "environmental" variables on behavior. Feldman (1999), who distinguished between intrapsychic or "proximal" causes of behavior and cultural or "distal" causes, has provided an explicit statement of this position, which is particularly popular among cognitive social psychologists. Once again, the effects of distal causes are thought to be mediated by intraindividual processes.

Models of this type are admirably efficient and work quite well within the worlds for which they were designed. The lack of consideration of culture–individual relationships, however, may significantly limit their applicability to specific cultural contexts. For example, the Fishbein and Ajzen model specifies two determinants of intentions: attitudes and subjective conceptions of normative behavior regarding a social object. In recent years, cross-cultural researchers have suggested that cultural norms are more likely to become internalized and thus more consistent with attitudes in collectivist cultures (Bontempo, Lobel, & Triandis, 1990). This finding implies that the two determinants identified by Fishbein and Ajzen (1975) are conceptually less distinguishable in collectivist cultures.

A further analysis of this issue suggests an even more complicated picture. Joan G. Miller's (1994) proposal that collectivist cultures have a duty-based moral code may mean that "moral obligation," a variable that is virtually indistinguishable from a subjective norm in monocultural (U.S.) research, plays a significant role in the formation of personal intentions in these cultures. In fact, Kidd, Litzner, and Adamopoulos (2006) have reported that moral obligation—distinct from a norm—appears to be related to collectivism even *within* an individualist culture like the United States. It is clear that culture plays a far more important role in the determination of individual behavior than has been traditionally assumed in Western psychology.

CULTURE AND THE INDIVIDUAL: INDEPENDENCE OR INTERDEPENDENCE OF LEVELS?

The argument at the heart of this chapter is whether or not we should expect isomorphism in individual-level and culture-level constructs and processes, and, by extension, whether or not such isomorphism reflects cross-level interactions. Both positions are reasonable and have been endorsed by a number of theorists through the years, including cultural and cross-cultural psychologists. In this section, I will consider the reasoning behind each position in turn and present several examples representing each point of view.

The basic thesis for independence of levels is simple: We should not expect *findings* at the individual level of analysis to mirror those at the cultural level because there is no compelling reason to expect such parallelism or isomorphism between the two levels (e.g., Bond, 1988; Leung & Bond, 1989; Shweder, 1973; Smith, 2002; see Polanyi, 1969, for a similar position in the biological sciences). This assumption necessitates the development of methodologies that allow the decoupling of phenomena under study at the two levels, as well as the construction of theoretical models appropriate for each level. As I have noted, there has been already quite a lot of activity in the methodological arena, but only some theoretical stirrings.

The statement that there is no necessary parallelism between individual and cultural levels implies that functional relationships among relevant variables at the two levels may be very different. Yet, as already described, in the same breath many cross-cultural researchers also assert that culture has a very strong influence on the individual—much stronger than the other way around (e.g., Smith, 2002). Lonner and Adamopoulos (1997) have pointed out that analyses that rely on the ecocultural framework (Berry et al., 2002)—and, indeed, most major theoretical approaches in cross-cultural psychology—also make such assumptions about the primacy of culture-to-individual processes, with culture typically considered an antecedent to individual behavior. While they are not logically inconsistent, these two assumptions taken together present a bit of a paradox, or, at the very least, an intellectual challenge: How does such a set of relationships develop? It is something of a mystery that one set of variables *strongly* and *directly* affects another, and yet the precise relationships between the two are rarely specified prior to analysis. We can feign ignorance, as has often—and justifiably—been done in discussions of biology–behavior connections and argue that analyses at different levels of abstraction complement but do not necessarily mirror each other (e.g., Rychlak, 1993). One can presumably deal with cognitive processes (e.g., decision making) without relying on explanations hinging on the functioning of neurons.

The situation is a bit different in cross-cultural psychology, however, because this discipline is *supposed* to bring the two levels together. Silverstein (1976) aptly observed that "in psychology, ignorance about behavior has been concealed, on occasion, by a retreat into the brain" (p. 411). More recently, we have seen a similar retreat from sociocultural explanations of behaviors like mate selection in favor of accounts based on evolutionary theory (e.g., Buss et al., 1990), even when the former appear quite likely (Lonner & Adamopoulos, 1997). Cross-cultural psychologists have no such luxury: They must confront phenomena related to individual behavior and cultural processes at the same time if they are to remain faithful to their aims. The complementarity of cross-level phenomena may lead to improved theoretical understanding (e.g., Raybeck, 2005), and, therefore, must be addressed—mystery or not. Heraclitus was quite likely correct— nature loves to hide—but this simply means that the problem of levels of analysis must be resolved through the formulation of theories that explain *at once* cross-level influences and interactions, as well as the emergence of different theoretical relationships among variables of interest at the individual and cultural levels. This has rarely been done in past years, though clearly such work is more frequently found today.

Independence or Decomposability of Levels

Let us consider further the argument that there is no compelling reason to expect isomorphism in the functional relationships between variables at the individual and cultural levels—in other words, that there is independence of levels. For the most part, this view has been based on empirical findings, rather than theoretical analysis. Shweder's (1973) statement of the problem appears to have been inspired by his empirical examination of several pairs of theoretical relationships. Similarly, Smith (2002) framed his argument about lack of isomorphism around specific examples. However, we must assume that at least some of the observed level differences are spurious and are due to artificial restrictions in the range of theoretical models, inappropriate or inadequate analytic techniques, and the like. Some examples may help explicate this problem.

In a holocultural investigation of the relationship between parental acceptance-rejection and artistic complexity, Rohner (1975) replicated findings of earlier research that, *at the cultural level*, there is a significant relationship between parental rejection and preference for complex artistic designs. In an attempt to clarify this puzzling relationship, Rohner and Frampton (1982) examined the same variables *at the individual level* within the United States and found exactly the opposite pattern: preference for complex art was correlated with perceived parental acceptance. Apparently what we have here is yet another "levels-of-analysis" puzzle.

It is likely, however, that the explanation is far more benign: Rohner's (1975) parental acceptance–rejection theory, which formed the theoretical foundation for the analysis of this phenomenon, is restricted to a single— albeit the most important—dimension of parental practices. It is quite possible that this empirical puzzle can be explained easily if we expand the theoretical framework to include additional dimensions—in this case parental dependence–independence training. In fact, Adamopoulos and Bontempo (1984) showed that such an expanded framework can easily reconcile the seemingly contradictory findings. At the cultural level, preference for artistic complexity is correlated both with severity of socialization and with independence training. Parental practices in the Unites States focus on the latter, but also involve parental acceptance. Thus, the case of the United States would contradict the culture-level results only if an important socialization dimension was not taken into consideration. The puzzle is not one of levels but one of restricted theoretical scope: A richer model does away with the problem.

A rather different explanation can be offered for an example used by Smith (2002) to illustrate the levels-of-analysis problem. Smith cited early social–psychological research that found a negative correlation between the frequency of individual lynchings of African Americans and the price of cotton in U.S. southern states over a period of approximately 50 years. The obvious explanation of this correlation is that low income from poor sales of cotton increased frustration, which in turn led to the lynchings. A different, county-by-county analysis, however, found that lynchings were most common in the counties with the fewest African Americans, and thus suggested that the presence of a visible minority explained the lynchings: Another levels-of-analysis puzzle?

Smith (2002) raised such a possibility by arguing that different causal mechanisms explained lynching behavior at two different levels. It is quite possible, however, that limited datasets and analytic techniques combined to create the illusion of two distinct explanations. In a much more recent reexamination of this problem, Hepworth and West (1988) used modern time-series techniques and confirmed the original economy-based explanation. Furthermore, they identified the same relationship between economic conditions and black as well as *white* lynchings. This quite possibly makes the aggregate (county)-level explanation questionable because it extends the economic frustration hypothesis to nonminority groups. At the very least, it suggests that we need to reconsider much more carefully the usefulness and accuracy of the aggregate-level hypothesis.

If we assume that we can always challenge the relevance of any one instance to the problem's resolution, and, therefore, question the ability of any set of converging empirical cases to make the point, it is perhaps necessary to reevaluate the problem's foundation. Are there possible theoretical arguments in favor of the proposition that there are no good reasons to expect cross-level isomorphism?

Simon (1965, 1973) developed a series of arguments that are skeptical of presumed cross-level continuities and, instead, approach complex social systems as hierarchies characterized by considerable independence among their components. He focused his ideas on the structure of what I would call production systems (e.g., a heat-exchange system, an economy), but his arguments are relevant to all hierarchies, broadly defined. Individual–culture relationships are, without a doubt, components of a social hierarchy.

Simon (1973) believed that the most successful natural systems are hierarchical (hence, "nature loves hierarchies") because there are evolutionary advantages to such structures: They can develop over long periods of time from very simple to highly complex forms and thus achieve great stability (see also James G. Miller, 1978). He cited as an example the Macedonian Empire built by Alexander the Great. Alexander received a smaller system (Macedonia) from his father, Philip, and added a number of subsystems reaching all the way to India. Upon his death, the system broke up into its subsystems (i.e., various geographical regions like Macedonia, Ptolemy's Egypt, the Old Persian Empire, etc.) instead of completely disintegrating. Regions acquired later in the campaign (e.g., near India) were far less stable upon the Empire's fragmentation, presumably because they did not have as much time to evolve within the system (Simon, 1965).

Following this line of reasoning, Simon (1973) was able to conclude that successful hierarchical systems are characterized by *near-independence* or *near-decomposability*. In other words, complex systems have an advantage if they are characterized by strong interactions *within* subsystems and weak interactions *among* subsystems. It should be obvious that a "loosely coupled" set of subsystems has a much greater chance of evolutionary success than a set of highly interdependent ones because in the latter case if a subsystem is damaged, the whole system suffers greatly. This adaptive property of hierarchical systems seems to be reflected in the ability of the brain to recover functions lost to injury or illness, a phenomenon known as plasticity (e.g., Ornstein, 1991). Naturally, the property of decomposability extends to vertical structures (i.e., across different levels of the hierarchy). It should be noted here that complete independence does not appear plausible to Simon because of "leakages" within various components of any system.

Simon's notion of near decomposability received a great deal of attention in subsequent discussions of multilevel systems because it seems to characterize a number of physical and social phenomena. However, it has also led to the development of antithetical points of view, reviewed in the next section, that emphasize the integration and cross-level interaction of system components, and predict the *emergence* of new system components that are often "indecomposable" (Hofstadter, 1979), or more "complex" than their constituent lower-level parts (Holland, 1998).

The evolutionary advantages of hierarchical systems should resonate with those cross-cultural psychologists who wish to argue that there is no reason to expect cross-level isomorphism in individual–culture relationships. Simon's (1973) line of reasoning could lead us to the conclusion that it is quite likely that different theoretical mechanisms operate at different levels of the system, and, therefore, that there is no reason to expect cross-level isomorphism. Put in a different way, if there is to be an evolutionary advantage for a hierarchy with individual psychological and cultural processes at distinct levels, these two sets of processes should proceed along more or less independent paths. That would maximize the availability of resources for dealing with environmental challenges to both the individual and the society. For example, cultural groups may develop collective coping mechanisms for a variety of reasons and in response to different sociohistorical forces, such as invasions from foreign enemies, civil conflicts, and economic conditions stemming from particularly constraining ecologies. Similarly, individuals may develop coping skills for dealing with intensely personal matters like grief from the loss of family members, psychic trauma, or professional success and failure to the extent that cultural mechanisms are not entirely effective in such cases. The net result of this development is that there will be no direct, one-to-one correspondence between individual and collective coping strategies, even though the system's overall capabilities are that much greater. It is quite possible that the outcome of such a process is what Kashima and Triandis (1986) captured with their finding that the self-serving bias, a coping skill manifested in internal attributions of success and external attributions of failures by actors, is observed in ability-related judgments in an individualistic culture like the United States. In a collectivist culture like Japan, however, this pattern is not observed, presumably because the Japanese culture has developed collective coping mechanisms that are available to the individual as needed within appropriate (i.e., in-group) contexts. This conclusion is supported—though not definitively—by recent statements confirming the greater prevalence of self-enhancement in individualistic, relative to collectivist cultures, and the importance of modesty in the latter (e.g., Heine, 2003; Heine & Lehman, 1999).

The individual human being is, of course, the beneficiary of coping strategies generated at the cultural level. Thus, we would expect to find some, or even significant, similarities ("leakages") across levels in coping strategies. The point of this example, however, is that there is an advantage to a hierarchical system in that different goals and processes at different levels maximize the coping mechanisms available to the individual or to the group.

Simon (1973) also proposed that near-decomposable systems have an additional evolutionary advantage because they can link different components of the system to distinct features of the system's environment—a process that allows them to evolve more rapidly. Thus, presumably, specific regions of Alexander's empire would be better able to deal with neighboring groups and border challenges than a monolithic structure that could not be responsive to local sensitivities. Similarly, the brain's plasticity may allow areas of the visual cortex to become dedicated to hearing in blind people, thus allowing them to hear better (Ornstein, 1991).

This process is well documented, though not identified as such, in cross-cultural research. For example, the analysis of individual conformity behavior based on the ecocultural framework explicitly takes into consideration the coupling of particular features of the ecology to certain attributes of the social system and to distinct patterns of socialization and individual behavior (e.g., Berry, 1979). Specifically, Berry assumes that ecologies that favor the development of agriculture-based subsistence economies encourage parental practices that emphasize training children to fulfill strict social role obligations and, therefore, result in high levels of conformity behavior in adults. Ecologies that promote the development of hunting–gathering economies, however, encourage parental practices that emphasize training children to be independent and self-reliant, and thus result in low levels of observed conformity among adults.

Decomposability: A Caveat

Simon's (1973) insightful analysis of the properties of hierarchical systems provides a theoretical argument for cross-cultural researchers who want to claim that there is no reason to expect isomorphism between cultures and individuals. However, Simon's account deviates in one important respect from such claims: There is nothing in his argument that supports the expectation—so widely shared by cross-cultural psychologists—that the influence of culture on the individual is much greater than the other way around. In fact, I suspect that if Simon had to argue one way or the other, he might support the opposite process. He believed, for example, that the pattern of each level is best understood through a process of abstraction from lower-level information (Simon, 1973). The implication appears to be that we should be better able to discern culture from the behavior of individual members than the other way around. If so, on what basis can one argue that the influence of culture on the individual is greater than that of the individual on the culture? A top-down process does not seem to be necessary or inevitable in this case, though it can be theoretically supportable. For example, Mead's (1932/1964) "social behaviorism" is founded upon the assumption that a mind—an individual self—could not possibly come to be without the prior existence of a social environment, which is a nexus of social relationships and interpersonal activity, or perhaps even a culture. This classical perspective has not had much success generating a receptive audience in experimental psychology and has not been used as the theoretical rationale for statements about the direction of culture–individual influence in cross-cultural psychology.

A somewhat similar approach has had considerable impact on cultural and, perhaps to a lesser extent, on cross-cultural psychology, however. Vygotsky's theory of intellectual development also is based on the notion that individual cognitive activity can only be understood as emerging within a complex of social relationships and cultural practices. Thus, the causal direction in the explanation of the development of mental activity in Vygotsky's approach appears to be from the sociocultural context to the individual (cf. Rogoff, 1990).

In general, a top-down process would have to assume that the transmission across generations of shared elements of culture (e.g., belief and value systems) is much more powerful, influential, or adaptive than the effect of individual activity on cultural practices and schemas. If this were the case, the individual psychological makeup could be revealed by a careful analysis of the interrelationships among the elements of culture. For example, by knowing the modal parental practices in a community a researcher ought to be able to predict individual behavior or personality traits. In contrast, a bottom-up process would assume the opposite: Individual decisions and actions determine to a large extent collective knowledge and cultural patterns. According to such a perspective, the behavior and cognitive activity of the individual reveal the belief system of the collective. Thus, for instance, the preponderance of individualistic values would predict the market-based economic model of the community.

Neither perspective has an obvious theoretical advantage because there are no clear criteria that can be used to select one type of process over the other—both seem perfectly reasonable. Therefore, it appears that it is only the bias of the discipline that shapes the very definite preferences of the cross-cultural community for a top-down process. After all, what distinguishes cross-cultural psychology from mainstream monocultural psychology is its ability to reach back—beyond the individual, the immediate situation, and the small group—to the culture and even to the ecology for explanations of human behavior.

CROSS-LEVEL GENERALIZATION

Just as a logically consistent argument can be developed for the decomposability of hierarchical systems, an equally compelling case can be made for interlevel generalization and, possibly, isomorphism. Scientists are always tempted to see relationships across levels of abstraction, and, in many instances, they may well be justified in doing so. Even Simon (1965), who was clearly of a different persuasion, admitted to the possibility of such relationships and, over a period of time, softened his arguments against this position.

It is not difficult to find examples of cross-level generalization in cross-cultural research. One interesting case that involves the possibility of isomorphism is found in discussions of individualism-collectivism—two culture–level constructs—and their personality correlates, idiocentrism and allocentrism (e.g., Triandis, 1995; Triandis, Leung, Villareal, & Clack, 1985). Despite the use of different terms, there is assumed to be strong correspondence across levels, such that idiocentrics are predominantly found in individualistic and allocentrics in collectivist cultures. In fact, the very definitions of the corresponding structures make use of each other (Triandis, 1995). To emphasize the correspondence further, Triandis (1995) has pointed to the fact that the two sets of constructs are highly correlated across a number of studies. Other researchers have also referred to connections between these constructs as well as related ones, but with greater caution (e.g., Schwartz, 1990).

The correspondence of individualism-collectivism and idiocentrism-allocentrism has been somewhat of a problem ever since Triandis et al. (1985) first proposed it. The different positions on this issue taken by the present chapter and that by van de Vijver, van Hemert, and Poortinga (this volume), which argues that the two sets of constructs are different enough to suggest nonisomorphism, is emblematic of the ambiguity of any cross-level relationship between them. However, it may well be that this divergence of opinion is based on the different orientations of the two arguments, with the former emphasizing isomorphism in theoretical terms and the latter focusing on empirical equivalence. As proposed elsewhere in this chapter, it may be useful for these two domains to employ different criteria for isomorphism.

Triandis et al. (1985) never defined what "correspondence" meant theoretically; they simply assumed that it must be there, even though they also acknowledged a need to keep individual-level and culture-level phenomena distinct from each other. Furthermore, this early statement of the psychological-level manifestation of individualism and collectivism implicitly assumed isomorphism. For example, Triandis et al. (1985) suggested that their approach could be used to develop "profiles" of predominant psychological tendencies in different cultures, so that in "a culture with a modal profile that is idiocentric, we would then be justified to use the label individualist culture," (p. 397). Implicit in this statement is the notion that individualism and collectivism at the cultural level are defined in terms of idiocentric and allocentric attributes, which necessarily means that individualism and idiocentrism, as well as collectivism and allocentrism, cannot possibly be theoretically all that different from each other. Some degree of isomorphism is taken for granted in this case.

The ensuing years of research on these constructs complicated this matter further because empirical findings did not always support the notion of isomorphism—or supported only a partial cross-level similarity. For example, Triandis (1995) argued that several major attributes of individualism-collectivism at the cultural level (e.g., "separation from in-group," "personal competence") were also found at the individual level, whereas one culture-level attribute ("family integrity") did not discriminate among individuals. However, this lack of correspondence was due to limits in the range of the variable within cultures, rather than to any theoretical differences between the two sets of constructs.

Over time, it became a matter of convenience to treat individualism and collectivism as opposite poles of a single dimension and idiocentrism and allocentrism as orthogonal dimensions (e.g., Triandis and Suh, 2002). In this fashion, cross-cultural researchers could contrast cultures while at the same time being able to maintain that any individual could have attributes of both types of culture. There was very little change, however, in our theoretical understanding of these cross-level relationships. Triandis and Suh (2002) maintained a "modal" approach, advocating that a sizable majority of individuals in collectivist cultures is allocentric, whereas in individualistic cultures a similar majority is idiocentric. Presumably, it continues to be the case that the psychological attributes shared by a majority of individuals in any culture are used to define the type of culture it is. What seems to be implied here is an isomorphism akin to that of a homology in evolutionary biology: The culture-level phenomenon is understood by reaching down to the level of individual processes.

Another example of cross-level isomorphism appears in an attempt to reconcile a number of psychological theories of social relations. I have described a process to explain the appearance of various forms of individualism and collectivism over time (Adamopoulos, 1999). This process is a member of a family of models that explain the emergence of interpersonal structure (e.g., Adamopoulos, 1991). These models begin with the assumption that the purpose of all human social behavior is to secure resources necessary for survival. They describe several types of affordances and constraints that typically operate on social exchange (e.g., the psychological characteristics of a resource or the nature of the interpersonal relationship). Over time, these constraints become integrated into psychological constructs that represent basic features of the meanings we attribute to our social environment (e.g., affiliation, dominance, or intimacy). In other words, this class of models describes various emergent structures of interpersonal relations.

The models implicitly describe cognitive processes that occur at the individual level: Their measurement across cultures has been at the individual level (e.g., Adamopoulos, 1984) and their diachronic predictions have been explored via systematic analyses of certain types of literary works (e.g., epic poetry) composed by single individuals (Adamopoulos, 1991; Adamopoulos & Bontempo, 1986). However, a basic assumption has been that cognitive processes are shared in a cultural community to the extent that its individual members need similar resources and are subject to similar constraints. Thus, authors of epic poems may be viewed as representing, in a very broad way, cultural knowledge and value systems. In other words, this approach has assumed that there is a strong congruence between individual and cultural systems.

Related culture-based theories of social relations include, of course, vertical and horizontal individualism and collectivism (Triandis, 1995) as well as Fiske's (1990) theory of the basic elements of sociality. Triandis (1995) has explicitly outlined the correspondence of the two theories, both of which are conceptualized at the cultural level. It is fairly easy to draw further direct connections between these two theories and the general model of interpersonal structure described above, even though the latter was conceptualized at the individual level. In other words, models that describe cultural patterns of social relations appear to map directly onto individual models of interpersonal interaction, indicating the possibility of substantial isomorphism across levels. Adamopoulos (1999) has provided a detailed description of this mapping.

General System Theory and the Argument for Isomorphism

Isomorphism in psychological structures existing at two distinct levels is, of course, not a novel idea. I have borrowed the term as used here from one of the best-known (and least understood) principles of Gestalt psychology, which concerns a hypothesized correspondence between experience and underlying brain events (Köhler, 1947). In broader terms, the notion that there exist strong relationships across levels of hierarchies that allow for generalizations from one level to another has been traced back at least to the middle of the 19th century (James G. Miller, 1978).

The intellectual force behind the logical possibility of cross-level generalizations and the basic assumption that processes at different levels are similar is *general system theory*. A major goal of this orientation was the description and explication of phenomena at different levels of abstraction using the same or similar theoretical mechanisms. In a very simple example, the same theory of growth can be applied to the understanding of the emergence of social organization in human societies and to the development of the structure of a production company (von Bertalanffy, 1968). Some social scientists saw in system theory an opportunity to represent formally heretofore vaguely understood behavioral and social phenomena by considering them analogous to more precisely described physical or physiological systems (e.g., Deutsch, 1968). The essence of this position is captured in the following statement (James G. Miller, 1971):

> What makes…interlevel formal identities among systems important
> and of absorbing interest, is that…very different structures, which
> carry out similar processes, may well turn out to carry out acts so
> much alike that they can be quite precisely described by the same
> formal model. (p. 287)

The success of this exceedingly ambitious perspective is at best dubious.
The desire for a nonreductionist unification of science is a lofty goal that
has proven particularly elusive to achieve. Even advocates of open system theory have cautioned against a simple assumption that individual
behavior can best be understood through processes found at different levels of abstraction, and have proposed instead a certain amount of level
independence (e.g., Katz & Kahn, 1966).

ISOMORPHISM OR NOT?

Both of the two major positions regarding isomorphism in multilevel systems that have been reviewed so far—one proposing the near independence of levels and the other advocating cross-level generalization and
isomorphism—are logically consistent and rich theoretical orientations.
There does not appear to exist at the present time an adequate set of formal criteria or empirical data that would allow us to select one approach
over the other, and, therefore, we cannot conclude with ease that either is
preferable.

It is quite possible that isomorphism in multilevel systems is content-
dependent. In other words, it is a phenomenon-driven characteristic of
natural systems. This possibility would explain the opposing positions
taken on the issue among cross-cultural researchers working in different theoretical domains, as described above, and is certainly supported
by findings that particular concepts do not necessarily have the same
meaning at the individual and national culture levels (e.g., Van de Vijver
& Poortinga, 2002). Obviously, there would be no reason to expect isomorphism if the meaning of a construct is different at two levels of a system.

The idea of content-driven isomorphism is also indirectly supported by
some of the general analyses of systems reviewed earlier. Simon (1965,
1973) described physical and social systems in which he believed cross-
level interactions are weak (i.e., they are nearly *decomposable*)—for example heat exchange systems or formal organizations. On the other hand,
Hofstadter (1979) described physical systems in which interactions among
components are so strong as to render them virtually indistinguishable
from each other (i.e., they are nearly *indecomposable*)—for example the
system of a proton constituted by strongly interacting quarks. It is quite

possible that isomorphism would not be found in the type of systems described by Simon, but would be found in the nearly indecomposable systems described by Hofstadter.

INDIVIDUAL–CULTURE RELATIONSHIPS REVISITED

There are several questions that are endemic to any discussion of the problem of levels of analysis in cross-cultural psychology. These include:

- What is the definition of a level? Are "culture" and "individual behavior" (broadly defined, of course) appropriate levels of the sort of theoretical system that cross-cultural researchers explore?
- What is the appropriate sequencing of levels in psychosocial systems that include the individual and culture?
- How can we conceptualize culture as a level of a system that also includes the individual as another level? What are the basic ingredients of such a conceptualization? Are there any available metaphors that might be useful in such an endeavor?
- What are major concerns in aggregating data to generate the level of culture?

Finding answers to these questions will go a long way toward clarifying the distinction between levels, describing their essential nature, and developing theoretical tools for the explanation of culture–individual interaction. These tasks far exceed the scope of this chapter; they will be mentioned here briefly only as a way of setting an agenda for future work.

What Is a Level?

It is not easy to find generally agreed-upon definitions of "levels" in discussions of hierarchical systems. It is a rather loose term that can be used to refer sometimes to vertical arrangements and at other times to horizontally distributed components of systems. Holland (1998) has offered an intuitively meaningful definition of levels in his discussion of the emergence of new patterns from a system's components. He proposed that levels involve the generation of a mechanism from some combination of simpler mechanisms. The definition ceases to be disturbing to most psychologists once the word *mechanism* is replaced with the words *process*, *unit*, and the like. However, this seemingly innocuous definition poses a tremendous challenge to cross-cultural researchers who work with constructs that involve individual–culture relationships. It requires that, to the extent that they treat individuals and cultures as levels, they specify the simple "mechanisms" that combine to produce more complex ones. As mentioned before, this is not done.

If we pursue the definitional challenge further, we run into an additional conceptual difficulty. By proposing that "[c]ulture is to society what memory is to individuals" or that "[c]ulture is to human collectivity what personality is to an individual," Triandis (1995, p. 4) and Hofstede (2001, p. 10), respectively, highlighted the difficulty with the assumption that "culture" and "individual" can be levels within the same hierarchical structure. In the world that Triandis's statement describes, culture would be preceded by some type of individual knowledge subsystem; only certain aspects of individual human beings and their behavior, which includes much more than knowledge structures, are parts of such a world. The very informality and intuitive nature of the term *level* generates a great deal of confusion as cross-cultural researchers go from the individual to the aggregate. What exactly is the appropriate aggregation in this context? I will return to this question later.

Appropriate Levels for Cross-Cultural Analysis

There is also considerable disagreement among social and behavioral scientists, including open system theorists, on what constitutes the proper sequencing of levels in any social system (e.g., James G. Miller, 1971). Even if we ignore for the moment the problem of a possible culture–behavior incompatibility (as levels of the same system), and we accept the term *culture* as a referent to a population, there are conflicting ideas about the structure of a relevant hierarchy. As much as we do not like to admit it, the standard practice in cross-cultural psychology is to use the words *society*, *nation*, and *ethnic group* as practically equivalent to *culture*, even though we have been properly chastised by our wiser colleagues on more than one occasion (e.g., Jahoda, 1984; Rohner, 1984).

A number of theorists have suggested that there are several levels that separate "nation" or "society" from "individual." For example, James G. Miller (1978; see also Hofstede, 2001) interposed the levels "group" and "organization" between "individual" and "society." It seems reasonable to argue that it is difficult to understand relationships among variables without examining relevant phenomena at all levels and *in their proper sequence*. The idea that we can discern what happens at the societal level without first understanding processes at the level of social organizations and institutions is at best hopeful. In fact, mature perspectives in cross-cultural psychology, like the ecocultural framework, take these steps for granted. Unfortunately, their dictates often cannot be followed because the process is exceedingly difficult, as can be seen in the work by Georgas,

Van de Vijver, and Berry (2004). In a complex application of ecocultural analysis, Georgas et al. related societal and ecological indices directly to individual behaviors. On the basis of theoretical considerations outlined so far, an argument can be made that there is a need to study individual and interindividual experiences *within the family and other social structures* before intrapsychic variables like values or subjective well-being can be understood. An argument can be made in this particular case that since individual behavior was measured at the aggregate level, there is no conflict with cross-level inferences. However, the point raised here is a conceptual one: Is it legitimate to explain individual behavior—however measured—from societal-level variables, or should one rely on intermediate structures like the family for a better understanding of how the whole system operates?

Along similar lines, "groups" in psychology typically consist of small, manageable numbers of individuals, gathered in close if not immediate proximity to each other, involved in specific relationships with each other, and communicating via particular channels (e.g., Levine & Moreland, 1995). Cultures are not "groups" as the latter are studied by social psychologists.

Cross-cultural psychologists have attempted to deal with problems of appropriate sequencing of levels in unique ways, including "doing away" with culture as a necessary concept (e.g., Segall, 1984) or introducing new terms like "national culture" (e.g., Hofstede, 2001). However, this strategic maneuvering only serves to emphasize the depth of the problem with levels in cross-cultural research. As mentioned earlier, in some approaches (e.g., cultural psychology) "culture" is seen as permeating *all* levels of a social system, and thus should not be viewed as a *separate* level that hovers above something like "behavior" or even "individual."

How Can Culture Constitute a Level of a System?

Cross-cultural psychology and related disciplines tend to define culture as a series of adaptations either "out there" or "in the mind" (Shore, 1996), which are shared by a fairly large number of people who happen to exist in relative (i.e., not necessarily immediate) geographical and historical proximity and are subject to particular affordances (McArthur & Baron, 1983) and constraints (Adamopoulos, 1991, 1999). In this context, "ecological" analyses of psychological phenomena attempt to *abstract* from the responses of individuals—who share these affordances, constraints, behavior patterns, worldviews, and values—some commonality or essential element that binds them all together. This process of abstraction is found in different forms in the work of a variety of scientists with distinct orientations. For example, Simon (1973) clearly viewed the ability to detect what happens at different levels of hierarchies as such an abstractive process. Valsiner (2004) developed a view of culture that emphasizes its functional representation within the individual psychological universe. Triandis (1993) generated the concept of a "cultural syndrome" by abstracting from the mass of attributes that are found in a group those that meet certain "sharedness" criteria. Finally, Fiske (1986) argued that individual proclivities and processes are manifested across levels of analysis in ways that differ in abstraction.

This process of describing, and ultimately measuring, culture as a psychological whole by extracting relevant themes shared by members of a group leads to a tacit construction. It generates inevitably a structure that can appropriately be included as a higher level in a hierarchical system that contains, at a lower level, the psychological makeup and behavior patterns of a single individual. For the lack of a better term I call such a construction a *virtual cultural participant* or, for those who prefer mixing the archaic with the modern, a *virtual denizen* of a culture. This virtual denizen is what culture means from a psychological point of view: *a distillation of adaptations to environmental challenges and to internal conflicts experienced and shared, however imperfectly, by individual members of a group.*

There are multiple manifestations of cultural knowledge and culturally appropriate behavior that appear in the real denizens of a society. My assumption is that underneath these various manifestations there exists a prototypical configuration of shared elements that can somehow capture the essence of what it means to be a participant of the specific culture. Shore (1996) calls such a configuration a "foundational schema." In my opinion, this is what a virtual denizen represents, and this is the point where the many different intellectual strands pursued in this chapter converge: The cross-level application of mathematical functions by system theorists, the wholeness of hierarchies advocated by Simon, the aggregation efforts by cross-cultural psychologists, even the "leakages" of near-decomposable systems. In a way, what cross-cultural researchers do by aggregating data to create a cultural construct is combing through idiographic (personal) manifestations of "foundational schemata" to generate a rather nomothetic (societal) view of specific behavioral domains (cf., Allport, 1937). This view can then be compared across instances generated by different affordances, constraints, ecologies, and the like. As a final note, it may be worth mentioning that such a construction is not subject to the problems associated with the ecological fallacy, reviewed earlier.

Aggregating Individual Instances

This line of argument at once clarifies the conceptual nature of "culture" as a level of a hierarchy and introduces a series of methodological considerations. In constructing such a virtual denizen for a given culture exactly *how* the individual data are aggregated becomes of paramount importance. The following two questions are central to this methodological puzzle:

What Procedures Should Be Used to Develop
Profiles of Virtual Denizens?

Cross-cultural researchers have used a variety of procedures to generate cultural profiles that approximate the present notion of a virtual denizen. These procedures range from simple means of cultural samples to far more complex data reduction and scaling techniques. I propose, however, that this problem is not merely statistical, but extends into the theoretical arena. In other words, a virtual denizen should be conceptualized as a complex cultural norm that is derived from the aggregation of a sampling of individual instances. Such a norm will reflect world knowledge accessible to a group of people and have implications for their cognitive and behavioral functioning. I suspect that a conceptual system analogous to norm theory (Kahneman & Miller, 1986) that can be extended beyond the intraindividual level may be necessary in this case. I find one element of norm theory particularly intriguing. Kahneman and Miller have argued that essential to the development of a norm about one's experience of reality is the construction of counterfactuals based on the principle of mutability: The individual experiences reality, counterfactuals are produced and, depending on their ability to change mutable aspects of reality, these counterfactuals will affect norm formation to a greater or lesser extent. In the case of the formation of a cultural index—a sort of cultural norm—individual instances of behavior that run counter to general expectation are viewed as "error" or "outliers" in standard treatments of the problem. However, such "counterfactuals" may in fact reflect individual variations or adjustments to the cultural norm or foundational schema, likely affect the experiences (and surprise) of others in the group, and, therefore, should be treated with much greater theoretical respect.

It is this emphasis on the importance of divergent perspectives that sets the notion of a virtual denizen apart from similar-sounding constructions, like "modal personality" from the culture-and-personality school or the notion of "citizen scores" advocated by some cross-cultural researchers (e.g., Smith, Bond, & Kagitcibasi, 2006). "Modal personality" is a statistical concept that relies on measures of central tendency to characterize the personality that is typical of a cultural group. It does not necessarily reflect interrelationships among traits or patterns of behavior (e.g., Wallace, 1970). Similarly, "citizen scores" are also statistical concepts; they refer to sample means on a particular variable, and also do not reflect patterns of relationships.

The virtual denizen is primarily a theoretical, rather than a statistical, construction. It should include not only information about central tendency, but also about dispersion—as a gauge of individual variation around the norm—and, most important, it should incorporate information about patterns of relationships among variables of interest (foundational schemata). Put in a different way, it may well be that the precise configuration of a virtual denizen should be context-dependent, and different procedures may need to be used for different research questions.

What Conceptual Criteria Should Be Used to Define an Appropriate Group of People for Aggregation?

In some ways this is similar to asking how many cultures there are, which is an unanswerable question (Triandis, 1994). The relatively sloppy sampling procedures employed in much cross-cultural research make it difficult to define populations to which findings can be generalized. An easy answer may be simply to demand that we specify the criteria used for the selection of individual cases that will be used in the construction of the virtual denizen. At the very least, this will enhance comparability across investigations.

CONCLUSION

In this chapter I attempted to summarize two major theoretical orientations with regard to individual–culture relationships, viewed from a systems perspective, along with concomitant issues and problems. At the risk of oversimplifying these complex orientations, they can be summarized as follows: Individuals and cultures (broadly defined) are levels of hierarchical systems that can be characterized as involving (1) strong interactions *within* levels but weak interactions *across* levels, or (2) strong interactions *both* within and across levels. In the first case we would expect to find a lack of *isomorphism* across levels. In other words, we would not expect that structural patterns and relationships among constructs would be similar at the levels of individuals and cultures. In the second case we would anticipate isomorphic relationships and structural similarities across levels.

Both orientations are reasonable and psychologically consistent, and there appear to be no absolute criteria that would lead us to prefer one over the other. In fact, multilevel systems of both types appear to be abundant in nature, from subatomic particles to economic and sociocultural hierarchies. This suggests the possibility that isomorphism across levels is phenomenon-specific, and it should come as no surprise that some cultural researchers find similar structural relationships across levels and some do not. Therefore, the choice of orientation cannot really be anticipated, but, rather, will *unfold* as researchers investigate particular domains of individual–culture relationships.

A critical issue in the examination of individuals and cultures within a system is the appropriate understanding of "culture" as a level of the system. Current definitions of culture in cultural and cross-cultural psychology, which typically focus on adaptations to environmental challenges by geographically bound groups, make it difficult to conceive how such an abstract configuration of ideas can be a higher level in a system with individual human beings at a lower level. It was proposed that we develop the concept of a "virtual cultural denizen" as a more appropriate level in such a system. Unlike the notions of "citizen score" and "modal personality," a virtual denizen is not a statistical concept. In fact, its measurement may well employ different procedures across investigations. Rather, the "virtual cultural denizen" is a theoretical construct that should convey what it means to be a member of a cultural group and, at the same time, reflect individual variations around basic cultural schemata, norms, and shared belief systems. A number of social and behavioral scientists have proposed similar ideas. However, cross-cultural psychologists have yet to consolidate and integrate their approaches into a generally agreed-upon concept of culture as a level of a multilevel system. I believe such a development is an important goal in the study of psychology and culture.

Author Note

I am grateful to Christine Smith and to the editors of this volume for helpful comments on an earlier version of this text.

REFERENCES

Adamopoulos, J. (1982). The perception of interpersonal behavior: Dimensionality and importance of the social environment. *Environment and Behavior, 14,* 29–44.

Adamopoulos, J. (1984). The differentiation of interpersonal behavior: Toward an explanation of universal interpersonal structures. *Journal of Cross-Cultural Psychology, 15,* 487–508.

Adamopoulos, J. (1991). The emergence of interpersonal behavior: Diachronic and cross-cultural processes in the evolution of intimacy. In S. Ting-Toomey & F. Korzenny (Eds.), *International and intercultural communication annual* (Vol. 15, pp. 155–170). Thousand Oaks, CA: Sage.

Adamopoulos, J. (1999). The emergence of cultural patterns of interpersonal behavior. In J. Adamopoulos & Y. Kashima (Eds.), *Social psychology and cultural context* (pp. 63–76). Thousand Oaks, CA: Sage.

Adamopoulos, J., & Bontempo, R. N. (1984). A note on the relationship between socialization practices and artistic preference. *Cross-Cultural Psychology Bulletin, 18*(2–3), 4–7.

Adamopoulos, J., & Bontempo, R. N. (1986). Diachronic universals in interpersonal structures: Evidence from literary sources. *Journal of Cross-Cultural Psychology, 17,* 169–189.

Adamopoulos, J., & Lonner, W. J. (1994). Absolutism, relativism, and universalism in the study of human behavior. In W. J. Lonner & R. Malpass (Eds.), *Psychology and culture* (pp. 129–134). Boston: Allyn & Bacon.

Adamopoulos, J., & Lonner, W. J. (2001). Culture and psychology at a crossroad: Historical perspective and theoretical analysis. In D. Matsumoto (Ed.), *The handbook of culture and psychology* (pp. 11–34). Oxford: Oxford University Press.

Adamopoulos, J., & Stogiannidou, A. (1996). The perception of interpersonal action: Culture-general and culture-specific components. In H. Grad, A. Blanco, & J. Georgas (Eds.), *Key issues in cross-cultural psychology* (pp. 263–275). Lisse, the Netherlands: Swets & Zeitlinger.

Ajzen, I. (1991). The theory of planned behavior. *Organizational Behavior and Human Decision Processes, 50,* 179–211.

Ajzen, I. (2001). Nature and operation of attitudes. *Annual Review of Psychology, 52,* 27–58.

Allport, G. W. (1937). *Personality: A psychological interpretation.* New York: Henry Holt.

Anderson, J. R. (1990). *The adaptive character of thought.* Hillsdale, NJ: Lawrence Erlbaum.

Berry, J. W. (1969). On cross-cultural compatibility. *International Journal of Psychology, 4,* 119–128.

Berry, J. W. (1979). A cultural ecology of social behavior. In L. Berkowitz (Ed.), *Advances in experimental social psychology* (Vol. 12, pp. 177–206). New York: Academic Press.

Berry, J. W. (1989). Imposed etics-emics-derived etics: The operationalization of a compelling idea. *International Journal of Psychology, 24,* 721–735.

Berry, J. W., Poortinga, Y. H., Segall, M. H., & Dasen, P. R. (2002). *Cross-cultural psychology: Research and applications* (2nd ed.). New York: Cambridge University Press.

Bond, M. H. (1988). Finding universal dimensions of individual variation in multicultural studies of values: The Rokeach and Chinese value surveys. *Journal of Personality and Social Psychology, 55,* 1009–1015.

Bond, M. H. (2002). Reclaiming the individual from Hofstede's ecological analysis—A 20-year Odyssey: Comment on Oyserman et al. (2002). *Psychological Bulletin, 128,* 73–77.

Bontempo, R., Lobel, S., & Triandis, H. C. (1990). Compliance and value internalization in Brazil and the U.S.: Effects of allocentrism and idiocentrism. *Journal of Cross-Cultural Psychology, 21,* 200–213.

Buss, D. M., Abbott, M., Angleitner, A., Asherian, A., Biaggio, A., Blanco-Villasenor, A., et al. (1990). International preferences in selecting mates. *Journal of Cross-Cultural Psychology, 21,* 5–47.

Cacioppo, J. T., Berntson, G. G., Sheridan, J. F., & McClintock, M. K. (2000). Multilevel integrative analyses of human behavior: Social neuroscience and the complementing nature of social and behavioral approaches. *Psychological Bulletin, 126,* 829–843.

Deutsch, K. W. (1968). Toward a cybernetic model of man and society. In W. Buckley (Ed.), *Modern systems research for the behavioral scientists: A sourcebook* (pp. 387–400). Chicago: Aldine.

Feldman, J. M. (1999). Four questions about human social behavior: The social cognitive approach to culture and psychology. In J. Adamopoulos & Y. Kashima (Eds.), *Social psychology and cultural context* (pp. 43–62). Thousand Oaks, CA: Sage.

Fishbein, M., & Ajzen, I. (1975). *Belief, attitude, intention, and behavior: An introduction to theory and research*. Reading, MA: Addison-Wesley.

Fiske, A. P. (1990). *Structures of social life: The four elementary forms of human relations*. New York: Free Press.

Fiske, D. W. (1986). Specificity of method and knowledge in social science. In D. W. Fiske & R. A. Shweder (Eds.), *Metatheory in social science* (pp. 61–82). Chicago: University of Chicago Press.

Georgas, J. (1993). An ecological–social model for indigenous psychology: The example of Greece. In U. Kim & J. W. Berry (Eds.), *Indigenous psychologies: Theory, method, and experience in cultural context* (pp. 56–78). Newbury Park, CA: Sage.

Georgas, J., Van de Vijver, F. J. R., & Berry, J. W. (2004). The ecocultural framework, ecosocial indices, and psychological variables in cross-cultural research. *Journal of Cross-Cultural Psychology, 35*, 74–96.

Goodson, F. E., & Morgan, G. A. (1976). On levels of psychological data. In M. H. Marx & F. E. Goodson (Eds.), *Theories in contemporary psychology* (2nd ed., pp. 394–407). New York: Macmillan.

Gould, S. J. (2002). *The structure of evolutionary theory*. Cambridge, MA: Harvard University Press.

Heine, S. J. (2003). Making sense of East Asian self-enhancement. *Journal of Cross-Cultural Psychology, 34*, 596–602.

Heine, S. J., & Lehman, D. R. (1999). Culture, self-discrepancies and self-satisfaction. *Personality and Social Psychology Bulletin, 25*, 915–925.

Hepworth, J. T., & West, S. G. (1988). Lynchings and the economy: A time-series reanalysis of Hovland and Sears (1940). *Journal of Personality and Social Psychology, 55*, 239–247.

Heraclitus (1960). Fragments. In P. Wheelwright (Ed. & Trans.), *The Presocractics* (pp. 69–79). Indianapolis: Bobbs-Merrill. (Original work published ca. 500 BCE)

Hofer, J., Chasiotis, A., Friedlmeier, W., Busch, H., & Campos, D. (2005). The measurement of implicit motives in three cultures: Power and affiliation in Cameroon, Costa Rica, and Germany. *Journal of Cross-Cultural Psychology, 36*, 689–716.

Hofstadter, D. R. (1979). *Gödel, Escher, Bach: An eternal golden braid*. New York: Vintage Books.

Hofstede, G. (1980). *Culture's consequences: International differences in work-related values*. Beverly Hills, CA: Sage.

Hofstede, G. (2001). *Culture's consequences: Comparing values, behaviors, institutions, and organizations across nations* (2nd ed.). Thousand Oaks, CA: Sage.

Holland, J. H. (1998). *Emergence: From chaos to order*. Reading, MA: Addison-Wesley.

Hox, J. J. (2000). Multilevel analyses of grouped and longitudinal data. In T. D. Little, K. U. Schnabel, & J. Baumert (Eds.), *Modeling longitudinal and multilevel data: Practical issues, applied approaches, and specific examples* (pp. 15–32). Mahwah, NJ: Lawrence Erlbaum.

Hox, J. (2002). *Multilevel analysis: Techniques and applications*. Mahwah, NJ: Lawrence Erlbaum.

Jahoda, G. (1984). Do we need a concept of culture? *Journal of Cross-Cultural Psychology, 15*, 139–151.

Kahneman, D., & Miller, D. T. (1986). Norm theory: Comparing reality to its alternatives. *Psychological Review, 93*, 136–153.

Kashima, Y., & Triandis, H. C. (1986). The self-serving bias in attribution as coping strategy: A cross-cultural study. *Journal of Cross-Cultural Psychology, 17*, 83–98.

Katz, D., & Kahn, R. L. (1966). *The social psychology of organizations*. New York: John Wiley.

Kidd, C., Litzner, K., & Adamopoulos, J. (2006, May). *The role of cultural and personality variables in the formation of intentions*. Paper presented at the Midwestern Psychological Association meeting, Chicago.

Klassen, R. M. (2004). Optimism and realism: A review of self-efficacy from a cross-cultural perspective. *International Journal of Psychology, 39*, 205–230.

Köhler, W. (1947). *Gestalt psychology: An introduction to new concepts in modern psychology*. New York: Liveright.

Kuhn, T. S. (1962). *The structure of scientific revolutions*. Chicago: University of Chicago Press.

Leung, K., & Bond, M. H. (1989). On the empirical identification of dimensions for cross-cultural comparisons. *Journal of Cross-Cultural Psychology, 20*, 133–151.

Levine, J. M., & Moreland, R. L. (1995), Group processes. In A. Tesser (Ed.), *Advanced social psychology* (pp. 419–465). New York: McGraw-Hill.

Little, T. D., Schnabel, K. U., & Baumert, J. (Eds.) (2000). *Modeling longitudinal and multilevel data: Practical issues, applied approaches and specific examples*. Mahwah, NJ: Lawrence Erlbaum.

Lonner, W. J., & Adamopoulos, J. (1997). Culture as antecedent to behavior. In J. W. Berry, Y. H. Poortinga, & J. Pandey (Eds.), *Handbook of cross-cultural psychology: Vol. 1. Theory and method* (pp. 43–83). Boston: Allyn & Bacon.

McArthur, L. Z., & Baron, R. M. (1983). Toward an ecological theory of social perception. *Psychological Review, 90*, 215–238.

Malpass, R. S. (1977). Theory and method in cross-cultural psychology. *American Psychologist, 32*, 1069–1079.

Markus, H. R., & Kitayama, S. (1991). Culture and the self. *Psychological Review, 98*, 224–253.

Mead, G. H. (1964). *Mind, self, and society from the standpoint of a social behaviorist*. Chicago: University of Chicago Press. (Original work published 1932)

Miller, James G. (1971). The nature of living systems. *Behavioral Science, 16*, 277–301.

Miller, James G. (1978). *Living systems*. New York: McGraw-Hill.

Miller, Joan G. (1984). Culture and the development of everyday social explanation. *Journal of Personality and Social Psychology, 46*, 961–978.

Miller, Joan G. (1994). Cultural diversity in the morality of caring: Individually oriented versus duty-based interpersonal moral codes. *Cross-Cultural Research, 28*, 3–39.

Miller, Joan G. (1997). Theoretical issues in cultural psychology. In J. W. Berry, Y. H. Poortinga, & J. Pandey (Eds.), *Handbook of cross-cultural psychology: Vol. 1. Theory and method* (pp. 85–128). Boston: Allyn & Bacon.

Nezlek, J. B. (2001). Multilevel random coefficient analyses of event and interval contingent data in social and personality psychology research. *Personality and Social Psychology Bulletin, 27,* 771–785.

Nisbett, R. E., Peng, K., Choi, I., & Norenzayan, A. (2001). Culture and systems of thought: Holistic versus analytic cognition. *Psychological Review, 108,* 291–310.

Ornstein, R. (1991). *The evolution of consciousness: The origins of the way we think.* New York: Touchstone.

Oyserman, D., Coon, H., & Kemmelmeier, M. (2002). Rethinking individualism and collectivism: Evaluation of theoretical assumptions and meta-analyses. *Psychological Bulletin, 128,* 3–72.

Polanyi, M. (1969). Life's irreducible structure. *Science, 160,* 1308–1312.

Prasolov, V. V. (1995). *Intuitive topology* (A. Sossinsky, Trans.). American Mathematical Society.

Raybeck, D. (2005). The case for complementarities. *Cross-Cultural Research, 39,* 235–251.

Richards, J. M., Gottfredson, D. C., & Gottfredson, G. D. (1990/1991). Units of analysis and item statistics for environmental assessment scales. *Current Psychology: Research and Reviews, 9,* 407–413.

Rogoff, B. (1990). *Apprenticeship in thinking: Cognitive development in social context.* New York: Oxford University Press.

Rohner, R. P. (1975). *They love me, they love me not.* New Haven, CT: HRAF Press.

Rohner, R. P. (1984). Toward a conception of culture for cross-cultural psychology. *Journal of Cross-Cultural Psychology, 15,* 111–138.

Rohner, R. P. (1986). *The warmth dimension: Foundations of parental acceptance-rejection theory.* Newbury Park, CA: Sage.

Rohner, R. P., & Frampton, S. B. (1982). Perceived parental acceptance-rejection and artistic preference. *Journal of Cross-Cultural Psychology, 13,* 250–259.

Rumelhart, D. E., & McClelland, J. L. (1986). PDP models and general issues in cognitive science. In D. E. Rumelhart, & J. L. McClelland (Eds.), *Parallel distributed processing: Explorations in the microstructure of cognition: Vol. 1. Foundations* (pp. 110–146). Cambridge, MA: MIT Press.

Rychlak, J. F. (1993). A suggested principle of complementarity for psychology: In theory, not method. *American Psychologist, 48,* 933–942.

Schwartz, S. H. (1990). Individualism-collectivism: Critique and proposed refinements. *Journal of Cross-Cultural Psychology, 21,* 139–157.

Schwartz, S. H. (1992). Universals in the structure and content of values: Theoretical advances and empirical tests in 20 countries. In M. Zanna (Ed.), *Advances in experimental social psychology* (Vol. 25, pp. 1–65). Orlando, FL: Academic Press.

Segall, M. H. (1984). More than we need to know about culture, but are afraid not to ask. *Journal of Cross-Cultural Psychology, 15,* 153–162.

Segall, M. H., Dasen, P. R. Berry, J. W., & Poortinga, Y. H. (1999). *Human behavior in global perspective: An introduction to cross-cultural psychology* (2nd ed.). Boston: Allyn & Bacon.

Shore, B. (1996). *Culture in mind: Cognition, culture, and the problem of meaning.* New York: Oxford University Press.

Shweder, R. A. (1973). The between and within of cross-cultural research. *Ethos, 1,* 531–545.

Shweder, R. A. (1986). Divergent rationalities. In D. W. Fiske & R. A. Shweder (Eds.), *Metatheory in social science: Pluralisms and subjectivities* (pp. 163–196). Chicago: University of Chicago Press.

Shweder, R. A. (1990). Cultural psychology—What is it? In J. W. Stigler, R. A. Shweder, & G. Herdt (Eds.), *Cultural psychology: Essays on comparative human development* (pp. 1–43). New York: Cambridge University Press.

Shweder, R. A. (1991). *Thinking through culture: Expeditions in cultural psychology.* Cambridge, MA: Harvard University Press.

Silverstein, A. (1976). On reductionism. In M. H. Marx & F. E. Goodson (Eds.), *Theories in contemporary psychology* (2nd ed., pp. 407–411). New York: Macmillan.

Simon, H. A. (1965). The architecture of complexity. *General Systems, 10,* 63–76.

Simon, H. A. (1973). The organization of complex systems. In H. H. Patee (Ed.), *Hierarchy theory: The challenge of complex systems* (pp. 1–27). New York: George Braziller.

Smith, P. B. (2002). Levels of analysis in cross-cultural psychology. In W. J. Lonner, D. L. Dinnel, S. A. Hayes, & D. N. Sattler (Eds.), *Online readings in psychology and culture.* Retrieved from Western Washington University web site: http://www.wwu.edu/~culture

Smith, P. B. (2004). Nations, cultures, and individuals: New perspectives and old dilemmas. *Journal of Cross-Cultural Psychology, 35,* 6–12.

Smith, P. B., Bond, M. H., & Kagitcibasi, C. (2006). *Understanding social psychology across cultures: Living and working in a changing world.* London: Sage.

Sperry, R. (1982). Some effects of disconnecting the cerebral hemispheres. *Science, 217,* 1223–1226.

Triandis, H. C. (1993). Collectivism and individualism as cultural syndromes. *Cross-Cultural Research, 27,* 155–180.

Triandis, H. C. (1994). *Culture and social behavior.* New York: McGraw-Hill.

Triandis, H. C. (1995). *Individualism and collectivism.* Boulder, CO: Westview Press.

Triandis, H. C., Hui, C. H., Albert, R. D., Leung, S. M., Lisansky, J., Diaz-Loving, R. et al. (1984). Individual models of social behavior. *Journal of Personality and Social Psychology, 46,* 1389–1404

Triandis, H. C., Leung, K., Villareal, M. J., & Clack, F. (1985). Allocentric versus idiocentric tendencies: Convergent and discriminant validation. *Journal of Research in Personality, 19,* 395–415.

Triandis, H. C., & Suh, E. M. (2002). Cultural influences on personality. *Annual Review of Psychology, 53,* 133–160.

Valsiner, J. (2004, August). *Functional culture: The central theme for theoretical constructs in human psychology.* Paper presented at the 28th International Congress of Psychology, Beijing, China.

Van de Vijver, F. J. R., & Poortinga, Y. H. (2002). Structural equivalence in multilevel research. *Journal of Cross-Cultural Psychology, 32,* 141–156.

von Bertalanffy, L. (1968). *General system theory: Foundations, development, applications.* New York: George Braziller.

Wallace, A. F. C. (1970). *Culture and personality* (2nd ed.). New York: Random House.

Part II

Methodological Issues

3

Traditional and Multilevel Approaches in Cross-Cultural Research: An Integration of Methodological Frameworks

Johnny R. J. Fontaine

Many of the challenges facing monocultural psychological research are intensified when comparing psychological functioning across cultures. Valid use of the same measurement instrument across cultural groups is problematic. Moreover, psychological constructs may be tied to a specific cultural context, which precludes generalizability of theories (usually developed and operationalized in Western settings) from one cultural group to another. Even if psychological constructs correspond across cultural groups and even if the position of individuals within cultures on a construct can be identified validly by means of the same indicators, there is still a host of method artifacts that can distort the meaning of quantitative differences in scores on measures across these groups. Examples include differences in social desirability and acquiescence tendency between cultural groups that affect score levels in a host of self-report instruments, but are rarely made explicit (see Smith & Fischer, this volume).

An extensive methodological framework has been developed to cope with these challenges (e.g., Berry, Poortinga, Segall, & Dasen, 2002; Poortinga, 1989; Poortinga & Van de Vijver, 1987; Van de Vijver & Leung, 1997a, 1997b), to which I will refer as the traditional methodological framework for cross-cultural psychology. This framework is mainly oriented toward the analysis of individual scores. However, individuals are nested in cultural groups, implying that cultural context has to be taken into account when analyzing and understanding behavior. The simultaneous analysis of individual data and cultural data requires a multilevel approach. The aim of the present chapter is to discuss how multilevel approaches can contribute to the elaboration of the traditional framework. Despite the many possible applications multilevel theorizing and statistical modeling are only slowly entering cross-cultural research. One of the reasons is that multilevel models are often seen as a set of statistical procedures. However, the innovations offered by multilevel modeling are both statistical in nature, and also conceptual. The use of multilevel approaches has implications for both the conceptualization of research questions and the way in which data are analyzed.

To clarify the contribution of multilevel approaches, I discuss first the traditional methodological framework underlying contemporary research in cross-cultural psychology. In the second section, I explain the multilevel approach and demonstrate how this approach throws a new light on methodological issues. In the third section, I present the development of a methodological framework that integrates the traditional with the multilevel approach. Finally, I derive from this integrated framework four prototypical types of comparability that implicitly or explicitly guide cross-cultural research.

THE TRADITIONAL METHODOLOGICAL
FRAMEWORK OF CROSS-CULTURAL PSYCHOLOGY

A basic distinction in the methodology and data analysis of the social sciences can be made between (1) the identification of differences between individuals and between groups on constructs, and (2) the explanation of these differences. This distinction is also central for cross-cultural research and I first present these issues in more detail.

First, measurement amounts to estimating the position of individuals or groups on a theoretical and often unobservable variable on the basis of a set of observable variables that are assumed to all give an indication of that underlying theoretical variable. Measurement issues are focused on two types of variables: theoretical variables (called constructs in conceptual approaches and latent variables in statistical approaches) and observed variables (also called indicators). The step from observed to latent variables is justified by examining associations among the observed variables. Only if the indicators are significantly associated with each other, can they be assumed to measure the same construct. This condition is investigated by an analysis of the internal structure of an instrument (i.e., an analysis of the interrelationships of the items in the instrument).

Various data-analytic models have been proposed to examine internal structure, such as multidimensional scaling (MDS), principal component analysis (PCA), exploratory and confirmatory factor analysis (EFA, CFA), and item response theory (IRT) models. These models differ in terms of the restrictions they impose on the associations among the indicators, with MDS being least restrictive and confirmatory latent variable models (CFA, IRT) imposing most restrictions. While MDS only maps relative differences in the associations among indicators, CFA and IRT models test statistically whether the observed relationships among the indicators can be fully accounted for by the underlying latent variable (which is called the assumption of local independence).

The second set of issues deals with the explanation of differences between individuals and between groups. This is done by examining causal antecedents that can account for the differences. These causal relationships can be deterministic or probabilistic. Almost all causal models in the social sciences employ the general linear model (GLM). There are many GLM models; the three most frequently used are also the most important for the present chapter, namely analysis of variance (ANOVA), multiple regression analysis, and analysis of covariance (ANCOVA).

In line with the distinction between measurement and explanation in the social sciences in general, there are two common aims in cross-cultural psychological research. The first is the valid identification of differences and similarities between cultural groups and between individuals belonging to different cultural groups. The second aim is the valid explanation of these differences and similarities in terms of cultural characteristics. The bias and equivalence framework deals with the first question and cultural sampling and cultural unpacking deal with the second question. Each is presented in more detail below.

Measurement: The Equivalence and Bias Framework

A major part of cross-cultural research consists of comparing samples from various cultural groups on psychological scales. Severe doubts have been cast on the validity of such comparisons. The concept of equivalence and the concept of bias have been developed to deal with the question whether measurements represent identical constructs on identical scales. Equivalence refers to the comparability of psychological variables, while bias points to incomparability. Four levels of equivalence and four main categories of bias have been distinguished in the literature (e.g., Fontaine, 2005; Poortinga, 1989; Van de Vijver & Leung, 1997a, 1997b). I will first present these levels of equivalence, then the categories of bias, and thereafter I will discuss how bias or a lack of equivalence is being dealt with in cross-cultural research.

Four Levels of Equivalence

The four levels of equivalence distinguished here are functional equivalence, structural equivalence, metric equivalence, and full score equivalence (Fontaine, 2005). These four forms of equivalence are hierarchically ordered, in the sense that a higher level also implies all the requirements of the lower levels. Three questions are relevant, namely: (1) Can the same construct be used to interpret data obtained in different cultural groups?

(2) Can the same instrument be used to measure that construct? (3) Is it possible to make comparisons of score levels between cultural groups?

The most fundamental question is whether the same construct can be used to account for test responses in different cultural groups. In other words, is it meaningful to assume that the same latent variable accounts for the reactions to the indicators in each of the cultural groups? Relevant evidence can be obtained by looking within each culture at the relationships of indices with each other and of entire instruments with measures of other constructs. The same construct can be said to be assessed (even though item content can be entirely different), if the measures, each in their own cultural group, have similar networks of associations with presumably related constructs and absence of associations with unrelated constructs. It is then appropriate to use the same construct label across those groups. The type of equivalence satisfying this condition is called "functional equivalence."

The second question is whether a single instrument can be used in different cultural groups to measure a given construct. Two conditions have to be satisfied: (1) The instrument has to be relevant and representative of the construct in terms of item content in each of the groups (e.g., Messick, 1989). (2) The internal structure (relationships between items) has to be similar across the groups. The evidence for the first condition is mainly obtained from judges or raters who indicate to which extent items, stimuli, questions, or tasks are relevant for the construct in each of the cultural groups included in a study. Only if the content of the instrument is deemed to be representative of the intended construct can scores be generalized. It has been amply demonstrated in the validity literature (e.g., Messick, 1989) that it is not sufficient to only have a good rationale for including items into an instrument; it should also be demonstrated that the stimuli indeed elicit the intended behavior. In psychometric terms, this means that there have to exist nontrivial relationships between indicators (reactions to items) and the latent variable they are supposed to measure. There is "structural equivalence" if the internal structure of the instrument shows correspondence across the cultural groups. This is the case when nontrivial relationships exist between the indicators and the underlying latent variable in each of the cultural groups. Thus, structural equivalence justifies the use of the same instrument within each of the cultural groups. Since the levels of equivalence are hierarchically ordered, it is implied that conditions for functional equivalence also have to be satisfied.

The third question is whether scores of individuals from different cultural groups or average cultural score levels are comparable. Traditionally, structural equivalence is treated in the bias and equivalence framework as a necessary but insufficient condition for justifying direct quantitative comparisons between cultural groups (Fontaine, 2005; Van de Vijver & Leung, 1997a, 1997b). Additional psychometric restrictions have to be satisfied before scores can be compared quantitatively across cultural groups.

A first restriction is that the association between indicator and construct should be the same across cultural groups. In a linear measurement model (e.g., CFA), this restriction means that the weight parameters linking the latent variable to the indicators are the same across cultural groups. Under this condition, a shift on the latent variable will lead to the same expected shifts on the indicators across cultural groups. This means that the indicators form a scale that has the same metric across cultural groups. Hence, this type of equivalence is called "metric equivalence." This kind of equivalence justifies comparisons of score patterns between cultural groups; for example, it can be investigated to what extent the difference between males and females in aggression is the same across cultures.

Direct comparisons of a single variable can only be made if in addition to equal metric, there is some standard value, such as the origin of the scale, which across cultural groups has an identical meaning in terms of the construct. In a linear measurement model, this means that the intercept of the regression function linking the latent variable to the indicator should be the same across cultural groups. A given position on a latent variable is reflected in the same expected position on an indicator if both the slope and the intercept are the same across cultural groups. When the items of a scale meet the conditions of equal metric and equal scale origin, there is said to be "full score equivalence" and scores obtained in each cultural group can be directly compared with one another.

Four Categories of Bias

The term *equivalence* is used to indicate the level of measurement on which scores can be compared between cultural groups. The term *bias* or *cultural bias* refers to incomparability or inequivalence. Somewhat similar distinctions as between levels of equivalence can be made for bias.

A first category of bias has been referred to in the literature as "construct bias." This bias occurs when a psychological construct only applies in a specific cultural context. In this case it is impossible to find a comparable pattern of "functional" relationships with other constructs across cultural groups, violating the condition of functional equivalence.

Second, construct bias can also refer to construct underrepresentation by the instrument in one cultural group compared to another group. Identical indicators cannot be used meaningfully across cultural groups because of large differences in behavioral repertoire associated with the construct.

The third category of cultural bias is referred to as "method bias." This includes all sources of variation that affect most or all indicators making up an instrument and that do not relate to the construct the instrument is supposed to measure. Examples include errors in the translation of the instruction, a response scale that elicits more acquiescent responding in one cultural group than in another, or sample characteristics that differ between the cultural groups (such as a difference in motivation to do well on a test). Depending on how method bias affects the scores, each of the four levels of equivalence can be threatened.

The fourth and final bias category is "item bias," involving a lack of equivalence in a separate indicator or item. Two forms of item bias have been distinguished in the literature, namely nonuniform and uniform item bias. The latter term means that an item shows a systematically higher or lower score in a cultural group than expected on the basis of the scores on the other items of an instrument. In terms of a linear measurement model this means that the intercepts differ between cultural groups. For respondents with the same position on the latent variable, the expected score on an indicator is systematically lower or higher in one than the other cultural group. Thus, uniform bias implies a violation of full score equivalence; it implies a shift in the origin of the scale. Nonuniform bias means that the association between the item and the latent variable is not the same in each cultural group. An item may be relatively easy for low-ability persons in one cultural group and relatively difficult for high-ability persons from the same group in comparison to the low-ability and highly-ability persons from another group. In a linear measurement model, this means that the slope relating the latent variable to the indicator is different between cultural groups. Nonuniform bias implies a violation of metric equivalence.

Dealing with Lack of Equivalence and with Bias

If evidence of bias is detected, the individual researcher is confronted with two risks, namely the risk of making type I errors as a consequence of relying on spurious cultural differences that are the result of bias, and the risk of making type II errors as a consequence of ignoring genuine cross-cultural differences because the presence of bias is taken as a reason for not making comparisons. Traditional analyses give little hold on what is the most reasonable choice once bias is detected. Depending on the intuitions and preferences of the individual researcher, reactions to the identification of bias go from just ignoring the presence of bias and taking the risk of misrepresentation of cross-cultural differences, via removing salient sources of bias (like the most biased items) before comparison, to avoiding all cross-cultural comparison.

We can conclude that although the bias and equivalence framework has been developed to justify cross-cultural comparisons, it has mainly served to make researchers aware of the pitfalls of such comparisons. The likely presence of bias in cross-cultural measurement instruments is the Achilles heel of most cross-cultural research. It leads to the identification of spurious cross-cultural differences on psychological variables. Moreover, it has been demonstrated that increasing the sample size, which normally increases the precision and power of a study, increases the likelihood of finding spurious cross-cultural differences as soon as there is bias in a data set (Malpass & Poortinga, 1986).

Explanation: Sampling and Unpackaging Culture

It is a frequent but mistaken practice in cross-cultural research to compare two or a few cultural groups by applying an analysis of variance (ANOVA) on the scores of some psychological scale (often without prior bias analysis) *and* to attribute the cross-cultural differences to cultural factors. In such a study the results of the ANOVA are treated as if the data were resulting from a true experiment with cultural contexts as the conditions. There is no basis for treating data from cross-cultural research as experimental data, because there is no random allocation of the participants (on the contrary, participants are fully nested, each in their own culture), and also because the researcher has control neither over the independent variable nor over most ambient factors (cultural groups differ from one another on a host of variables) (see Berry et al., 2002). The ANOVA only helps to estimate differences between cultural groups, if the scores can be taken to be unbiased. It does not offer an explanation for the identified differences.

Systematic Sampling of Cultural Groups

One approach toward examining the meaning of cross-cultural differences is to sample cultural groups systematically on the basis of a presumed explanatory cultural variable that lies at the basis of these differences. For example, in typical studies of individualism-collectivism or independence-interdependence a few cultural groups are sampled that are either high or low on the target dimension. Such an approach is problematic. The cultural groups most likely will differ on a host of other variables some of which may well account for the difference in the dependent variable. Better estimates of cultural variability can be obtained by drawing a random sample of cultural groups that are high on individualism and a random sample of cultural groups that are high on collectivism, and apply a completely randomized hierarchical ANOVA design (e.g., Kirk, 1995). Such a design is capable of establishing a relationship between the cultural syndrome and the psychological variable, but it is still not capable of demonstrating that the postulated antecedent is the most important variable underlying observed differences in the dependent variable, and it is certainly not possible to demonstrate a causal link.

Unpackaging Cultural Differences

A second approach toward explaining cross-cultural differences is to measure the presumed explanatory variables and investigate whether statistically controlling for the effects of these variables can account for the cross-cultural differences on the dependent variable. The cultural difference on the dependent variable is then unpackaged in terms of the explanatory variables. This can be done by means of an ANCOVA. The presumed explanatory variables are treated as covariates and the cultural groups as the independent variable. It is examined whether the differences between the cultural groups on the dependent variable disappear (or at least become smaller), when the covariates have been controlled for. As in the case of systematic sampling of cultural groups, unpackaging is not without problems (unless, as we shall see below, multilevel models are relied on).

The problems a researcher faces with the unpackaging approach in part depend on the number of cultural groups studied. With only a few cultural groups unpackaging can be threatened in three ways: First, the approach does not work if the explanatory variables are situated at the culture level (e.g., level of democratization); with few cultural groups the culture-level variables that could possibly account for the differences are just too many in number. A second threat is the presence of cultural bias in the dependent or in the explanatory variables. Cultural bias can lead to spurious explanation of cultural differences (e.g., when both the dependent and explanatory variables share the same bias) or to the failure of identifying a genuine relationship (e.g., when the dependent and explanatory variables are biased in opposite directions). Finally, statistical inferences based on an ANCOVA are inadequate if the associations (slope parameters) between the covariates and the dependent variable differ between the cultural groups (Kirk, 1995). Thus, with a few cultural groups this approach can be used to explain cross-cultural differences on the dependent variable only under very restrictive conditions: covariates are measured at the individual level, dependent variable and covariates are measured bias free, and their association (slope parameter) is the same in each of the cultural groups.

When a large sample of cultural groups is studied, explanatory psychological variables can be identified and measured meaningfully at both the individual (e.g., personality traits) and culture level (e.g., level of democratization). However, both statistical and conceptual problems emerge when the data are analyzed with classical analysis methods, such as ANCOVA and multivariate regression (Snijders & Bosker, 1999). These methods only operate at one level of analysis at a time: either individual or culture level. In individual-level analyses all participants from the same culture are attributed the same value for variables measured at the culture level. From a statistical point of view the problem is that this equal score assigned to all individuals of a single cultural group is treated as if it was derived from statistically independent observations at individual level. This is both overly lenient when one looks at the relationships among the cultural variables and overly conservative when on looks at the relationships between the individual- and the culture-level variables. Conceptually, there is the problem that variables measured at culture level are not necessary meaningful at individual level. For instance, a culture-level variable such as level of democratization refers to a characteristic of a political system. It is not a summary score of individual-level characteristics. Thus, by attributing the same democratization score to each individual participant of a group, one makes a conceptual disaggregation error.

If analyses are done at the culture level, individual-level measurements are averaged per cultural sample. This averaging leads mainly to conceptual problems. The meaning of a variable at an individual within-culture level can be very different from its aggregated meaning at the culture level. For example, being pregnant or not at the individual level means something very different from the proportion of pregnant women in a cultural group. Thus, through aggregation of scores the meaning of variables can change. Moreover, as will be made clear later, computing summary scores at culture level on the basis of individual-level constructs could be meaningless. Thus, by doing all analyses at culture level, one runs the risk of making aggregation errors.

In general, the assumption with analysis of cross-cultural data is that the relationships found at one level can be applied to the other level. Since the meaning of variables can shift between the two levels, this assumption may not be correct. For instance, a positive correlation has been found at culture level between the proportion of divorces and the average self-rated well-being (Van Hemert, Van de Vijver, & Poortinga, 2002). At individual level, however, being involved in a divorce is considered to be a major stressor leading to negative affect. The unwarranted generalization of a relationship from culture level to individual level has been called the "ecological fallacy" (Robinson, 1950).

We can conclude that the conceptually very interesting approach of unpacking culture creates major statistical and conceptual problems with traditional analysis techniques. The approach can only be used under very restrictive conditions; that is, using individual-level explanatory variables, establishing full score equivalence, and parallel slopes in regression functions linking explanatory and dependent variables.

METHODOLOGICAL FRAMEWORK
FOR MULTILEVEL MODELING

Five fundamental characteristics can be identified in multilevel modeling (e.g., Goldstein, 2003; Hox, 2002; Raudenbush & Bryk, 2002; Snijders & Bosker, 1999). First, a distinction is made between different levels of analysis. A well-known example comes from educational research where levels include the individual pupil, the classroom and the school. Second, the levels are hierarchically ordered; the pupils are nested in classrooms, and the classrooms are nested in schools. Third, each level is treated as a population on its own from which a random sample is drawn in a multistage sampling procedure. A random sample of schools is first drawn from the population of schools, followed by a random sample of classes within the sampled schools, and thereafter a random sample of students within the sampled classes. Fourth, relationships are analyzed at each of the hierarchically ordered levels. Student achievement is related to student characteristics, such as intelligence. Average class achievement is related to class characteristics, such as class size. Average school achievement is related to school characteristics, such as the affluence of the neighborhood in which the school is situated. Finally, interaction effects are investigated between the hierarchically ordered levels of analyses. For instance, it is examined whether the relationship between intelligence and school achievement at student level is affected by class and school characteristics.

I only discuss models with two levels, where one level refers to cultural groups and the other level to individuals belonging to a cultural group. As in cross-cultural research, a distinction can be made between measurement and explanatory issues. Multilevel measurement is discussed first, because measurement at both the individual and the culture level precedes issues of causal explanation.

Measurement: Multilevel Analysis of Internal Structure

The possibility that the definition of a construct at an individual level is not the same as at a culture level was recognized already by Robinson (1950), and was introduced by Hofstede (1980) in cross-cultural psychology. Hofstede identified the four culture-level dimensions of individualism-collectivism, power distance, masculinity-femininity, and uncertainty avoidance based on the cultural averages of work values. In his model, these dimensions were only valid at culture level and not at individual level. Later, Triandis, Leung, Villareal, and Clack (1985) developed a scale to measure the individual-level counterpart of culture-level individualism-collectivism. To avoid confusion with the culture-level construct, they introduced the terms *idiocentrism* and *allocentrism* for the individual-level constructs (cf. Adamopoulos, this volume). Schwartz (1992, 2004) has developed a theory of value priorities both at the individual and the culture level. He has argued that there are different principles that structure the mutual compatibilities between values at the individual level and at the culture level. In line with his expectations he found a different geometrical representation of the value structure at both levels. While 10 value types were identified at the individual level, only seven rather different value types were identified at the culture level.

The central issue of measurement is to demonstrate that presumed indicators are positively associated with one another, and that these associations can be attributed to an underlying construct. Multilevel equivalence deals with the question of whether the individual-level associations among the indicators (such as covariances or correlations) reveal the same internal structure as the culture-level associations (i.e., associations among the cultural means of the indicators). The question is addressed whether the same latent variables account for the associations among the indicators at both levels of analysis. Three prototypical answers can be given to this question, namely isomorphism, non-isomorphism, and interaction (see also the introductory chapter by the Editors). I use a multilevel confirmatory factor model to clarify these three outcomes. There are two basic equations for each indicator in the multilevel confirmatory factor model, one at individual level and one at culture level. The equation at individual level is:

$$A_{i(j)} = a_j + b_j K_{i(j)} + e_{i(j)} \tag{1},$$

where $A_{i(j)}$ is the score of individual i nested in cultural group j on indicator A; a_j is the intercept of cultural group j; b_j is the slope between latent variable K and indicator A in cultural group j; $K_{i(j)}$ is the position of individual i nested in cultural group j on the latent variable K; and $e_{i(j)}$ the error term for individual i nested in cultural group j.

The equation at culture level is:

$$A_j = a + b L_j + e_j \tag{2},$$

where A_j is the average score on indicator A in cultural group j; b is the slope between latent variable L and indicator A at culture level; L_j is the position of cultural group j on latent variable L; and e_j is the error term for cultural group j.

Isomorphism

There is measurement isomorphism when the same measurement model holds in each of the cultural groups both at the individual and the culture level. In terms of multilevel CFA, this means (1) that latent variable K has a nontrivial association with indicator A in each of the cultural groups ($b_1 > 0, b_2 > 0, ... b_j > 0$ in Equation 1), (2) that the same latent variable can be used at the individual and the culture level (L and K are exchangeable), and (3) that latent variable K has a nontrivial association with indicator A at the culture level ($b > 0$). When these nontrivial associations hold for all indicators, the associations among the indicators at the individual and culture level reveal the same internal structure and the same constructs can be used to describe individual and culture-level variation.

The demonstration of isomorphism is highly important for cross-cultural research. Isomorphism is a necessary condition for comparability at an individual and culture level.

An example of multilevel isomorphism can be found in the work of Kuppens, Ceulemans, Timmerman, Diener, and Kim-Prieto (2006). They demonstrated with multilevel component analysis that two dimensions of positive and negative affect can be identified in both the individual- and the culture-level structure of self-reported frequencies of emotions.

Nonisomorphism

There is nonisomorphism when the same measurement model holds in each of the cultural groups, but differs between the individual and the culture level. In terms of multilevel confirmatory factor analysis, nonisomorphism means (1) that variable K has a nontrivial association with the indicator A in each of the cultural groups (nontrivial b_j in all cultural groups in Equation 1), and (2) that a different latent variable has to be used at the individual and the culture level (L and K in Equation 2 are not exchangeable). The relations among the indicators are different at the two levels of analysis in the case of nonisomorphism. As a consequence, a different internal structure at each of the two levels will be found. In the case of nonisomorphism the use of cultural averages derived from individual-level psychological scales cannot be justified.

The individual-level and culture-level value theory of Schwartz (1992, 2004) is a case in point. As predicted, he found a different internal structure of the value domain at the two levels of analysis. One of the most salient shifts was in the relationship between the items "humble" and "social power." These items tended to be negatively related at the individual level and positively at the culture level. At individual level the items are indicators of two different value types; "humble" is an indicator of the value type of tradition and "social power" of the value type of power. However, the cultural means of both items turned out to be indicators of the culture-level value type of hierarchy. Thus, it makes no sense to apply the individual-level value types at culture level. Values have a different meaning at both levels.

Interaction

There is a third scenario, namely that the relationships among the indicators at individual level interact with culture-level characteristics. The within-culture internal structure varies then systematically as a function of a culture-level variable. In terms of multilevel confirmatory factor analysis, this means that the association between latent variable K and indicator A differs in a systematic way between cultural groups. Thus each cultural group has its own specific b_j, with the size of this parameter being dependent on culture-level characteristics.

A recent example can be found in the work of Van de Vijver and Poortinga (2002). In a reanalysis of the data from 39 cultural groups on Inglehart's materialism–postmaterialism dimension, they found higher loadings of the indicators on this dimension for more affluent countries. The individual-level materialism–postmaterialism factor was more salient in more affluent countries.

Consequences for Equivalence and Bias

Multilevel modeling of internal structure has direct and important implications for the bias and equivalence framework. First, *nonisomorphism* necessarily implies the presence of uniform bias. Applying an individual-level measurement model will lead to overestimation or underestimation of cultural averages of indicators if the associations among the indicators are not the same between the individual and the culture level. Second, *interaction* will lead to nonuniform item bias at individual level. The more salient a factor or dimension becomes in a cultural group, the stronger the slope or discrimination parameters of the indicators for that dimension. Third, *isomorphism* does not necessarily exclude item bias. Multilevel isomorphism only implies similarity of the internal structures between cultural groups and between the individual and the culture level. Slight shifts in the meaning of translated items (which are most probably unavoidable with large samples of cultural groups), or slight shifts in the context of the research (e.g., due to differences in sampling, or in motivation of the participants) are likely to lead to uniform and nonuniform item bias. However, shifts that are unrelated to the underlying cultural constructs can have two effects that are compatible with measurement isomorphism. First, they can increase the nonexplained variance in the indicators at culture level. In terms of multilevel factor analysis, this means that the shifts increase the size of the error term in the factor equation at culture level (i.e., e_j in Equation 2). Second, they can lead to a random fluctuation of the association parameter linking the latent variable to the indicator between the cultural groups (i.e., b_j in Equation 1).

With the multilevel measurement approach in mind, we can go back to the three possible reactions to deal with bias in the traditional bias and equivalence framework, namely (1) ignoring bias, (2) correcting the bias, and (3) making no comparison. One does not run a big risk of identifying spurious cross-cultural differences by just denying the bias, provided three conditions are met. First, there is measurement isomorphism. Second, the association parameters linking the latent variable to the indicators are identical (or at least very similar) between cultural groups (see term b_j in Equation 1). Third, the error term is zero (or very small) at culture level (see term e_j in Equation 2) for each of the indicators (which means that there is little variance unexplained in the indicators at culture level). The risk is bigger when measurement isomorphism is combined with sizable error term at culture level (see term e_j in Equation 2) for one or more indicators (which means that there is much variance unexplained in the indicators at culture level) or a sizable variation of the association parameters linking the latent variable to the indicators (see term b_j in Equation 1). Correcting for bias is a sensible option in this case. However, cross-cultural comparisons are meaningless, if there is measurement nonisomorphism. The indicators then refer to different constructs at the individual and culture levels, which preempts the comparison of cultural groups on individual-level constructs. It can be concluded that the impact of item bias on validity is much easier assessed in a multilevel measurement framework. Depending on whether there is measurement isomorphism or nonisomorphism, the detection of item bias means imprecision or meaninglessness of cultural comparisons.

Explanation: Multilevel Regression Analysis

With measurement isomorphism between the culture level and the individual level, the question arises how individual and culture level variation can be explained. Conceptually, this question can be answered through the unpackaging of culture as discussed for monolevel analysis. The influence of presumed causal antecedents (predictors) at the individual and the culture level can be identified through multilevel regression analysis (hierarchical linear models, random coefficient models) (e.g., Goldstein, 2003; Hox, 2002; Raudenbush & Bryk, 2002; Snijders & Bosker, 1999). Such a procedure amounts to conducting regression analyses at both the individual and the culture level. There are at least two types of regression equations, namely one at individual, within-culture level and one at the culture level. At the individual level, the individual-level criterion is being regressed on the individual-level predictors. At the culture level, the culture-level criterion is being regressed on the culture-level predictors. To deal with the basic issues in multilevel regression modeling it is sufficient to present the bivariate regression model at individual and at culture level.[1] The individual-level regression equation can be written as follows:

$$X_{i(j)} = a_j + b_j Y_{i(j)} + e_{i(j)} \tag{3},$$

where $X_{i(j)}$ is the score of individual i nested in group j on criterion X; a_j is the intercept in cultural group j; b_j is the regression weight of predictor Y with criterion X in cultural group j; $Y_{i(j)}$ is the score of individual i nested in group j on predictor Y, and $e_{i(j)}$ is the error term of individual i nested in group j. The culture-level regression equation is:

$$X_j = a + b\,Z_j + e_j \tag{4},$$

where X_j is the average score of cultural group j on criterion X; a is the intercept; b is the regression weight of predictor Z with criterion X, Z_j is the score of cultural group j on predictor Z, and e_j is the error term of cultural group j. In cross-cultural psychology the multilevel regression model can have three types of predictors, namely (1) predictors that are measured and used only at the culture level; (2) predictors that are measured and used at the individual level; and (3) predictors that are measured at the individual level and that are both used at the individual and the culture level (under the condition that they have demonstrated measurement isomorphism).

As in the case of multilevel measurement, there are three prototypical scenarios in the case of multilevel explanation, namely isomorphism, nonisomorphism, and interaction.

Isomorphism

Isomorphism means that the same regression model accounts for the variation at each of the two levels of analysis. Isomorphism has three major characteristics: First, the relationships between predictors and criterion are nontrivially positive (or negative) in each of the cultural groups. In terms of the regression equation this means that the slopes are nontrivially positive (or negative) in each of the cultural groups (the values of the b parameters in Equation 3 are nontrivially larger (or smaller) than zero across cultural groups). Second, the same predictors can be used at the individual and the culture level (Z in Equation 4 is interchangeable with Y in Equation 3). Third, the predictor–criterion relationships are nontrivially positive (or negative) at culture level as at individual level (the values of all the individual-level b_j parameters in Equation 3 and of the culture-level value of b in Equation 4 are nontrivially larger (or smaller) than zero).

Imagine, for example, a study of the impact of calorie intake and physical exercise on body weight across cultures. A positive effect of calorie intake and a negative effect of physical exercise on body weight can be expected within each cultural group. Moreover, the same relationships can be expected at culture level. In cultural groups where people consume on average more calories and have less physical exercise the average body weight can be expected to be higher than in cultural groups where people consume on average fewer calories and have more physical exercise.

Nonisomorphism

Nonisomorphism shares with isomorphism the condition that the relationships of the predictors on the criterion are nontrivially positive (or negative) in each of the cultural groups. Thus, the slopes of the regression functions are nontrivially larger (or smaller) than zero for each of the cultural groups (the values of b_j in Equation 3 are nontrivially larger (or smaller) than zero). However, the regression models that account for the individual- and the culture-level variation differ from each other in the case of nonisomorphism. There are four ways in which nonisomorphism can emerge. First, culture-level predictors may not be applicable at the individual level (there is no correspondence between Z in Equation 4 and Y in Equation 3). For instance, characteristics of the political system (such as level of democratization) or the economic system (planned versus liberal economic system) have no individual-level counterpart. Second, individual-level predictors may not be applicable at the culture level. Schwartz's individual-level value scales, for instance, cannot be applied at the culture level, because there is no measurement isomorphism between the two levels. Third, although there is measurement isomorphism, a predictor may only be relevant at one level of analysis (b equals zero at one level of analysis). Fourth, there is also a case for nonisomorphism when the same predictors can be meaningfully used at the individual and the culture level, but relate in opposite ways to the criterion at both levels (the value of the slope parameter shifts from positive to negative or vice versa between the individual and the culture level). For example, it has been found that the proportion of divorced people is positively related to the average self-rated well-being at culture level, while at the individual level being involved in a divorce is a stressor that tends to negatively affect well-being (e.g., Van Hemert et al., 2002).

Interaction

The individual-level predictors can also be related differently to the criterion depending on a culture-level characteristic. In this case, the explanatory model at the individual level interacts with the culture level. In terms of the regression equations this means that the slopes of the regression functions vary systematically between cultural groups (each group has its own value of b_j in Equation 3) as a function of culture-level variables. In the analysis this means that a third type of regression equations is added in which individual-level slopes are regressed on culture-level predictors. For instance, Van de Vliert, Huang, and Levine (2004) found that there was a positive relationship between self-serving and altruistic motivations to help among voluntary workers in high-income countries with uncomfortably hot and cold climates, while self-serving and altruistic motivations to help were negatively related in low-income countries with uncomfortably cold climates.

Multilevel regression models are not just a new fancy statistical technique for cross-cultural psychology; they are of essential interest. It is only with the development of these models that it has become possible to fully unpackage culture and to understand differences in psychological variables in terms of cultural variables. Most of the problems that have been identified in the previous section can be solved by the application of multilevel regression models. First, the statistical problem of being overly lenient or overly conservative in interpretation dissipates because each variable can be treated at the level on which it has been measured. Second, one does not run the risk anymore of making disaggregation errors, since culture-level variables can be entered at the culture level. Third, it is possible to identify possible aggregation errors. It can be empirically investigated whether an individual-level predictor that is averaged at the group level does or does not shift in meaning. Fourth, one does not need to assume parallel slopes for individual-level predictors in all cultures, as in ANCOVA; the multilevel regression model offers the possibility to investigate interaction effects between both levels. Finally, provided measurement isomorphism has been demonstrated first, item bias can be treated in a multilevel regression model as random error at culture level. It increases the error term of the culture-level regression functions (e.g., see e_j in Equation 4). While item bias leads to the identification of spurious cross-cultural differences and explanations for these differences in a design with culture as a fixed factor, it can lead to the reverse effect in a design with culture as a random factor, namely the possible non-identification of existing culture level causal relationships.

AN INTEGRATED METHODOLOGICAL FRAMEWORK FOR CROSS-CULTURAL PSYCHOLOGY

There are three reasons to expect that the advantages of multilevel analysis do not make traditional approaches outdated. First, cross-cultural researchers will remain interested in cultural groups with specific psychological features, for instance when comparing minorities with the majority group in a multicultural society. In this case, the multilevel framework is not applicable because it requires a hierarchical design with a random sampling of cultural groups. Second, the assessment of individuals from different cultural groups plays an important role in applied cross-cultural psychology, for example in clinical diagnosis or job and educational selection. What can be treated as random error at culture level becomes a source of unfair treatment in the context of college admission and job selection. Thus, the requirement of full score equivalence remains important in applied contexts. Finally, genuine multilevel research with a random selection of cultural groups is a time-intensive and costly undertaking, even with advancing globalization and further developments in worldwide communication facilities. A random sampling of cultural groups becomes especially costly if criticisms of cultural psychologists and anthropologists are taken seriously implying that steps have to be taken to assure the relevance and representativeness of measurement instruments and concepts in each of the cultural groups sampled. All these problems make it likely that cross-cultural research with only a few cultural groups will remain important in the foreseeable future. Therefore, I propose an integration of traditional analyses and multilevel models into a comprehensive methodological framework.

There are two organizing principles in this framework, namely (1) measurement and explanation, and (2) random versus fixed sampling of the cultural groups. The first principle implies that measurement logically precedes explanation. The second, sampling of groups, is a major focus for multilevel models. Conclusions are difficult to generalize to the population of all cultural groups with a research design that includes only a few groups. In a multilevel approach, groups are randomly sampled, making interpretations feasible about the parent population. From a statistical perspective this distinction amounts to treating cultural groups either as a fixed factor or as a random factor in the research design.

By combining these two organizing principles, four prototypical types of cross-cultural research can be identified (see Table 3.1), namely (1) research focused on measurement with culture as a random factor; (2) research focused on explanation with culture as a random factor; (3) research focused on measurement with culture as a fixed factor; and (4) research focused on explanation with culture as a fixed factor. For each of these four research types, I briefly discuss after mentioning the main research question: (1) the conditions data have to meet to meaningfully conduct the analyses needed for answering the research question; (2) the data-analytic techniques that are suitable to address these conditions; and (3) the data-analytic techniques that can be used to address the research question.

TABLE 3.1

Four Prototypical Types of Research in Cross-Cultural Psychology

		Sampling of cultural groups	
		Random	**Fixed**
	Measurement issues	Measurement issues with a random sample of cultural groups	Measurement issues with a fixed sample of cultural groups
Research focus			
	Explanatory issues	Explanatory issues with a random sample of cultural groups	Explanatory issues with a fixed sample of cultural groups

Measurement: Culture as a Random Factor

It is important to establish whether and to what extent cultural groups differ from one another on a psychological variable before it makes sense to look for explanations of cross-cultural differences. The initial question in multilevel research is which proportion of the variation can be attributed to individual within-cultural differences and which proportion can be attributed to culture-level differences. For example, Poortinga and Van Hemert (2001) presented proportions of variance in personality traits that could be attributed to the culture level as compared to the individual level.

Prior Conditions

There are two main conditions that have to be met before the research question can be meaningfully addressed. First, the instrument should demonstrate structural equivalence at the individual level (which, as argued before, also implies functional equivalence, and relevance and representativeness of the items in the instrument) in each of the cultural groups. The second condition is that there is measurement isomorphism between the individual and the culture level of analysis. The examination of cultural averages of individual-level psychological scales (constructs) presupposes measurement isomorphism.

Data-Analytic Methods to Address the Prior Conditions

The prior conditions can be investigated with the structure-oriented data-analytic methods that are often used to investigate structural equivalence, namely multidimensional scaling (MDS), principal component analysis (PCA), exploratory factor analysis (EFA), and confirmatory factor analysis (CFA) (see Fischer & Fontaine, in press, and Fontaine & Fischer, in press, for an overview of these methods). As mentioned before, the four methods differ in the restrictions they impose on the data and on the internal structure model. MDS only requires ordinal information and represents associations between stimuli as distances between points in a low-dimensional space in such a way that the rank order of the associations is represented as accurately as possible by the rank order of the distances. PCA looks for a limited number of weighted sums of the original variables that represent as much of the total variance as possible. EFA searches for the underlying common factors that determine the associations between the observed items. CFA deals with a priori models about the underlying factors that account for the relationships among the items.

The approach that has been introduced by Van de Vijver and Poortinga (2002) in cross-cultural psychology, based on the work of Muthén (1994), can be used with all these analysis techniques. In a first step, the average individual-level internal structure is established, based on the pooled-within variance-covariance, or distance or correlation matrix. Thereafter it is investigated whether and to what extent the internal structure within each cultural group is equivalent with the average individual-level structure (using generalized Procrustes analysis for MDS configurations, orthogonal Procrustes rotations for PCA and EFA, and multigroup CFA for CFA analysis). The size of the cultural differences on the indicators can be examined subsequently, if the internal structure is stable in each of the cultural groups (structural equivalence). It is meaningful to look for a culture-level structure only if the indicators show sufficient variation across cultural groups; Muthén (1994) has proposed that at least 5% of the score variation in the dependent variables should be explained by country before the structure at country level can be meaningfully addressed. In a next step, a culture-level association matrix is computed on the basis of the average item scores (a dissimilarity matrix for MDS, a correlation matrix for PCA and EFA, and a variance-covariance matrix for CFA). The culture-level structure is then established on the basis of the culture-level association matrix. In the last step, measurement isomorphism is investigated by comparing the average individual-level structure with the culture-level structure, using one of the techniques that are used to examine structural equivalence at an individual level, such as Procrustes rotation.

The scales that are used to study individual within-cultural differences can be used for the study of cross-cultural differences when isomorphism has been established between the two levels of analysis. A separate analysis to establish the culture-level structure is indicated when there is no measurement isomorphism (the internal structure turns out to be different at culture level).

Data-Analytic Methods To Address the Research Question

Provided prior conditions are met, the proportion of within- and between-culture variability can be estimated by means of multilevel regression analysis or an ANOVA in which cultural groups are treated as a random design factor (Kirk, 1995). The proportion of within- and between-culture variability can also be estimated with multilevel regression software, such as HLM (e.g., Raudenbush & Bryk, 2002) and ML-Win (e.g., Goldstein, 2003).

Explanation: Culture as a Random Factor

The main research question in this type of research is to account for both individual and cultural variation in psychological variables. This type of research question imposes constraints on the design of the study; explanatory variables at both the individual and the culture level need to be included. For instance, based on Maslow's (1970) theory of well-being which states that "degree of basic need gratification is positively correlated with degree of psychological health" (p. 67), Veenhoven (1991) has investigated and confirmed three hypotheses about individual- and cultural-level differences in life satisfaction. He used a large data set containing individual-level data from many countries. The first hypothesis was that individual-level life satisfaction was positively correlated with individual-level income. The second hypothesis was that cultural-level life satisfaction was positively correlated with Gross National Product (GNP) per capita. The third hypothesis stated that the relationship between income and life satisfaction at the individual level would be weaker in countries with a high GNP compared to countries with a low GNP. Basic needs would be a less salient source of life satisfaction in countries with a high GNP, where basic needs are more likely to be satisfied. In these countries, life satisfaction would become more based upon the gratification of higher needs.

Prior Conditions

All individual-level variables should demonstrate structural equivalence across the cultural groups. Moreover, the individual-level variables that are aggregated at the culture level and are used as predictors at this level should demonstrate measurement isomorphism.

Data-Analytic Methods To Address the Prior Conditions

The data analytic procedures that can be used are the same as those mentioned in the previous subsection.

Data-Analytic Methods To Address the Research Question

Multilevel regression models can be applied to investigate the research question (e.g., Goldstein, 2003; Hox, 2002; Raudenbush & Bryk, 2002; Snijders & Bosker, 1999). The statistical analyses amount to the simultaneous application of regression models at the individual and the culture level.

Measurement: Culture as a Fixed Factor

The main question here is to estimate differences between a few cultural groups in which one is particularly interested (culture as a fixed factor) or between individuals from these cultural groups on a psychological variable. There is much cross-cultural research that fits in this category. The aim is often to explore cross-cultural differences by comparing relatively small number of cultural groups on psychological variables, such as personality traits, value priorities, and emotions.

Prior Conditions

Full score equivalence is required for the psychological variable (and by implication also metric, internal structure, functional equivalence, and relevance and representativeness of the items), if the goal is to compare score levels.

Data-Analytic Methods To Address the Preconditions

The number of countries involved in this type of study is too small to meaningfully address measurement isomorphism; with only a few countries analyzing the country-level structure of the construct under study is not meaningful. Therefore, structural equivalence is examined only at individual level by applying MDS, PCA, EFA, or CFA to compare the structure in each pair of cultural groups (Fischer & Fontaine, 2007). Once structure equivalence has been demonstrated, a range of psychometric techniques can be applied to identify nonuniform and uniform bias, such as conditional ANOVA, logistic regression, the Mantel Haenszel statistic, Item Response Theory, and CFA on Mean-Variance-Covariance Matrices (e.g., Van de Vijver & Leung, 1997a, 1997b).

Data-Analytic Methods To Address the Research Question

The traditional analysis of differences between cultural groups is a one-way ANOVA with cultural group as fixed factor, which presumes full score equivalence. This analysis tests the significance of cross-cultural differences in observed scores. There are also techniques for testing cross-cultural differences in latent means. Multigroup CFA can simultaneously test the equivalence of a measure in different cultural groups as well as the significance of latent mean differences between the cultural groups (see Selig, Card, & Little, this volume). It can be noted here that ANOVA or the multi-group CFA with latent means only identify cultural differences, they do not explain them.

Explanation: Culture as a Fixed Factor

The main aim here is to explain cross-cultural differences or patterns of differences on a psychological variable between specific cultural groups in terms of one or more explanatory variables. In an applied perspective the question is to account for differences between individuals belonging to different cultural groups.

An example of this research question can be found in social psychological research on social loafing (working less hard in a group than alone). It has been observed that people in the United States are more susceptible to social loafing than in China. Earley (1989) has investigated whether differences between U.S. and Chinese management trainees in social loafing can be accounted for by their individual-level differences in individualistic versus collectivistic orientation.

Prior Conditions

There are three conditions that have to be met, namely (1) explanatory variables have to be at the individual level (this condition is a consequence of the impossibility to evaluate the effects of culture-level variables properly in studies involving only a few cultural groups); (2) all variables have to meet conditions for full score equivalence (or metric equivalence if patterns of scores are to be explained); and (3) the associations (slope parameters) between the explanatory variables (covariates) and the criterion have to be equal across cultural groups.

Data-Analytic Methods To Address the Preconditions

The kinds of analyses needed to justify equivalence have been discussed previously. Identity of the slope parameters can be investigated within the ANCOVA framework (e.g., Kirk, 1995).

Data-Analytic Methods To Address the Research Question

The research question can be examined by means of an ANCOVA with the explanatory variables as covariates and the cultural groups as independent variable.

THREE PROTOTYPICAL SCENARIOS

In this final section I return to the two central questions of cross-cultural psychology, namely (1) comparability of psychological variables for cultural groups, and (2) comparability of psychological variables for individuals belonging to different cultural groups. These two questions are not distinguished in traditional cross-cultural research; full score equivalence is taken to mean that both individuals and cultural groups can be compared on one and the same psychological variable. A systematic comparison of the traditional and the multilevel framework shows that the two questions are to be distinguished. Comparability of psychological variables at culture level can, but need not, imply comparability of individuals from different cultural groups (i.e., when there is no measurement isomorphism between the two levels of analysis). Depending on the answers to the two questions, three scenarios in cross-cultural psychology can be distinguished, namely

(1) absence of comparability; (2) comparability of cultural groups; (3) comparability of individuals from different cultural groups.

Absence of Comparability

Absence of comparability can be a (meta-)theoretical postulate or an empirical finding. Cultural groups cannot be compared in either case and, by implication, it is impossible to compare individuals nested within cultural groups with one another. The theoretical position is taken by cultural psychologists who have a relativistic stance on culture–behavior relationships: Culture and psychological phenomena are seen as coconstructed entities that cannot be disentangled. Examples include indigenous concepts, such as the Japanese emotion concept of *amae* and the Indian personality concept of *jiva* (for more examples see Berry et al., 2002). Absence of comparability can also be the result of empirical research that is originally aimed at comparing cultural groups. Operationalizations and antecedent–consequent relationships of a construct can be fundamentally unreplicable across cultural groups, resulting in the absence of structural equivalence and functional equivalence. Such a cultural specificity could be a consequence of differential relevance and representativeness of item content for the cultures studied. No scores can be compared across cultures in such cases; comparing scores of individuals with one another is only sensible within a specific cultural context.

Comparability of Cultural Groups

Cultural groups, but not individuals from different groups, can be compared validly when the structure of variables differs between the individual and the culture level (i.e., when there is measurement nonisomorphism between both levels of analysis). As noted earlier, the best known example in cross-cultural psychology is the distinction between individualism-collectivism at the culture level and idiocentrism-allocentrism at the individual level (Triandis et al., 1985; see also the introductory chapter by the Editors and the chapter by Adamopoulos, this volume). Only recently have researchers begun to fully grasp the implications. The Schwartz value instrument is a case in point: The average within-cultural structure is rather stable, but differs systematically from the between-culture value structure (Schwartz, 1992, 2004). The implication is that different value scales have to be computed for studying individual differences and for studying cross-cultural differences in value priorities.

Comparability of Individuals from Different Cultural Groups

The two questions regarding comparability of cultural groups and of individuals both can be answered positively when the same psychological construct can be measured with the same measurement instrument in each cultural group, and when there is measurement isomorphism between the individual and the culture level. A major distinction can be made within this type of comparability between (1) measurement comparability of individuals from different cultural groups and (2) complete comparability of individuals from different cultural groups depending on whether there is multilevel isomorphism of the explanatory model.

There is only *measurement comparability* of individuals from different cultural groups if the individual-level and the culture-level explanations differ from one another. The cross-cultural comparability is restricted to the construct. A thought experiment proposed by Lewontin (1974) can clarify this point. In the context of culture–comparative intelligence research, Lewontin gave the example of grains from a single harvest that are sowed on two different plots, one with fertile and the other with infertile soil. All differences in the length of the grain stems within each plot should be accounted for by genetic differences between grain kernels, while the average differences in stem length between the two plots have to be attributed to differences in the fertility of the soil. Even though there is no doubt that the same construct is measured in each of these two plots (namely the length of the grain stems), differences in individual stem length within plots and in average length between plots cannot be attributed to the same underlying cause.

Complete comparability of individuals across cultural groups requires that individual-level and culture-level explanatory models are isomorphic. Not only can the same construct be used to describe all individuals and all cultural groups, but also the same explanations hold. A high or a low score refers to the same antecedent variables irrespective of the cultural background of the individual, if constructs are embedded in the same pattern of convergent and discriminant relationships at both levels of analysis. This state of affairs is assumed to exist, for example, by intelligence researchers who hold a strong genetic theory on intelligence. Actual test scores on intelligence tests are assumed to be largely caused by genetic factors. Differences between cultural groups on intelligence tests are attributed to differences in gene pools between the cultural groups.

CONCLUSION

The juxtaposition of the traditional monolevel framework with the multilevel framework has helped to clarify fundamental issues in the methodology of cross-cultural psychology. I mention three points. First, it is only with the development of multilevel regression models that the unpackaging approach to explaining cultural differences can be fully applied.

Variables that are defined at the culture level, such as democratization, and interactions between the cultural and the individual level can only be properly handled with statistical multilevel regression models.

Second, multilevel measurement models can help to clarify the threat of item bias. If there is measurement isomorphism, item bias points to imprecision of the cross-cultural comparisons. If there is measurement nonisomorphism, item bias points to the cross-cultural incomparability of individual-level scales. Different concepts and different scales have then to be used to describe individual- and culture-level differences.

Third, when there is both item bias and measurement isomorphism, the impact of the bias is different in a design with culture as a fixed factor, compared to a design with cultural as a random factor. Spurious cross-cultural differences and spurious relationships between variables are likely to emerge in a study involving only a few cultural groups. The methodological problems of a design with culture as a random factor are different. The more imminent danger in such designs is not to identify relationships that are actually present. Bias and equivalence remain a main concern for cross-cultural psychology, but their meaning and consequences can be put in a larger perspective with multilevel approaches.

Author Note

I would like to thank Ronald Fischer and especially Ype H. Poortinga for their constructive comments on earlier versions of this chapter.

Note

1. These equations assume that the predictors are first centered within each cultural group. Under this condition the individual-level intercept corresponds with the cultural average on the criterion. Since this is often a sensible thing to do, I restrict the discussion to this case (e.g., Snijders & Bosker, 1999).

REFERENCES

Berry, J. W., Poortinga, Y. H., Segall, M. H., & Dasen, P. R. (2002). *Cross-cultural psychology: Research and applications* (2nd ed.). Cambridge: Cambridge University Press.

Earley, C. (1989). Social loafing and collectivism: A comparison between the United States and the People's Republic of China. *Administrative Science Quarterly, 34*, 565–581.

Fischer, R., & Fontaine, J. R. J. (in press). Methods for investigating structural equivalence. In D. Matsumoto & F. J. R. van de Vijver (Eds.), *Cross-cultural research methods*. New York: Oxford University Press.

Fontaine, J. R. J. (2005). Equivalence. In K. Kempf-Leonard (Ed.), *Encyclopedia of social measurement* (Vol. 1, pp. 803–813). San Diego, CA: Academic Press.

Fontaine, J. R. J., & Fischer, R. (in press). Multilevel internal structure equivalence. In D. Matsumoto & F. J. R. van de Vijver (Eds.), *Cross-cultural research methods*. New York: Oxford University Press.

Goldstein, H. (2003) *Multilevel statistical models* (3rd ed.). London: Edward Arnold.

Hofstede, G. (1980). *Culture's consequences: International differences in work-related values*. Beverly Hills, CA: Sage.

Hox, J. (2002). *Multilevel analysis: Techniques and applications*. Mahwah, NJ: Lawrence Erlbaum.

Kirk, R. E. (1995). *Experimental design: Procedures for the behavioral sciences* (3rd ed.). Pacific Grove, CA: Brooks/Cole.

Kuppens, P., Ceulemans, E., Timmerman, M. E., Diener, E., & Kim-Prieto, C. (2006). Universal intracultural and intercultural dimensions of the recalled frequency of emotional experience. *Journal of Cross-Cultural Psychology, 37,* 491–515.

Lewontin, R. C. (1974). The analysis of variance and the analysis of causes. *American Journal of Human Genetics, 26,* 400–411.

Malpass, R. S., & Poortinga, Y. H. (1986). Strategies for design and analysis. In W. J. Lonner & J. W. Berry (Eds.), *Field methods in cross-cultural research* (pp. 47–84). Beverly Hills, CA: Sage.

Maslow, A. H. (1970). *Motivation and personality*. New York: Harper & Row.

Messick, S. (1989). Validity. In R. L. Linn (Ed.), *Educational measurement* (3rd ed., pp. 13–103). New York: Macmillan.

Muthén, B. O. (1994). Multilevel covariance structure analysis. *Sociological Methods & Research, 22,* 376–398.

Poortinga, Y. H. (1989). Equivalence in cross-cultural data: An overview of basic issues. *International Journal of Psychology, 24,* 737–756.

Poortinga, Y. H., & Van de Vijver, F. J. R. (1987). Explaining cross-cultural differences: Bias analysis and beyond. *Journal of Cross-Cultural Psychology, 18,* 259–282.

Poortinga, Y. H., & Van Hemert, D. A. (2001). Personality and culture: Demarcating between the common and the unique. *Journal of Personality, 69,* 1033–1060.

Raudenbush, S. W., & Bryk, A. S. (2002). *Hierarchical linear models: Applications and data analysis methods* (2nd ed.). Thousand Oaks, CA: Sage.

Robinson, W. S. (1950). Ecological correlations and the behavior of individuals. *American Sociological Review, 15,* 351–357.

Schwartz, S. H. (1992). Universals in the content and structure of values: Theoretical advances and empirical tests in 20 countries. In M. Zanna (Ed.), *Advances in experimental social psychology* (Vol. 25, pp. 1–65). Orlando, FL: Academic Press.

Schwartz, S. H. (2004). Mapping and interpreting cultural differences around the world. In H. Vinken, J. Soeters, & P. Ester (Eds.), *Comparing culture: Dimensions of culture in a comparative perspective* (pp. 43–73). Leiden, the Netherlands: Brill.

Snijders, T. A. B., & Bosker, R. J. (1999). *Multilevel analysis. An introduction to basic and advanced multilevel modeling.* London: Sage.

Triandis, H. C., Leung, K., Villareal, M. J., & Clack, F. L. (1985). Allocentric versus idiocentric tendencies: Convergent and discriminant validation. *Journal of Research in Personality, 19,* 395–415.

Van Hemert, D. A., Van de Vijver, F. J. R., & Poortinga, Y. H. (2002). The Beck Depression Inventory as a measure of subjective well-being: A cross-national study. *Journal of Happiness Studies, 3,* 257–286.

Van de Vijver, F. J. R., & Leung, K. (1997a). *Methods and data analysis for cross-cultural research.* London: Sage.

Van de Vijver, F. J. R., & Leung, K. (1997b). Methods and data analysis of comparative research. In J. W. Berry, Y. H. Poortinga, & J. Pandey (Eds.), *Handbook of cross-cultural psychology: Theory and method* (Vol. 1, pp. 85–128). Needham Heights, MA: Allyn & Bacon.

Van de Vijver, F. J. R., & Poortinga, Y. H. (2002). Structural equivalence in multilevel research. *Journal of Cross-Cultural Psychology, 33,* 141–156.

Van de Vliert, E., Huang, X., & Levine, R. V. (2004). National wealth and thermal climate as predictors of motives for volunteer work. *Journal of Cross-Cultural Psychology, 35,* 62–73.

Veenhoven, R. (1991). Is happiness relative? *Social Indicators Research, 24,* 1–34.

4

Latent Variable Structural Equation Modeling in Cross-Cultural Research: Multigroup and Multilevel Approaches

James P. Selig, Noel A. Card, and Todd D. Little

The focus of this chapter is on latent variable structural equation modeling (SEM) of cross-cultural data. Within the context of SEM, two general approaches for modeling between-culture differences and similarities exist. The first approach is multiple group mean and covariance structures (MACS) modeling (e.g., Browne & Arminger, 1995; Card & Little, 2006; Sörbom, 1982), and the second is multilevel SEM (ML SEM; e.g., Cheung & Au, 2005; Hox, 2002; Mehta & Neale, 2005). As we will elaborate in more detail below, the first approach is generally utilized when the number of cultures under consideration is small or relatively finite (e.g., <20 or so) and one is generally interested in comparing structural relations across specific groups (e.g., tests of measurement invariance; see below).

In contrast to the MACS approach, the ML SEM approach is useful for situations in which a large number of cultural groups is considered and one feels comfortable treating these cultural groups as random selections from the population of cultural groups; in other words, one is interested in general (and generalizable) across-group similarities and differences without attention to specific similarities and differences between particular groups. Under this condition, the cultural group that individuals are in can be treated as a higher-level effect that can vary randomly across the cultures under investigation. In multilevel modeling parlance, this situation would be described as a person model (level 1) nested within a culture (level 2) model. The primary difference between ML SEM and multilevel regression modeling is that the variables being assessed and modeled in ML SEM are latent; that is, the latent variables, or constructs, have multiple manifest indicators. Having multiple manifest indicators is advantageous for most analytic endeavors because the validity of the constructs can be established and the construct-level information is assessed without measurement error (Jöreskog, 1988). In the following, we will discuss the relative merits of these approaches as well as key issues that need to be considered when applying them. We turn first to multiple group MACS analyses.

ISSUES IN MULTIPLE GROUP MACS ANALYSES

Because a number of detailed didactic treatments of MACS modeling across groups exist (e.g., Card & Little, 2006; Little, 1997; Little, Card, Slegers, & Ledford, 2007), we will not provide a thorough description of this approach. Instead, we will discuss a number of important issues related to MACS modeling, particularly as they apply to cross-cultural research.

Perhaps the most critical, yet most often misunderstood, issue in the context of Multiple Group MACS modeling is the question of measurement invariance. Measurement invariance refers to the idea that an assessment tool and resultant latent variable representation provide equivalent measurement information across different groups. Meredith (1964, 1993) provides one important foundation for discussions of measurement invariance. Meredith's perspective on the issue of invariance is that of selection. That is, if one selects groups (randomly or purposefully) from a common population in which a common factor model holds for that population, then the factor structure (in terms of the relations of the indicators to the factors) will be invariant across the selected subgroups. In cross-cultural research, this theorem assumes that the common population is humanity and that the selection operator is culture. Some cross-cultural psychologists may find it difficult to agree with the adequacy of this assumption; it is, however, a statistically testable assumption. Meredith's selection theorem posits that the underlying indicator-to-construct relations will be invariant if the selection influence has affected only the common variance of each indicator, even under extreme selection (e.g., comparing non-Western vs. Western cultures as opposed to comparing a well-defined subset of Western cultures).

There are a number of conditions under which factorial invariance would fail given the guidelines of the selection theorem. First, the assumption of a common population may not be tenable; the selected samples may reflect distinctly different populations with distinctly different factor structures. In this case, cross-cultural analysis is no longer a quantitative comparison but rather a qualitative description that is more of the *emic* variety (i.e., understanding the nature of cultural groups on their own terms). Second, the factor model for the population may be misspecified. Here, empirical knowledge may not be sufficient to inform the appropriate theory. Such misspecification can also occur, for example, if, in the presence of sampling error, the factor structure is derived on one subpopulation and then transported to another subpopulation. In such situations, one or more factors may "fall apart" in the other subpopulations (see, e.g., Little, Miyashita et al., 2003). Third, the theorem limits the extremity of selection such that there needs to be enough common variance in the indicators to lead to a significant amount of variance in the construct. Lastly, invariance will fail if the selection operator differentially influences the specific variances of the indicators (Little, Preacher, Card, Selig, & Lee, 2006). Specific variance is the portion of an item's variance that is reliable but unique to the indicator in question. If this portion of an item is responded to in a culturally specific way then the common variance relations among a set of indicators may no longer remain invariant.

Levels of Measurement Invariance

Invariance is often discussed in terms of a hierarchy of increasingly stringent tests of the invariance assumption (Widaman & Reise, 1997). In the general parlance of invariance testing, configural invariance refers to pattern similarity across subpopulations. Here, having the same pattern of zero and nonzero loadings on the constructs and having no (or similar) constraints among the constructs' relations is sufficient to conclude that the factor pattern is configurally invariant. Figure 4.1 depicts a two culture model; configural invariance refers to the fact that the six measured variables (Y_1–Y_6) have the same pattern of loadings in both culture A and culture B.

The second level of invariance is often referred to as weak measurement invariance, sometimes also called loading invariance (Widaman & Reise, 1997). This test of invariance means that the parameter estimates for loadings can be constrained to have the same value. Loading invariance is illustrated in Figure 4.1 by the fact that the values for the loadings ($\lambda_{(1,1)}$–$\lambda_{(6,2)}$) are equated across the two cultures. Conceptually, this level of invariance implies that the relative loadings of indicators to constructs are equivalent across cultures. Here, indicators that are central to the construct in culture A are also central to the construct in culture B (i.e., their factor loadings are high and equivalent in both cultures), and those that are less central (have low factor loadings) in one culture are also less central in the other culture(s). Equivalence of the loadings, however, does not mean that the total amount of reliable variance implied by the loading is mathematically equal across cultures because the variances of the constructs are unconstrained across the groups. That is, any differential amounts of reliable variance would be carried up to the constructs and the estimated variances would reflect the true estimates of common factor variance in both groups. This estimated construct-level variance also functions as a

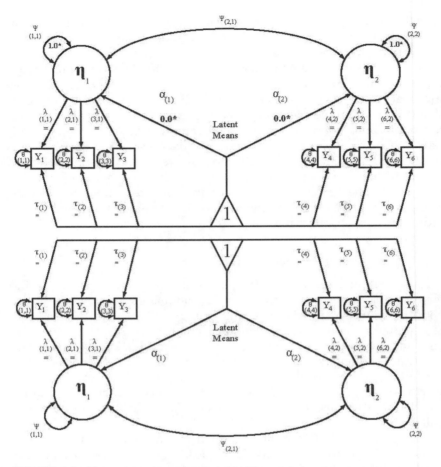

FIGURE 4.1 Illustration of a two-group MACS model showing strong measurement invariance. Note. α = latent variable means; λ = loadings of observed variables on latent variables; ψ = latent variable variance/covariances; τ = observed variable intercepts; θ = observed variable residual variances.

proportional weighting for the loadings that allows the model to reproduce the observed variance and covariance patterns among the indicators (see Little, 1997; Little, Preacher et al., 2006).

The third level of invariance (i.e., strong invariance) refers to equivalence of the intercepts of the indicators' regressions onto the construct. Here, the test of weak invariance (i.e., equality of factor loading) must be deemed tenable before evaluating this more stringent level of invariance (i.e., relative equality of indicator intercepts). If so, these constraints remain in place and additional constraints on the intercepts are added. The equality constraints on the intercepts ($\tau_{(1)}$–$\tau_{(6)}$) in Figure 4.1 shows this additional level of invariance. As with the loadings, this level of invariance implies that the *relative* intercept values are equivalent across groups (i.e., the pattern of high and low scores on a set of indicators is the same in both cultures). Here, the observed differences between groups in all indicators' means are carried up to the level of the latent means of the constructs. This level of invariance is referred to variously as strong measurement invariance, scalar invariance, or measurement equivalence. We prefer strong invariance because when *both* the intercepts and the loadings of a set of indicators for a construct are invariant across subpopulations, then one has sufficient evidence to claim that the indicators are measuring the same underlying construct and that any differences in the constructs are veridical differences (Little, 1997).

The fourth level of invariance of the measurement parameters is termed strict invariance and focuses on cross-group equality of the residuals of the indicators across groups. Figure 4.1 depicts the recommended strong invariance model; a strict invariance model would require that the residual variances ($\theta_{(1,1)}-\theta_{(6,6)}$) also be equated across groups. Although this test of invariance has a certain appeal, it is not a requirement to conclude that constructs are measured equivalently; it is, indeed, a level of invariance that we do not recommend. Instead, it is simply a test of whether the sum of the specific variance and the random error of a given indicator is equal across groups. Some have interpreted this test as implying equal precision of measurement (Cheung & Rensvold, 2002). Although precision may be a reasonable term to describe this level of invariance, the nature of the "precision" of measurement cannot be determined. That is, the total amount of residual variance may be equal across two groups, but for one group the residual variance may be primarily error variance whereas in another group the residual variance may be primarily indicator-specific variance. The latter is a reliable variance that is specific to a given indicator. As Little and colleagues (Card & Little, 2006; Little, Card, et al., in press; Little & Slegers, 2005) have argued, this test is generally an unreasonable level of invariance to impose across groups because if the residual variance is not exactly equal across groups, the invariance constraint will force some amount of error into other estimated parameters of a given model.

A Hypothetical Example for Extreme Differences in Loadings

Because the issue of extreme differences between two populations is very often construed as noninvariance, we feel that it is important to walk the reader through a more technical treatment of the reasons why (i.e., the mathematical basis) measurement invariance will hold even in situations that may seem on the surface to be unlikely. Real data examples can be found in the literature (e.g., Grob, Little, Wanner, Wearning, & Euronet, 1996; Little & Lopez, 1997; Stetsenko, Little, Gordeeva, Grasshof,

& Oettingen, 2000). Using a hypothetical scenario, we will show that it is possible to get extreme selection influences yet still expect and obtain strong measurement invariance. For this hypothetical example, we will assume that the observed variances of the indicators in two subpopulations are about equal and that we can safely describe the process in a standardized metric within each subpopulation (this is for didactic purposes; it is not a necessary assumption if one uses an unstandardized metric). Assume that in the configural invariance model one obtains loadings of .8 for each indicator of a construct in the first culture (culture A in Figure 4.1), and in a second culture the observed loadings are .5. In this idealized example, the .8 loadings (in standardized metric) lead to correlations of .64 (.80 * .80) among the indicators in culture A. For culture B, the loadings lead to correlations of .25 (.50 * .50) among its indicators.

If the method of identification used to establish the scale of the estimates fixes the latent variance at 1.0, the model is estimated in standardized metric (see Little, Slegers, & Card, 2006, for a discussion of methods of scale setting). In Multiple Groups MACS models, it is common to refer to group 1 as the reference group and group 2 as the comparison group. In our hypothetical example, we will use culture A as the reference group. When loading invariance is specified, the scale for the estimates is established by fixing the latent variance of the construct in this group to be 1.0. Because of the cross-group equality constraints on the loadings (i.e., weak invariance is specified), the estimates of the parameters in the second group are also in reference to the 1.0 latent variance metric established in the reference group. This scaling implies that the loadings in group 2 will be estimated as .8 (equal to the loadings in group 1), but the latent variance will no longer be 1.0. Instead, the latent variance will be adjusted to reflect the true amount of latent variance relative to the 1.0 scale-defining value used in group 1. That is, it will equal the interindicator correlation divided by the product of any two loadings on the construct; that is, .25/(.80 * .80) = .39. This value reflects the amount of common variance among the observed indicators in the second group relative to the amount observed in the reference group.[1]

If one fits the configural invariance model in both groups and sets the factor variance to 1.0 for scaling purposes, the resulting factor loadings are .8 in culture A and .5 in culture B. Alternatively, if one chooses to fix the loading of a marker variable to 1.0, the estimated latent variances are .64 in culture A and .25 in culture B. This example implies that the amount of common variance associated with the construct in culture A is .64 and for culture B the value is .25. Culture A has more reliable construct information (i.e., common variance among indicators) than culture B (this can be formally tested via a nested-model comparison). According to Meredith (1964, 1993), this outcome can result from (extreme) selection that has only influenced the common variance of the indicators of each respective construct. In other words, no assumption is made that the construct variances are homogeneous in each population under the selection theorem. Therefore, uniform differences among the indicators are consistent with selection on the common factor variance. By way of interpretation, one would conclude that the measurement of the construct has more measurement error in culture B than in culture A.

Even if the observed variances of the indicators differed in cultures A and B, however, this would only lead to a proportional difference in the amount of common variance implied by a .8 loading versus a .5 loading. For example, begin with setting the scale for the latent variable by fixing its variance at 1.0. If the observed variances of the indicators in culture A are 2.0 and the observed variances of the indicators in culture B are 1.0, then the residual variance estimates in subpopulation 1 would be 1.36 and in subpopulation 2 they would be .75 (the variance of a variable is reproduced as the square of the loading times the estimated variance of the construct plus the residual: $.8 * .8 * 1.0 = .64; .64 + 1.36 = 2.0$). When one imposes invariance of the loadings across the groups, the loadings in culture B would become .8 and the latent variance would become a proportional rescaling value that would solve $.8^2 * p = .5^2 * 1.0$ (in this case, p is the estimated latent variance in culture B which would turn out to be .39), and the residuals in both groups would be unchanged. That is, the "true" latent variance in culture B would be .39 and in culture A it would be 1.0. If the difference is significant according to nested-model comparison, one would conclude that variability in the latent construct in culture B is smaller than in culture A.

This outcome, which is not uncommon in cross-cultural research, would result in covariances among constructs that are on significantly different metrics and comparing unstandardized relationships among the constructs would not be very defensible. Little (1997) describes how one can introduce Rindskopf's (1984) phantom-construct approach to estimate the model such that the associations among the constructs are estimated in a standardized metric (for an example, see Little, Oettingen, Stetsenko, & Baltes, 1995). It is possible that observed loadings of .8 vs. .5 would violate the invariance assumption. Such a situation could materialize, if the selective influence impacted the specific variance components of one or more of the indicators in some correlated manner. Such a selection process could result, therefore, in (one or more) indicators that (1) cannot be considered as identical across each subpopulation (i.e., show evidence of differential item functioning and may be only partially invariant; see Reise, Widaman, & Pugh, 1993); (2) require a dual loading in one subpopulation but not the other; or (3) require a number of correlated residuals in one subpopulation, but not the other. In this hypothetical example, the likelihood of such violations of selection is largest for culture B because the ratio of common factor to specific factor variance is smaller than for culture A.

Are Constructs Unbiased if Measurement Equivalence Holds?

A key question for researchers is whether one can claim that constructs are unbiased if measurement equivalence holds. In cross-cultural research this issue relates directly to questions about acquiescent response style, social desirability, and the like. Measurement equivalence rules out differential effects of these sources of bias; this has been a topic of considerable interest in the measurement field and has been referred to as item bias, test item bias, and differential item functioning (e.g., McDonald, 1999; Osterlind, 1983). However, strong measurement invariance does not rule out sources of bias if the source of bias impacts the common factor variance of a construct. In this case, all items of a construct would have the same behavior and would not show a differential pattern. For example, the difference in the latent construct variances outlined in our hypothetical example could be due to a common acquiescent response style in culture B. However, when one interprets the findings for such a construct, one has to keep in mind that the acquiescent response style is a characteristic of the cultural influences that embody the subpopulation (cf. Cheung & Rensvold, 2000). In this case, one needs to specify one or more response style constructs to remove this common source of bias from the common factors (e.g., Billiet & McClendon, 2000).

Acquiescent response style would be a tremendously biasing problem if one analyzes relationships among variables using a manifest variable approach because the degree of measurement error caused by the bias is not accounted for in the manifest variables. In the latent variable space, on the other hand, the change in the latent variances due to the set of cultural influences is represented explicitly in the model and one can account for this influence to still make veridical comparisons across groups (Billiet & McClendon, 2000). If the construct variances are significantly different across cultures, even after response style corrections, one can compare associations between constructs on a standardized metric by using a phantom variable approach described by Little (1997; see also Rindskopf, 1984). In addition, the estimates of the latent means can be directly compared because tests of latent means in multiple group MACS models make no assumptions about the homogeneity or heterogeneity of the variances between samples (instead, these are directly estimated and homogeneity is testable). Finally, the observed differences in the variances across groups represent the true variance differences in the cultures, and any such differences then must be interpreted in light of what is known about the set of possible cultural variables that influence each of the groups.

Scale-Setting Issues

Perhaps the most common scale-setting approach is to arbitrarily choose a marker variable of the construct and fix its loading to 1.0. As Little,

Slegers, and Card (2006) argue, this arbitrary approach has many unsatisfying consequences in terms of the interpretability of the model parameters. Other authors point out that using the marker variable method of identification is unsatisfying when it comes to determining which indicators are noninvariant in situations where the omnibus test of invariance is deemed unreasonable (Hancock, Stapleton, & Arnold-Berkovits, 2005; Little, Preacher et al., 2006). The other common method of identification that was mentioned in the hypothetical example above is to fix the latent variance of a construct to be 1.0 and thereby freely estimate each of the loadings of the indicators on a construct. A key feature of this approach is that when one is testing the invariance of loadings, one must free up the latent variance in the comparison groups else one is also assuming equal latent variances across groups when loadings are equated (Little, 1997). Little, Slegers, and Card (2006) introduced a nonarbitrary method of scale setting for latent constructs. This technique adds a third approach for scale setting beyond the two traditional ones. In their approach, which they termed the *effects coded method*, one places a constraint on the set of indicators of a construct such that the average of the loadings is constrained to be 1.0. If each indicator is measured on a similar metric, this method has the advantage of estimating the latent parameter estimates in the metric of the observed indicators, and the estimated variance is a weighted average of the common factor information contained in each indicator of a construct (for details, see Little, Preacher et al., 2006; Little, Slegers, & Card, 2006).

Evaluating the Tenability of Invariance Constraints

The final issue in this discussion of Multiple Group MACS comparisons across cultures relates to how one evaluates tests of invariance. Fundamentally, two approaches can be distinguished. The first approach, based on a statistical rationale, is to employ a strict null hypotheses testing perspective in which the tenability of invariance constraints would be evaluated using the χ^2 difference test. That is, the model χ^2 and degrees of freedom of a less constrained model is subtracted from the χ^2 and degrees of freedom of a more constrained (and nested) model. Under the null hypothesis, the difference in χ^2s is distributed as a χ^2 with degrees of freedom equal to the difference in degrees of freedom between the two models. If this χ^2 value is significant, then the researcher might conclude that one or more of the constraints across the groups differs significantly and the set of constraints would not be considered tenable. Some researchers have argued that this strict statistical test is overly sensitive to violations of the invariance assumption (Cheung & Rensvold, 2002; Little, 1997) for at least two reasons. First, the χ^2 is a very sensitive measure, particularly with the large sample sizes that are typically needed for estimating MACS models and, second, the measurement parameter estimates that are the focus of the weak and strong invariance tests are a key source of noise in the system.

A second approach to evaluating measurement invariance is from a modeling rationale (in which one considers the tenability of invariance rather than strictly considering the absolute, statistical truth of invariance). From this perspective, numerous recommendations have been offered for using practical fit statistics for making such determinations instead of relying on the χ^2 difference test. Cheung and Rensvold (2002), for example, advocated using the absolute change in three relative fit statistics: the Comparative Fit Index (CFI) (change less than or equal to .01), McDonald's noncentrality parameter (change less than or equal to .02), and Gamma hat (change less than or equal to .001). In addition to these criteria, Little, Card et al. (in press) have suggested that one could also evaluate the change in the RMSEA (Browne & Cudeck, 1993). Specifically, if the point estimate of the RMSEA for a more restricted model falls within the 90% confidence interval of the less constrained model, this would indicate that the degradation in fit is a nonsignificant loss (also see MacCallum, Browne, & Cai, 2006; Preacher, Cai, & MacCallum, 2007). Finally, Preacher and Wirth (2006) argue that model selection criteria, such as the expected cross-validation index, be used to determine the level of invariance that is likely to cross-validate the best across repeated sampling.

As mentioned, we will not provide a didactic example of this type of modeling because other sources provide detailed examples of how to conduct such tests (Card & Little, 2006; Little, 1997; Little, Card et al., in press). A relatively new extension of latent variable SEM for use with multiple populations is the multilevel SEM approach (ML SEM). Unlike multigroup models, where cultural groups are treated as fixed effects and point estimates are compared across the finite set of groups, in ML SEM the cultural groups are treated as random effects (that the cultural groups studied are a representative sample of a large number of cultures). In the following, we review the specifics of ML SEM and provide a didactic example of this relatively new approach to modeling cross-cultural differences in latent variables.

MULTILEVEL STRUCTURAL EQUATION MODELING

Generally speaking, any model that can be depicted as a multiple-group SEM can also be defined as a ML SEM, given that the data are hierarchically clustered as individuals within groups. ML SEM integrates the benefits of both multilevel models (producing unbiased estimates in the presence of nested data structures) and those of SEM (correcting for measurement error and the ability to test complex hypotheses). Although several methods for estimating ML SEMs have been proposed for over two decades (e.g., Goldstein & McDonald, 1988; McDonald & Goldstein, 1989), the application of these methods is relatively new and many questions regarding the use of such models remain unanswered. After briefly describing the ML SEM by means of a cross-cultural data example and giving an overview to three different, but very similar approaches to conducting such an analysis, we present a detailed ML SEM analysis of the sample data. Finally, we review some of the unanswered questions in the area of ML SEM.

The Multilevel Structural Equation Model

We will explain the ML SEM using data from the International Social Survey Program (ISSP; 2002) Family and Changing Gender Roles III. A full explanation will be provided before the example analysis, but for now we will focus on the construct Life Satisfaction. Life Satisfaction is indicated by responses to two questions answered by over 25,000 individuals within 35 different countries. Since the groups in the data are based upon countries, rather than culture (culture is not specifically addressed here but could be addressed by having a three-level model with cultures nested within countries or countries nested within cultures, depending upon the definition of cultural groups), the following description of the model will refer to countries.

The model we are using is the SEM analogue to the random intercepts model in multilevel modeling. This model implies that there is mean-level variation in Life Satisfaction across countries. Though it is also possible to incorporate random slopes into a ML SEM model, for simplicity, we will only show the random intercepts model (see Bovaird, 2007; Mehta & Neale, 2005 for examples of ML SEM with random slopes). Following Muthén (1994), we can describe scores from the Life Satisfaction indicators in the ML SEM with the following formula:

$$y_{gi} = v + \lambda \eta_{gi} + \varepsilon_{gi} \tag{1}$$

where y_{gi} is a vector of the two measured Life Satisfaction variables for person i in country g (we have used subscripts i and g for consistency with more traditional notation for individuals within group), v is a vector of the Life Satisfaction indicator intercepts, λ is the factor loading of the Life Satisfaction indicators on the latent Life Satisfaction factor, η_{gi} is the Life Satisfaction factor score for person i in country g, and ε_{gi} is a vector of residuals for person i in country g. Applying the above equation to our data example, we may explain the response to a Life Satisfaction question of an individual within a particular country by the average response to that question across all persons within all countries plus the Life Satisfaction factor score for that individual plus some residual variance. We can then describe an individual's Life Satisfaction factor score as:

$$\eta_{gi} = \alpha + \eta_{Bg} + \eta_{Wgi} \tag{2}$$

where α is the overall latent Life Satisfaction mean across all countries, η_{Bg} is the variation of country g from this overall mean (a random variable), and η_{Wgi} is the deviation of person i from the mean within his or her country (also a random variable). So, the Life Satisfaction factor score for an individual within a country is equal to the overall mean Life Satisfaction across countries plus the degree to which one's country departs from that overall mean plus the degree to which one departs from the mean for one's country. Variance in η_{Bg} represents the amount that countries do in fact differ in levels of Life Satisfaction (i.e., between-country variance), and is typically represented as Ψ_{Bg}. Similarly, the variance of η_{gi} within each country measures the degree to which members of the same country vary in levels of Life Satisfaction (i.e., within-country variance).

Equations (1) and (2) above describe how mean-level information about individuals within countries can be represented. Similarly, it is central to ML SEM to separate variances and covariances into within- and between-country components. In Confirmatory Factor Analysis (CFA; a specific SEM in which no directional paths are specified; Brown, 2006), a model-based variance-covariance matrix is specified by the following formula:

$$\Sigma = \Lambda\Psi\Lambda' + \Theta \tag{3}$$

where Σ is the implied variance-covariance matrix among manifest variables (estimated by the variance-covariance matrix of one's sample), Λ is a matrix of factor loadings (of observed variables onto underlying latent factors), Ψ is the variance-covariance matrix of the latent variables, and Θ is the matrix of residual variances, or specific variance and/or covariance attributable to the indicators (note that SEM with directional paths is simply an elaboration on this model, $\Sigma = \Lambda (I - B)^{-1} \Psi (I - B')^{-1} \Lambda + \Theta$, in which B is a matrix of directional, or regression, paths among latent variables, which we will not describe here for simplicity). Similar to other multilevel models (e.g., Raudenbush & Bryk, 2002), the components of the CFA model (Equation 3) can be decomposed into level-1 (i.e., person-level) and level-2 (i.e., country-level) components.

As described in more detail by Muthén (1994), we can model within- and between-country variances and covariance with separate structural models:

$$\Sigma_B = \Lambda_B \Psi_B \Lambda'_B + \Theta_B \tag{4}$$

$$\Sigma_W = \Lambda_W \Psi_W \Lambda'_W + \Theta_W \tag{5}$$

where Equation (4) models variances and covariances that exist between countries, and Equation (5) models variances and covariances within countries. This parameterization assumes, due to the fitting of one within-country equation to represent all countries, that the same factor model fits the data across countries (i.e., configural invariance), and that this param-eterization uses a common matrix of loadings (Λ_W) across all countries (weak factorial invariance). Researchers would be well advised to conduct preliminary multiple-group analyses (i.e., analyses where data from each country are modeled as a separate group) to evaluate measurement invari-ance, as described above, before conducting the ML SEM described here.

Just as parameter estimates of SEM are often obtained via maximum likelihood, available estimation methods for ML SEM typically rely on variations of this criterion. However, these estimation methods are com-plex and beyond the scope of this chapter. Interested readers can consult an accessible treatment of estimators in Bovaird (2007) or Muthén (1994); a number of more advanced treatments are also available (e.g., Bentler & Liang, 2003; Goldstein & McDonald, 1988; Lee, 1990; Lee & Poon, 1998; McDonald & Goldstein, 1989).

Issues of Invariance in ML SEM

When we move from multigroup SEM to ML SEM, we still must be mind-ful of issues of measurement and structural invariance, however, the mul-tilevel nature of the model adds appreciably to the complexity of these issues. As alluded to before, any ML SEM necessarily assumes weak mea-surement invariance given that only one set of loadings is estimated for the within group portion of the model. Because the grouping variable is a random rather than a fixed variable, there is no straightforward way to conduct formal tests of measurement invariance (i.e., testing invariance with a 30-group MACS model is unwieldy at best and pairwise compari-sons of even a small number of parameters across groups would lead to extreme levels of type I error inflation), so we are left with the ad hoc solution of separately testing small numbers of groups for invariance. In addition to invariance across groups, there is also the issue of invariance across levels; that is, the between- and within-portions of the model. For example, we can ask whether a construct is measured the same way at the individual and group levels and whether constructs related to one another similarly at these two levels. To further complicate the assess-ment of invariance, it is possible to establish cross-level invariance while simultaneously failing to establish cross-group invariance (Van de Vijver & Poortinga, 2002). See Mehta and Neale (2005) and Zyphur and Preacher

(2006) for discussions of the promise and complexity of cross-level invariance testing.

Approaches to Multilevel Structural Equation Modeling

Next, we present approaches to establish the need for building and testing a ML SEM. We will discuss three such approaches. Though we will recommend one of these over the others, our goal is not so much to advocate for one approach but to point out the similarities and also to alert the reader to these helpful tools for dealing with a complex analysis.

Muthén's (1994) approach is the most commonly used for building and testing a ML SEM (Cheung & Au, 2005; Heck, 2001; Heck & Thomas, 2000; Kaplan & Elliott, 1997). Muthén presents a four-step strategy in which it is assumed that the researcher has already computed the between-group and pooled within-group covariance matrices. The first step is an analysis of the total covariance matrix without regard to the nested structure. The results from this initial model are incorrect in the presence of multilevel effects so this step is used only to give an approximation of model fit. The second step is to determine whether there is any between-level variation. This step can be carried out in the context of a ML SEM by estimating a model without between-level variation, and comparing that model to one in which between-level variation is estimated. Muthén (1994) suggests using the intraclass correlations (ICCs) for each variable as a simple way to assess the amount of between-level variation. Large ICCs indicate that cluster membership is accounting for a large proportion of variance, but it is not clear how small an ICC must be before the nested structure can be ignored. The third step is an analysis of the within-group structure in which a model is imposed on the pooled within-group covariance matrix. The fourth and final step in this process, the estimation of the between-groups structure, can be the most challenging because the estimate for the covariance matrix to be modeled (Σ_B) is often not definite. Muthén (1994) notes that using S_B for this analysis, which is an unbiased estimate of $\Sigma_W + c\Sigma_B$ where c is a constant reflecting average group size, will often produce results similar to the analysis of Σ_B. After completing these steps, the investigator can proceed to the final ML SEM.

Hox (2002) outlines a related but different set of steps for building a ML SEM. In his method, Hox establishes a number of "benchmark" models as a means of testing the ML SEM. A benchmark model, in this context, is any model designed to test the key assumptions (i.e., whether there is between-group variance or covariance) of the ML SEM. All models described by Hox (2002) can be tested within the context of a ML SEM. First a null model is estimated in which only the within-groups structure is estimated. If this model fits, we assume that there is no meaningful between-level variation among the variables in the model. If the model does not fit, a second model, called the independence model, is estimated in which between-group variation is estimated, but the variables at the between-group level are not allowed to covary. If this second model fits, it shows that there is variation around the group means, but there is no meaningful structure to be modeled. As a third step, a saturated model is estimated in which all the between-group variables are allowed to freely covary. This model should show the best fit as it is limited only by the level of misfit in the within-group portion of the model. The saturated model can be used as a standard by which to judge further restrictions made on the between-group part of the model. Subsequent steps will be guided by theory about the constructs in the model. For example, Hox (2002) tests a model of intelligence and whether the data support a one- or two-factor solution. However, if an investigator has no such hypotheses, it would be reasonable to proceed to an estimation of the final model to assess how much fit is lost by imposing restrictions on the between part of the model.

A third approach is introduced by Mehta and Neale (2005). In this approach, a univariate random intercepts model is first fitted to the data. This analysis provides estimates of between-group variance as well as ICCs, and is used to assess the amount of variability at the between-group level. The second step is to fit a multivariate random intercepts model to obtain the between- and within-group covariance matrices. This step shows the pattern and amount of covariation. It can also be used as a first step in determining whether there can be similar models at the between- and within-group levels. As a third step, Mehta and Neale conduct a multilevel confirmatory factor analysis. At this point it is possible to test a number of additional hypotheses, such as whether there is measurement invariance across the between and within portions of the model and whether constructs are uni- or multidimensional.

All three of the above methods have in common that they seek to establish whether there exists variation among the means at the between level. In addition, all explore and test models at both the between- and within-group levels. Finally, all approaches test a ML SEM at some stage and allow for further hypothesis testing using that model. Although all three approaches can be fruitfully employed, we find the Hox (2002) approach to be the most straightforward and easiest to implement.

The Muthén (1994) approach is based on the calculation of the between and within covariance matrices, a necessary step in implementing Muthén's Maximum Likelihood (MUML) solution pioneered as a forerunner to the Full Information Maximum Likelihood (FIML) estimation of ML SEM models. Because of this, Muthén's method places a heavy emphasis on preliminary analyses of the individual between- and within-groups covariance matrices. However, since a number of software packages (such as M*plus*, LISREL, Mx, and AMOS) now make FIML estimation available, it is unnecessary to estimate the matrices and model them separately. We are not saying that it is not useful to inspect these matrices, but only that it is not necessary to estimate and model them separately as part of conducting a ML SEM.

The approach of Mehta and Neale (2005) is elegant in that it clearly shows the continuity between the family of multilevel models and ML SEMs. It is well designed to acquaint those who are familiar with multilevel modeling with how these models can be applied to situations with latent variables. However, the Mehta and Neale approach requires the user to conduct the first two steps in a different software package, such as SAS Proc Mixed (which also requires the data to be structured in a "long" format necessary for many multilevel software packages instead of the "wide" format used by SEM packages). Though this formatting issue may be a minor consideration for some, it is certainly more time consuming than a method that can be conducted seamlessly within a single model using a single software package. The method of Hox (2002) has the advantage that it can be executed within one package and additionally it proceeds in a way that will be quite familiar to practitioners of SEM who are accustomed to building and testing models in a stepwise fashion. Therefore, we chose to present the data example for this chapter using the benchmark models described by Hox (2002).

Data Example

As mentioned, we will demonstrate the methods of ML CFA described above using data from the International Social Survey Program (ISSP; 2002) Family and Changing Gender Roles III. Data from this program, but a different survey, were previously used by Cheung and Au (2005) who provide an excellent introduction to ML SEM using Muthén's aforementioned steps and the MUML estimator. The Family and Changing Gender Roles III survey was the third in a series conducted by the ISSP to explore issues such as family relations, gender roles at home and work, and job stress and satisfaction. The total sample size (with listwise deletion) is 25,468 individuals from 35 countries. We employ listwise deletion only to simplify the example. For any substantive analysis, we would strongly recommend missing data imputation (Schafer, 1997; R. J. Little & Rubin, 2002). Participating countries and associated sample sizes are shown in Table 4.1. In order to demonstrate the use of a level-two predictor, we drew from the work of Hofstede (1983) who aggregated data from a large international database to define four cultural dimensions at the country level. These dimensions reflect work-related values defined at the country level. For this data example, we used the Uncertainty Avoidance Index (UAI), which assesses how tolerant a country is of uncertainty and ambiguity.

TABLE 4.1

Participating Countries and Associated Sample Sizes

Country	Sample size
Australia	754
Austria	879
Brazil	1,275
Bulgaria	352
Cyprus	655
Czech Republic	746
Denmark	806
Finland	827
Flanders	667
France	1,209
Germany (East)	204
Germany (West)	496
Great Britain	1,023
Hungary	429
Ireland	616
Israel (Jews, Arabs)	773
Japan	700
Latvia	611
Mexico	962
Netherlands	714
New Zealand	618
Northern Ireland	433
Norway	924
Philippines	645
Poland	472
Portugal	514
Republic of Chile	734
Russia	833
Slovak Republic	622
Slovenia	568
Spain	1,139
Sweden	756
Switzerland	548
Taiwan	1,160
United States	804
Total sample size	25,468

Model

The model for this example was built from our own exploratory factor analysis (EFA) of the ISSP data. Again, we would not advocate the use of exploratory analyses in constructing a SEM and only did so for the purposes of arriving at a useful data example. The results of the EFA suggested two easily interpretable constructs, namely Life Satisfaction and Overwork. Indicators of Life Satisfaction are v52 "If you were to consider your life in general, how happy or unhappy would you say you are, on the whole?" and v54 "All things considered, how satisfied are you with your family life?" Indicators of Overwork are v46 "There are so many things to do at work, I often run out of time before I get them all done," v48 "In the past three months it has happened that I have come home from work too tired to do the chores which need to be done," and v49 "In the past three months it has happened that it has been difficult for me to fulfill my family responsibilities because of the amount of time I spent on my job." Item v46 is scored on a 5-point ordered integer scale with values ranging from "strongly agree" to "strongly disagree." Items v48 and v49 are scored on a 4-point ordered integer scale with values ranging from "several times a week" to "never." Item v52 is measured on a 7-point ordered integer scale with values ranging from "completely happy" to "completely unhappy." Finally, item v54 is also measured on a 7-point scale with values ranging from "completely satisfied" to "completely dissatisfied."

Analysis

All analyses were conducted in M*plus* 3.11 which allows for the full maximum likelihood estimation of ML SEMs and can also provide robust standard errors and a χ^2 test of model fit (Muthén & Muthén, 2004). Prior to estimating any of the benchmark models we used M*plus* to calculate ICCs and the between and within covariance and correlation matrices. These matrices are presented in Tables 4.2 and 4.3. Intraclass correlations range from .04 to .05. Relatively speaking, the level of variance accounted for by country is not large; however, this does not necessarily mean that we should ignore the nested design. Gulliford, Ukomunne, and Chin (1999) used a large health survey to describe ICCs found at various levels of nesting ranging from household to postal code, and found that ICCs varied inversely with cluster size. Gulliford and colleagues (1999) went on to state that even when ICCs are low, the design effects $(1 + (n - 1)\rho)$ or the impact of the nested design, where n is the cluster size and ρ is the ICC, could still be large when the cluster size is large. As further evidence that even small ICCs should not be ignored, Julian (2001) showed in a simulation study of ML SEMs that ICCs between .05 and .15 can result in an inflated model χ^2 statistic and biased estimates of both parameters and standard errors, especially when the group-to-member ratio is small as is the case with the current data set. Visual inspection of the between and within correlation matrices shows support for a two-factor model at both levels, however, correlations among the variables both within and between factors are stronger at the between-level.

Next we estimate the benchmark models as well as the final model (see Table 4.4 for model fit statistics for all models). None of the models tested fitted the data based on the χ^2 test of model fit. Given that the χ^2 statistic

TABLE 4.2

Covariances and Correlations at the Individual (within) Level

	1	2	3	4	5
1. Gen sat	0.87	0.61	-0.06	–0.14	–0.13
2. Fam sat	0.58	1.04	-0.04	–0.13	–0.12
3. Time work	–0.06	–0.05	1.47	0.31	0.33
4. Tired chore	–0.13	–0.13	0.38	0.99	0.55
5. Fam resp	–0.11	–0.12	0.40	0.53	0.97

Notes. Correlations are shown above the diagonal, variances on the diagonal, and covariances below the diagonal. Gen sat: general satisfaction ("If you were to consider your life in general, how happy or unhappy would you say you are, on the whole?"). Fam sat: family satisfaction ("All things considered, how satisfied are you with your family life?"). Time work: not enough to me to do work ("There are so many things to do at work, I often run out of time before I get them all done'"). Tired chore: too tired to do household chores after work ("In the past three months it has happened that I have come home from work too tired to do the chores which need to be done"). Fam resp: not enough time for family responsibilities ("In the past three months it has happened that it has been difficult for me to fulfill my family responsibilities because of the amount of time I spent on my job")

for model fit is overly sensitive to even minor model misfit when sample sizes are large, we also assessed model fit based upon a number of the practical fit indices mentioned before. These indices included the Comparative Fit Index (CFI), the Root Mean Squared Error of Approximation (RMSEA), as well as the Standardized Root Mean Residuals (SRMR) for both the between- and within-groups models. While the CFI and RMSEA give us an assessment of global fit, the SRMRs assess fit separately for the

TABLE 4.3

Covariances and Correlations at the Country (between) Level

	1	2	3	4	5
1. Gen sat	0.04	0.83	0.18	–0.43	–0.46
2. Fam sat	0.04	0.05	0.29	–0.26	–0.31
3. Time wrk	0.01	0.02	0.05	0.16	0.17
4. Chores	–0.02	–0.01	0.01	0.06	0.76
5. Fam resp	–0.02	–0.02	0.01	0.04	0.05
Means	2.68	2.46	2.79	2.51	2.95
ICCs	0.05	0.05	0.04	0.05	0.05

Note. Correlations are shown above the diagonal, variances on the diagonal, and covariances below the diagonal. See Table 4.2 for an explanation of the items in the first column.

TABLE 4.4

Model Fit Statistics

	χ^2	df	p	CFI	RMSEA	SRMR Between	SRMR Within
Null model	4148.507	19	< .001	.837	.092	.366	.011
Independence model	122.830	14	< .001	.996	.017	.366	.010
Saturated model	39.636	4	< .001	.999	.019	.000	.010
Two-Factor model	44.945	8	< .001	.999	.013	.113	.010
Loadings equated	52.287	11	< .001	.998	.012	.196	.010

between- and within-levels of the model and for that reason can be particularly useful in ML SEM. Based on all indices of model fit, the null model specifying the two-factor model for the within-level but fixing all values in the between model to zero did not fit the data, leading us to conclude that there is between-level variation that should be modeled. This result is in accord with the ICCs we found for the variables in the model. We proceeded to the independence model in which variances, but not covariances, are modeled at the between-level. Though the independence model shows a vast improvement in fit over the null model and reasonably good fit overall, we proceeded with the saturated model to assess how much fit is improved by allowing the between-country means to covary. Since any model misfit in the saturated model is due exclusively to the within portion of the model, the saturated model is expected to show very good fit and it does in this case. Our use of the saturated model is as a best-fitting model with which we can compare our final two-factor model. Next we tested the two-factor solution on both the between and the within levels. The two-factor model, fitted nearly as well as the saturated model ($\Delta\chi^2(4) = 5.31$; $p = .26$). Unstandardized loadings and residual variances are shown in Table 4.5 for the two-factor model. In this model, one residual variance (v52) has a negative estimate. A simulation study by Hox and Maas (2001) shows that this is not an uncommon problem in ML SEM when sample sizes at the highest level are small. In our experience, this type of estimate problem is fairly common and can be addressed by allowing the estimate to be negative, constraining it to be zero, or placing a restriction that the estimate must be nonnegative.

The next question we addressed was that of cross-level invariance, whether the two constructs in the model were being measured in the same way at the within- and between-levels. We addressed this question with a measurement invariance model in which the factor loadings were

TABLE 4.5

Unstandardized Estimates from the Two-Factor Model

	Within			Between		
	Loadings satisfaction	Loadings overwork	Residual variances	Loadings satisfaction	Loadings overwork	Residual variances
Gen sat	0.76		0.29	0.23		−0.01
Fam sat	0.76		0.46	0.17		0.03
Time wrk		0.53	1.19		0.04	0.05
Chores		0.72	0.48		0.21	0.01
Fam resp		0.74	0.41		0.21	0.01

equated across the two levels. If this model holds, it is reasonable to conclude that the constructs are similarly measured across levels. Additionally, it is feasible to compare the latent variances across levels as they are on the same scale when factor loadings are equated. In order to compare the latent variances, we estimated the latent variances by fixing the first factor loading to 1.0. This model fit the data well and did not result in a significant loss of fit as compared to the unconstrained model ($\Delta\chi^2(3) = 7.34$; $p = .06$). As mentioned above, equating the loadings allowed us to directly compare the latent variances, which in turn, allows us to calculate a latent variable ICC for our two constructs as $\psi_B/(\psi_B + \psi_W)$. The latent ICC for Satisfaction is $0.094/(0.094 + 1.353) = 0.06$ and the latent ICC for Overwork is $0.105/(0.105 + 1.052) = 0.09$.

In the final step of this example, we introduced two predictors into the model. The first is a level-1 predictor, sex of the respondent, and the second is a level-2 predictor, each country's score on Hofstede's Uncertainty Avoidance Index (UAI). For a more comprehensive approach to the introduction of multiple predictors into a ML SEM, including the use of random intercepts of level-1 variables as level-2 predictors, see Bovaird (in press). The results from the present model showed that being female is a significant predictor of higher Satisfaction ($t = 6.78$) and of less Overwork ($t = -18.99$). In addition, the degree to which residents of one's country avoid uncertainty and ambiguity (UAI) was a significant predictor of lower levels of Overwork ($t = -2.53$) but not related to Satisfaction ($t = 0.69$).

Unresolved Issues in ML SEM

In ML SEM, sample size is complicated by the fact that there are multiple sample sizes to consider. We can consider the number of level-1 units (e.g., individuals), the number of level-2 units (e.g., cultures), and even the average number of level-1 units nested within each level-2 unit (e.g., average number of individuals sampled from each cultural group studied). The issue of level-2 sample size is particularly relevant to cross-cultural research. As Cheung and Au (2005) point out, there are a finite number of countries to sample, and many of these are developing countries in which it would be difficult if not impossible to draw a sample. Information from simulation studies using the MUML estimator suggests that the minimum level-2 sample size needed to avoid estimation errors is 100 (Hox & Maas, 2001). In addition, the simulation study of Cheung and Au (2005), also using MUML, found that increasing the sample size at the individual level does not compensate for smaller sample sizes at the second level. Given the relatively recent implementation of FIML estimation for ML SEMs, information is not available regarding the necessary sample size when using this estimator.

Also related to sample size is a further complication of assessing model fit. Although model fit statistics are provided by software packages (e.g., M*plus* calculates a χ^2 statistic, CFI, SRMR, and RMSEA; LISREL calculates a χ^2 statistic, SRMR, and RMSEA), little is known about the accuracy of these indices as they apply to ML SEM. As Mehta and Neale (2005) point out, the χ^2 test of model fit (and therefore the CFI, RMSEA, and any fit indices based upon χ^2) is likely to be affected by three aspects of sample size mentioned above: the total number of individuals, the total number of clusters, and the average number of individuals per cluster. It is also unclear in some cases which sample size should be used in the computation of fit indices in ML SEM.

CONCLUSION

The latent variable modeling approaches discussed here have great promise to allow researchers to explore the fundamental similarities and differences among cultural groups. When the constructs under investigation are assumed to transcend culture-specific definitions, both variations of the latent variable modeling approach have numerous advantages over traditional manifest variable approaches. The choice of one model over another will largely be determined by one's research questions and whether the investigator is treating the cultures in a study as levels of a fixed variable or a sample from a random variable. The difficulty entailed in the second choice is that the number of cultures is in fact finite and it is cost-prohibitive to obtain a sample of more than a few cultural groups. Multiple Groups MACS models are very useful for detailed analyses with a relatively small number of groups. The MACS model allows for clear tests of invariance as well as tests of specific hypotheses such as whether cultures differ on levels of variation in, or relations among constructs. Though the tradition of MACS analyses is well established, we focused on a number of issues that remain unresolved. For example, we demonstrated that even under strong selection influence (i.e., selecting culture with very different levels of common variance), we can still find strong measurement invariance.

In contrast to Multiple Groups MACS models, ML SEM requires larger numbers of cultures and assumes rather than tests for measurement invariance. Though the history of ML SEM spans over two decades, the ability to readily conduct such analyses is a relatively recent occurrence, and therefore our goal was simply to demonstrate the logic of such an analysis with attention to each step in the process. We are still learning about many of the subtleties of these models including cross-group and cross-level invariance, as well as issues of sufficient sample size and the assessment of model fit. The issues that arise when using ML SEM are complex, but they allow us to test theories about both group-level and individual-level phenomena that we would otherwise be unable to test. Rather than arguing for one latent variable approach to cross-cultural research over another, we hope we have shown that both approaches can be fruitfully employed in the appropriate situation.

Author Note

This work was supported in part by grants from the NIH to the University of Kansas through the Mental Retardation and Developmental Disabilities Research Center (5 P30 HD002528), the Center for Biobehavioral Neurosciences in Communication Disorders (5 P30 DC005803), an Individual National Research Service Award (F32 MH072005) to the second author while at the University of Kansas, and a NFGRF grant (2301779) from the University of Kansas to the third author. The views expressed herein are not necessarily those of the sponsoring agencies.

Note

1. Another way to consider this estimated value is in terms of the amount of reliable variance implied by .64 correlations relative to .25 correlations. Specifically, because the observed correlations in the second group are .25, the implied common variance among the indicators in this group is $.25^2 = .06$. In the reference group, the common variance is $.64^2 = .41$. The ratio of 1.0 to .39 (the fixed and estimated latent variables in groups 1 and 2) is the same as the square root of the ratio of .06 to .41 (i.e., $\sqrt{.15} = .39$). That is, $1.0/.39 = .64/.25 = \sqrt{(.06/.41)}$.

   The observed variance of a variable i on construct f in group g is reproduced by $\sigma^2_{ifg} = \lambda_{ifg} \Psi_{fg} \lambda_{ifg} + \theta_{ifg}$ and the observed covariance between variables i and j as indicators of the same construct is reproduced by $COV(i,j) = \lambda_{ifg} \Psi_{fg} \lambda_{jfg}$. Using these formulae, we can substitute values of .8 for both of the loadings (e.g., λ_{ifg} and λ_{jfg}) in group 1 and set the scale of the estimates of the construct by fixing the variance of the construct (Ψ_{fg}) at 1.0. If the data are unstandardized, the resulting loadings would reproduce covariances (i.e., correlations when the data are standardized) of .64 and the amount of residual variance for each indicator would be .36. In group 2, if the loadings are .5, the resulting covariances (i.e., correlations when the data are standardized) would be .25 and the residual variances would be .75. When invariance of the loadings is specified and the latent variance in group 2 is estimated, the equations would change such that $\sigma^2_{ifg} = \lambda_{if} \Psi_{fg} \lambda_{if} + \theta_{ifg}$ and $COV(i,j) = \lambda_{if} \Psi_{fg} \lambda_{jf}$. Note that λ_{if} no longer is subscripted with a g but the variance of the construct (Ψ_{fg}) would vary across groups. This latent variance would be fixed at 1.0 in group 1 to set the scale, but would become an estimated value in group 2 because the scale is set via the equality constraints on the factor loadings (λ's). Here, the loadings in group 2 would be .8 but the estimated variance of the latent construct would be estimated to be .39 in order to reproduce the observed covariance of .25 between the indicators. The residuals would be the same values in both solutions. If the observed variances are not standardized but differ across groups, the equations would still hold but the implied magnitude of covariation would depend on the metric of the observed variables.

REFERENCES

Bentler, P. M., & Liang, J. (2003). Two-level mean and covariance structures: Maximum likelihood via an EM algorithm. In S. P. Reise & N. Duan (Eds.), *Multilevel modeling: Methodological advances, issues, and applications* (pp. 53–70). Mahwah, NJ: Lawrence Erlbaum.

Billiet, J. B., & McClendon, M. J. (2000). Modeling acquiescence in measurement models for two balanced sets of items. *Structural Equation Modeling, 7,* 608–628.

Bovaird, J. A. (2007). Multilevel structural equation models for contextual factors. In T. D. Little, J. A. Bovaird, & N. A. Card (Eds.), *Modeling contextual effects in longitudinal studies.* Mahwah, NJ: Lawrence Erlbaum.

Brown, T. A. (2006). *Confirmatory factor analysis for applied research.* New York: Guilford.

Browne, M. W., & Arminger, G. (1995). Specification and estimation of mean- and covariance-structure models. In G. Arminger, C. C. Clogg, & M. E. Sobal (Eds.), *Handbook of statistical modeling for the social and behavioral sciences* (pp. 185–241). New York: Plenum.

Browne, M. W., & Cudeck, R. (1993). Alternative ways of assessing model fit. In K. A. Bollen & J. S. Long (Eds.), *Testing structural equation models* (pp. 136–162). Newbury Park, CA: Sage.

Card, N. A., & Little, T. D. (2006). Analytic considerations in cross-cultural research on peer relations. In X. Chen, D. C. French, & B. Schneider (Eds.), *Peer relations in cultural context* (pp. 75–95). New York: Cambridge University Press.

Cheung, G. W., & Rensvold, R. B. (2000). Assessing extreme and acquiescence response sets in cross-cultural research using structural equation modeling. *Journal of Cross-Cultural Psychology, 31,* 187–212.

Cheung, G. W., & Rensvold. R. B (2002). Evaluating goodness-of-fit indexes for testing measurement invariance. *Structural Equation Modeling, 9,* 233–255.

Cheung, M. W. L., & Au, K. (2005). Applications of multilevel structural equation modeling to cross-cultural research. *Structural Equation Modeling, 12,* 598–619.

Goldstein, H., & McDonald, R.P. (1988). A general model for the analysis of multilevel data. *Psychometrika, 53,* 455–467.

Grob, A., Little, T. D., Wanner, B., Wearing, A. J., & Euronet. (1996). Adolescents' well-being and perceived control across fourteen sociocultural contexts. *Journal of Personality and Social Psychology, 71,* 785–795.

Gulliford, M. C., Ukomunne, O. C., & Chin, S. (1999). Components of variance and intraclass correlations for the design of community-based surveys and intervention studies. *American Journal of Epidemiology, 149,* 876–883.

Hancock, G. R., Stapleton, L. M., & Arnold-Berkovits, I. (2005). *The tenuousness of invariance tests within multisample covariance and mean structure models* (CILVR Paper No. 1). College Park, MD: University of Maryland, Center for Integrated Latent Variable Research.

Heck, R. H. (2001). Multilevel modeling with SEM. In G. A. Marcoulides & R. E. Schumacker (Eds.), *New developments and techniques in structural equation modeling* (pp. 89–128). Mahwah, NJ: Lawrence Erlbaum.

Heck, R. H., & Thomas, S. L. (2000). *An introduction to multilevel modeling techniques.* Mahwah, NJ: Lawrence Erlbaum.

Hofstede, G. (1983). National cultures revisited. *Behavioral Science Research, 18,* 285–305.

Horn, J. L., & McArdle, J. J. (1992). A practical and theoretical guide to measurement invariance in aging research. *Experimental Aging Research, 18,* 117–144

Hox, J. J. (2002). *Multilevel analysis: Techniques and applications.* Mahwah, NJ: Lawrence Erlbaum.

Hox, J. J., & Maas, C. J. M. (2001). The accuracy of multilevel structural equation modeling with pseudobalanced groups and small samples. *Structural Equation Modeling, 8,* 157–174.

International Social Survey Program, (2002). *International social survey program: Family and changing gender roles III, 2002* [Computer file]. ICPSR version. Cologne, Germany: Zentralarchiv fur Empirische Sozialforschung.

Jöreskog, K. G. (1988). Analysis of covariance structures. In J. R. Nesselroade & R. B. Cattell (Eds.), *Handbook of multivariate experimental psychology* (2nd ed., pp. 207–230). New York: Plenum.

Julian, M. W. (2001). The consequences of ignoring multilevel data structure in nonhierarchical covariance modeling. *Structural Equation Modeling, 8,* 325–352.

Kaplan, D., & Elliott, P. R. (1997). A didactic example of multilevel structural equation modeling applicable to the study of organizations. *Structural Equation Modeling, 4,* 1–24.

Lee, S. Y. (1990). Multilevel analysis of structural equation models. *Biometrika, 77,* 763–772.

Lee, S. Y., & Poon, W.Y. (1998). Analysis of two-level structural equation models via EM type algorithms. *Statistica Sinica, 5,* 749–766.

Little, R. J., & Rubin, D. B. (2002). *Statistical analysis with missing data* (2nd ed.). New York: Wiley.

Little, T. D. (1997). Mean and covariance structures (MACS) analyses of cross-cultural data: Practical and theoretical issues. *Multivariate Behavioral Research, 32,* 53–76.

Little, T. D., Card, N. A., Slegers, D. W., & Ledford, E. C. (in press). Modeling contextual effects with multiple-group MACS models. In T. D. Little, J. A., Bovaird, & N. A. Card (Eds.), *Modeling contextual effects in longitudinal studies* Mahwah, NJ: Lawrence Erlbaum.

Little, T. D., & Lopez, D. F. (1997). Regularities in the development of children's causality beliefs about school performance across six sociocultural contexts. *Developmental Psychology, 33,* 165–175.

Little, T. D., Miyashita, T., Karasawa, M., Mashima, M., Oettingen, G., Azuma, H. et al. (2003). The links among action-control beliefs, intellective skill, and school performance in Japanese, U.S., and German school children. *International Journal of Behavioral Development, 27,* 41–48.

Little, T. D., Oettingen, G., Stetsenko, A., & Baltes, P. B. (1995). Children's action-control beliefs and school performance: How do American children compare with German and Russian children? *Journal of Personality and Social Psychology, 69,* 686–700.

Little, T. D., Preacher, K. J., Card, N. A., Selig, J. P., & Lee, J. (2006). *Revisiting the question of factorial invariance.* Manuscript in preparation.

Little, T. D., & Slegers, D. W. (2005). Factor analysis: Multiple groups. In B. Everitt & D. Howell (Eds.), & D. Rindskopf (Section Ed.), *Encyclopedia of statistics in behavioral science* (Vol. 2, pp 617–623). Chichester, UK: Wiley.

Little, T. D., Slegers, D. W., & Card, N. A. (2006). A non-arbitrary method of identifying and scaling latent variables in SEM and MACS models. *Structural Equation Modeling, 13,* 59–72.

MacCallum, R. C., Browne, M. W., & Cai, L. (2006). Testing differences between nested covariance structure models: Power analysis and null hypotheses. *Psychological Methods, 11,* 19–35.

McDonald, R. P. (1999). *Test theory: A unified treatment.* Mahwah, NJ: Lawrence Erlbaum.

McDonald, R. P., & Goldstein, H. (1989). Balanced versus unbalanced designs for linear structural relations in two-level data. *British Journal of Mathematical & Statistical Psychology, 42,* 215–232.

Mehta, P. D., & Neale, M. C. (2005). People are variables too: Multilevel structural equation modeling. *Psychological Methods, 10,* 259–284.

Meredith, W. (1964). Notes on factorial invariance. *Psychometrika, 29,* 177–185.

Meredith, W. (1993). Measurement invariance, factor analysis and factorial invariance. *Psychometrika, 58,* 525–543.

Muthén B. O. (1994). Multilevel covariance structure analysis. *Sociological Methods & Research, 22,* 376–398.

Muthén, L. K., & Muthén B. O. (1998–2005). *Mplus user's guide* (3rd ed.). Los Angeles, CA: Muthén & Muthén.

Osterlind, S. J. (1983). *Test item bias.* Newbury Park, CA: Sage.

Preacher, K. J., Cai, L., & MacCallum, R. C. (2007). Alternatives to traditional model comparison: Strategies for covariance structural models. In T. D. Little, J. A. Bovaird, & N. A. Card (Eds.), *Modeling contextual effects in longitudinal studies* (pp. 33–62). Mahwah, NJ: Lawrence Erlbaum.

Preacher, K. J., & Wirth, R. J. (2006). *A model selection approach to assessing cross-group factorial invariance.* Manuscript in preparation.

Raudenbush, S. W., & Bryk, A. S. (2002). *Hierarchical linear models: Applications and data analysis methods* (2nd ed.). Thousand Oaks, CA: Sage.

Reise, S. P., Widaman, K. F., & Pugh, R. H. (1993). Confirmatory factor analysis and item response theory: Two approaches for exploring measurement invariance. *Psychological Bulletin, 114,* 552–566.

Rindskopf, F. (1984). Using phantom and imaginary latent variables to parameterize constraints in linear structural models. *Psychometrika, 49,* 37–47.

Schafer, J. L. (1997). *Analysis of incomplete multivariate data.* London: Chapman & Hall.

Sörbom, D. (1982). Structural equation models with structured means. In K. G. Jöreskog & H. Wold (Eds.), *Systems under direct observation* (pp. 183–195). New York: Praeger.

Stetsenko, A., Little, T. D., Gordeeva, T. O., Grasshof, M., & Oettingen, G. (2000). Gender effects in children's beliefs about school performance: A cross-cultural study. *Child Development, 71,* 517–527.

Van de Vijver, F. J. R., & Poortinga, Y. H. (2002). Structural equivalence in multilevel research. *Journal of Cross-Cultural Psychology, 33,* 141–156.

Widaman, K. F., & Reise, S. P. (1997). Exploring the measurement invariance of psychological instruments: Applications in the substance use domain. In K. J. Bryant, M. Windle & S.G. West, (Eds.), *The science of prevention: Methodological advances from alcohol and substance abuse research* (pp. 281–324). Washington, D.C.: American Psychological Association.

Zyphur, M. J., & Preacher, K. J. (2006). *Assessing construct comparability across levels of analysis: The logic, application, and implications of cross-level measurement and structural invariance.* Manuscript submitted for publication.

Part III

Multilevel Models
and Applications

5

Levels of Control across Cultures: Conceptual and Empirical Analysis

Susumu Yamaguchi, Taichi Okumura, Hannah Faye
Chua, Hiroaki Morio, and J. Frank Yates

Control over one's physical and social environment is essential for one's psychological well-being. Weisz and Rothbaum (1984), in their seminal work on the notion of control, proposed a distinction between primary and secondary control. The former type of control refers to control over one's physical environment, whereas the latter refers to control over one's internal states, such as emotion and interpretations about one's environment. Weisz and Rothbaum further argued that primary control is a dominant control style in the U.S., whereas secondary control is more dominant in East Asia including Japan. In this chapter, we will argue that we need to extend our conceptual framework to understand Asian control orientations, based upon Yamaguchi (2001). Then, we will show how research on control orientations from an extended framework will benefit from multilevel analysis. Implications for future research as well as policy making will be discussed.

Throughout human history, control over the physical and social environment has been essential for our survival and well-being. Natural disasters (e.g., earthquakes, floods, typhoons, and more recently global warming) and pandemics (e.g., the plague in the medieval period, Spanish flu following the First World War) are probably the two most important targets of our control attempts. No less important is control over our social environment. Most of us need to work with others and thus control our relationships with them, so that we can be comfortable in our work situations. Even in personal situations, individuals exert control over their environment. For example, individuals control room temperature by switching on and off an air-conditioner or, when such equipment is unavailable, opening or closing windows. Thus, control is ubiquitous in our lives, whether it is in response to a large-scale disaster or just a small rise in room temperature.

In this chapter, we focus on how individuals' control attempts are mainly exercised in group or collective settings. As will be shown, multi-level analysis provides the most appropriate data analysis strategy. Before we present more details on how such analyses should be conducted, an overview of the concept of control is needed. The concept of control is much more complex in cross-cultural psychology than it may appear at first glance.

CULTURE AND TYPOLOGY OF CONTROL

The concept of control has attracted psychologists' theoretical and empiri-cal attention (e.g., Morling & Evered, 2006; Rothbaum, Weisz, & Snyder, 1982; Skinner, 1996; Weisz, Rothbaum, & Blackburn, 1984; Yamaguchi, 2001). It is known by now that forms of control can be appropriately clas-sified according to their target (i.e., what one would like to control) and agent (i.e., who actually exerts control over the target).

Target of Control

Individuals may attempt to control external realities, like a person who switches on an air conditioner to cool down the room. Alternatively, the person in a hot room may take off clothes to cool him- or herself down. Rothbaum et al. (1982) and Weisz et al. (1984), in their seminal work, intro-duced a distinction between primary control and secondary control. The former refers to control over existing external realities in one's physical and social environment. In this kind of control, individuals attempt to "enhance their rewards by actively influencing existing realities (e.g., other people, circumstances, symptoms, or behavior problems)" (Weisz et al., 1984, p. 955). On the other hand, secondary control refers to control over the self (see Morling & Evered, 2006, for a review). In secondary control, individuals attempt to "enhance their rewards by accommodating to exist-ing realities and maximizing satisfaction or goodness of fit with things as they are" without changing the existing realities (Weisz et al., 1984, p. 955). In the case of room temperature, a person with primary control orientation will attempt to cool down the air in the room by using an air conditioner, whereas another person with secondary control orientation will just take off clothes without attempting to change the room temperature.

In the literature, unfortunately, this excellent dichotomy has been con-fused, partly because Weisz et al. (1984) did not mention explicitly that a person could have a choice regarding the agent of control, especially in what they termed primary control. They assumed that in primary control individuals attempt to control external realities by means of "personal agency, dominance, or even aggression" (p. 955). For this reason, target and agency have been confused in the subsequent literature. The agent in primary control has often been assumed to be a person who wishes to exert control over the target, although, as the next section will elaborate, the agent in primary control is not restricted in this way.

Agent of Control

Yamaguchi (2001) proposed that there are at least three possibilities for the agent of control regardless of the type of control target: the self, collective, and someone else. Depending on the agent(s), control attempts can be classified into three kinds: personal, collective, and proxy. In *personal control*, a person who wishes to control a target, either existing external realities or the self, attempts to exert control over the target. In *collective control*, the person attempts to control the target along with others who can be helpful in exerting control. In *proxy control*, the person asks someone else who is powerful to control the situation on his or her behalf. For example, a businesswoman can fix problems that she is facing on her own (personal control), with her colleagues (collective control), or through her supervisor (proxy control).

Other researchers have also attempted to clarify the concept of control by introducing additional dimensions on which control orientation varies. For example, Spector, Sanchez, Siu, Salgado, and Ma (2004) introduced a control concept named "socioinstrumental" control, which is said to characterize a type of control typically found among Asians. According to Spector et al., socioinstrumental control is defined as "active attempts to influence the environment through social means" (p. 43), which is obviously a kind of primary control. In our view, the essential difference between primary control and socioinstrumental control is in the agency of control. Because people are supposed to exercise socioinstrumental control by maintaining and maximizing the utility of interpersonal relationships (Spector et al.), it will amount to proxy control if a specific individual acts as an agent for other people, or collective control when a group or community they belong to act as an agent collectively. Spector et al.'s discussion of expected cultural differences between Eastern and Western cultures in socioinstrumental control is similar to collective control that we have discussed. In East Asia, getting along with others in a group is not only valued, but also often instrumental in achieving goals in organizational settings. Personal outcomes are often deemphasized and group outcomes become the focus of attention.

It is quite reasonable, therefore, that Spector et al. (2004) expected that Asians would be higher in both secondary and socioinstrumental control. In order to test this hypothesis, they developed two scales to measure individuals' secondary and socioinstrumental orientations respectively and administered them to students in the United States, People's Republic of China (PRC), and Hong Kong. Although some significant cultural differences were found, the obtained pattern was not straightforward. For socioinstrumental control, the mean score for the PRC sample was higher than that for Hong Kong and the United States, indicating that people in the PRC felt a stronger sense of socioinstrumental control than those in the United States and Hong Kong. On the other hand, for secondary control, people in Hong Kong scored lower than those in the United States and PRC.

Another control construct, "harmony control," was proposed by Morling and Fiske (1999) as an attempt to clarify the concept of secondary control. Harmony control was introduced as a separate construct, independent of primary and secondary control, and it was defined as "an active, intentional endeavor in which people recognize the agency in contextual, social, or spiritual forces and attempt to merge with these forces" (Morling & Fiske, 1999, p. 381). This definition addresses agency but it does not specify the differences among the three types of agency: contextual, social, or spiritual forces. Harmony control was operationally defined as and measured by a scale with five factors. Of the five factors, three factors, Friends Care, Anticipate Others, and Merge with Others, are essentially measuring one's willingness to cooperate with unspecified others in a person's surroundings, so that the person will exercise control with others. From the present perspective, these factors correspond to the sense of collective control. The remaining factors, Higher Power and Wait on Luck, tap one's tendency to rely on supernatural power or sheer luck without any human agency. Because there is no agent involved in the individual differences assessed by these factors, it remains uncertain if these two factors can be called "control," as the authors themselves admit (Morling & Fiske, 1999, p. 409).

More recently, Morling and Evered (2006) incorporated the construct of harmony control into the concept of secondary control. They argue that it is possible to classify the definitions and operationalization of secondary control in the literature into two groups: *control-focused secondary control* and *fit-focused secondary control*. The conceptual and operational definition of the control-focused secondary control is in line with the initial theoretical framework provided by Rothbaum et al. (1982), who coined the term *secondary control*, emphasizing that it could be considered as a form of *control*. The operationalization of fit-focused secondary control, which includes harmony control proposed by Morling and Fiske (1999), is characterized by one's acceptance of specific circumstances as they are. The thorough review of the relevant literature by Morling and Evered is quite informative and no doubt sheds light on the nature of secondary control. However, they did not address the issue of agency, which has also been neglected by most researchers in the field. It is unfortunate that Morling and Evered's definition of fit-focused secondary control leaves the agent of control unidentified. In our view, there remains room for further conceptual clarification.

Culture and Control

Weisz et al. (1984) were the first to claim a relationship between culture and control. In their now classic work, they insisted that primary control is more important in everyday life in the United States, whereas secondary control is more important for Japanese everyday life. This argument is based on their observation that primary control is both less feasible and less desirable for Japanese as compared with Americans. For this reason, they suggested that secondary control is more prevalent than primary control in Japan, whereas the opposite is the case in the United States.

In the U.S. value system, in which independence and self-sufficiency are valued, individuals would attempt to acquire abilities to keep important societal and material resources under their control, so they can claim their independence and self-sufficiency. The primacy of primary control as proposed by Weisz et al. (1984) is consistent with such orientations, because primary control essentially refers to personal control over existing external realities. One can assert independence and autonomy when one controls the environment personally. For example, if a businesswoman can solve problems that her company is facing on her own, she can definitely claim her autonomy to the management. Her attempt to solve the problem on her own is risky, however, from the perspective of interpersonal harmony in her company. Her business strategy may not be liked by her colleagues and thus cause a conflict with them. On the other hand, if she attempts to solve the problem along with her colleagues (i.e., collective control), she can avoid the disruption of interpersonal harmony but she will be unable to claim autonomy in this kind of control. Also, if the businesswoman asks her boss to handle the situation and obtains her supervisor's approval, then her attempt to control the situation through the boss (i.e., proxy control) will allow her to keep a harmonious relationship with this supervisor, although obviously she cannot claim autonomy and independence.

Thus, Yamaguchi (2001) concluded that personal control, in which an individual can assert personal agency and thus autonomy, would be more prevalent in the United States as compared with Japan, whereas collective control, in which an individual can maintain interpersonal harmony, would be preferred by Japanese. Although Weisz et al. (1984) claimed that Japanese would attempt to exert secondary control, in which the target of control is the self, it does not make sense for the businesswoman in the above example to just think about the meaning of the problem or just attempt to control her feelings. This must be the case with businesspeople in any culture, including Japan. Thus, the dichotomy between primary and secondary control is not enough to understand cultural differences in control orientations (for a review of relevant research, see Yamaguchi, 2001). With this extended framework, we can now predict that collective control would be more prevalent in Japan as compared with the United States, whereas personal control would be more prevalent in the United States than in Japan. However, this does not mean that Japanese would never attempt to exert personal control or North Americans would never attempt to exert collective control. Rather, both types of control are necessary in any culture.

More recent studies appear to support Yamaguchi's (2001) conclusion that the primary–secondary distinction alone cannot fully explain cultural differences in control orientations. For example, Lam and Zane (2004) found significant cultural differences between Asian and European Americans in primary and secondary control assessed by a self-report measure. Asian Americans were found to endorse items corresponding to the sense of primary control less, and to endorse the sense of secondary control more, as proposed by Weisz et al. (1984). However, the aforementioned study by Spector et al. (2004) found that the effect of culture on the sense of secondary control was significant, yet the pattern was not straightforward. As explained before, they found the sense of secondary control among North Americans and Chinese in the PRC to be higher than that of Chinese in Hong Kong. Such a significant difference was not found between North Americans and Chinese in the PRC. This perplexing result suggests that it is essential to take agency of control into consideration in order to understand the cultural differences in perception and practice of primary and secondary control. In all, the foregoing literature review suggests that cultures may well differ on the dimension of personal–collective control orientations when the targets of control are external realities.

EMPIRICAL EVIDENCE ON THE SENSE OF COLLECTIVE CONTROL

Group Diffusion Effect

The foregoing conceptual analysis suggests that collective control can be an option when individuals attempt to control external realities. It is quite reasonable that individuals attempt collective control in response to large-scale threats such as natural disasters and pandemics. Indeed, we have seen a lot of collective control attempts that turned out to be successful in our history. For example, many modern cities are much better protected from floods than was once the case and smallpox has been totally eradicated. Thus, individuals would expect that they are more in control in the presence of others as compared with when they are alone.

The sense of collective control, as conceptualized here, is different from a similar concept of "perceived collective efficacy" (Bandura, 1997). The sense of collective control refers to individuals' sense of effectiveness in collective control, whereas "perceived collective efficacy" refers to a group's shared belief "in its conjoint capabilities to organize and execute the courses of action required to produce given levels of attainments. The collective belief centers on the group's operative capabilities" (Bandura, 1997, p. 477). In other words, the sense of collective control refers to an individual-level sense of the capabilities of a group, a view that is not necessarily shared by group members.

Yamaguchi (1998) focused on the sense of collective control at the individual level and confirmed the above expectation that individuals feel more in control in the presence of others than when they are alone. This effect was named *group diffusion effect*. In this research, Japanese female students felt safer as the number of their risk companions, who were exposed to the same risk source, increased. In one study, participants were presented with scenarios including a risk situation and they were asked to estimate the risk level involved. As expected, the estimated risk level decreased as the number of risk companions increased. For example, the participants estimated that their chance of getting stomach cancer due to water contaminated by a carcinogen would be lower as more people drank the water on a daily basis. This tendency was confirmed in Hong Kong by Ho and Leung (1998).

The fact that East Asians feel safer in groups does not exclude the possibility that North Americans too feel safer in a group. Rather, people need to exert collective control when it comes to large-scale threats to well-being such as natural disasters. However, North Americans presumably would be less inclined to feel safe in a group. A replication study conducted at the University of Michigan answers at least a part of the question (Chua, Yamaguchi, & Yates, 2001). We explain the study in detail as it has not been published.

So far, three reasons for the sense of collective control have been examined. First, as Yamaguchi (1998) hypothesized, the risk diffusion effect may be due to the comfort provided by presence of others in a fearful situation (cf. Schachter, 1959). However, Ho and Leung (1998) found that risk diffusion was just as strong when participants were provided with an alternative source of comfort and security in a fearful situation (i.e., providing insurance coverage to participants) as when they were not. Second, there is also a possibility that the risk diffusion effect rests on the collectivism of the cultures in which it previously has been demonstrated to occur (Japan and Hong Kong). The argument is that, because collectivists see the group rather than the individual as the basic unit of survival (Hui & Triandis, 1986), they draw great comfort from the presence of others. Yet, Ho and Leung (1998) found no evidence that the risk diffusion effect is especially pronounced among those who have strong collectivist orientations.

The third possibility, which was tested by Chua et al. (2001), is concerned with overgeneralization. Risk diffusion may rest at least partly on overgeneralization, and this may have to do with "shallow reflection." Suppose that late one night you are walking down a dark street in a dangerous neighborhood. Your chances of being robbed are significantly less if you are walking with a group of 19 friends than if you are walking alone. After all, as a sizable group, you and your friends collectively could do a variety of things that would protect each of you from being relieved of your belongings. The underlying principle is that there is "safety in numbers," a principle that everyone recognizes and accepts. The proposition at issue is that people tend to overgeneralize the "safety in numbers" principle to situations where it does not actually apply. In particular, they overgeneralize to the kinds of situations where the risk diffusion effect has been observed (e.g., the previous carcinogen scenario). They overgeneralize for two reasons: First, in many real-life situations that are superficially similar (e.g., the dangerous neighborhood scenario), the principle really *does* apply. Second, in ordinary discourse, including experimental procedures, they do not feel compelled to think deeply. Thus, they engage in mere "shallow reflection."

In the Chua et al. (2001) study, 104 males and 108 females from the United States, aged 18 to 23 years old, participated. The experiment was a 2 (list vs. control) × 2 (alone vs. group) between-participants design. Participants were given booklets with six hypothetical scenarios typical of those used in the previous research (Yamaguchi, 1998), where the presence of others in the group should not objectively decrease one's level of risk. Two orders of presentation of scenarios were made. Participants in the "control" conditions, "alone-control" and "group-control," were asked to read each scenario, imagine themselves in that situation, and then report their perceived risk in the situation. Prior to reporting their perceived risk, participants in the "list" conditions (alone-list and group-list) were asked whether there are things that can be done to reduce the pertinent risk, and if so, what. In each scenario in the "alone" conditions, the participant was described as being the only one exposed to the relevant hazard. In contrast, in the "group" conditions, the participant was described as being accompanied by numerous risk companions, who were other people also exposed to the hazard in question. Appendix A shows, respectively, the alone-control, group-control, and group-list versions of one of the scenarios; the alone-list condition is easy to derive.

A two-way ANOVA with planned comparisons was conducted for each of the scenarios. Out of the six scenarios we presented, risk diffusion occurred to a significant degree for only two of the scenarios, "Carcinogenic Additive" (as shown in Figure 5.1) and "Carcinogenic Water" (Figure 5.2). The remaining analyses were applied to those two instances in which the risk diffusion effect actually was demonstrated. Two-way ANOVAs indicated significant interactions of the alone-versus-group and control-

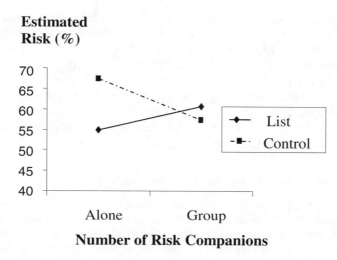

FIGURE 5.1 Perceived risk level for carcinogenic additive.

versus-list factors for the Carcinogenic Additive scenario, $F(1, 208) = 4.71$, $p < .05$ (see Figure 5.1), and for the "Carcinogenic Water" scenario, $F(1, 208) = 4.94$, $p < .05$ (see Figure 5.2). As predicted by the overgeneralization proposition, differences in estimated risk between the alone and group conditions were smaller when participants were required to list actions that might reduce risk than when they were not. Also consistent with the proposal, planned comparisons showed that the differences between the alone and group-condition risk estimates in the list condition were non-significant for the Carcinogenic Additive scenario, $F(1, 208) = 1.25$, *ns*, and also for the Carcinogenic Water scenario, $F(1, 208) = 2.28$, *ns*.

The fact that the risk diffusion was found only for the two carcinogen scenarios suggests two things. First, a possibility of collective control, even

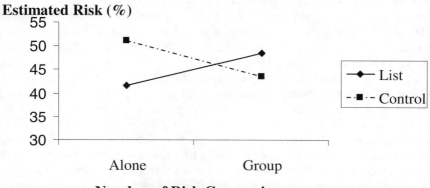

FIGURE 5.2 Perceived risk level for carcinogenic water.

though it can be illusory, affects people's risk perception. Second, in the United States, where the data were collected, the group diffusion effect is limited to the carcinogen scenario, which may have to do with a collective control orientation. Perhaps because people are oriented toward personal control they are less susceptible to the illusion of collective control. It is possible in the United States, where collective effort is under way to prevent and control cancer, people have an illusion of collective control over cancer. Possible cultural differences were tested in Yamaguchi, Gelfand, Ohashi, and Zemba (2005).

Primacy of Personal or Collective Control

We have seen in the previous sections that collective control, in addition to personal control, is an available choice for individuals in any culture. On the other hand, it was expected that the value system in the United States would lead people to prefer and rely on personal control over collective control, whereas in Japan collective control is beneficial for the maintenance of interpersonal harmony and thus people would prefer and rely on collective control. More specifically, it was expected that American men would overestimate their ability to exert control over their outcomes personally, whereas Japanese men would overestimate their ability to control their outcomes in collective terms. To test this prediction, American and Japanese college students were asked to estimate the result of a lottery drawing either in the alone condition or the group condition (Yamaguchi et al., 2005). The participants were told in the laboratory setting that the experiment was concerned with the effect of prior experience on subsequent learning. They were further told that there were two (fictitious) conditions, a control and an "unpleasant" condition. The difference between the two conditions was that in the unpleasant condition the participants had to have an unpleasant experience, which would be induced by taking a bitter drink before they solved puzzles. The participants were told that they would be assigned to the control or unpleasant condition, depending on the result of a lottery: If the sum of numbers given in a lottery exceeded a certain value they were to be assigned to the control condition in which they did not have to take a bitter drink.

In the alone condition, the participants were told to draw four lottery tickets by themselves. In the group condition, the participants were told that they were a member of a four-person group and that each of the four members would draw one lottery ticket. In the group condition, there were not actually the three group members in the other rooms. The most important issue in this manipulation is that there is no rational ground to believe that one can have a better outcome when one is alone or with others. The rational judgment is that there should be no difference no matter who draws the lottery tickets. But if individuals believe in their ability to exert personal control relative to collective control, they would show bias in judgment in favor of personal control. On the other hand, if individuals hold belief in their ability in the opposite direction, they would show bias in favor of collective control. Thus, it was expected that Americans, especially men, would show bias in judgment in favor of personal control, whereas Japanese would show the bias in the opposite direction. To measure the participants' judgment, they were asked to estimate the outcome by answering two questions: (1) the chance that they would be assigned to the control group as a percentage and (2) the same on a 7-point scale. Because the participants' answers were highly correlated, a composite variable was produced and analyzed in an ANOVA.

The results indicated that American men tended to predict a better result (being assigned to the control group) in the alone condition, whereas Japanese participants tended to predict a better result in the group condition, indicating that American men overestimate their ability to control outcome in personal control, whereas Japanese overestimate their ability to control outcome in collective control (Figure 5.3). This result indicates that there is a cultural difference in individuals' belief in their ability of personal and collective control. It is also interesting that such a difference is found only among men in the United States. As Gilligan (1982/1993) has aptly argued, the value system in which autonomy is valued to the extent that one has

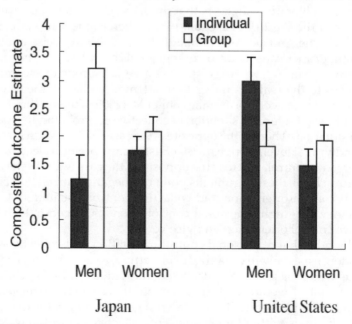

FIGURE 5.3 Mean composite outcome estimate by condition and sex. Notes: Higher bars indicate higher estimated probability of being assigned to the condition without the negative experience. Vertical lines depict standard errors of the means. (Reproduced with permission from the *Journal of Cross-Cultural Psychology, 36,* p. 756. © by Sage Publication, Inc., USA.)

biased belief in the ability of personal control, may be unique to American men. Women, on the other hand, may value interpersonal relationships.

In sum, our research has provided evidence that we should extend our framework to include collective control in addition to personal control. The latter has been considered mainly in the previous literature influenced by Weisz et al. and Rothbaum et al.'s conceptualization. An important implication of the distinction between personal and collective control is highlighted when considering organizational settings, such as companies. Employees in any culture are assumed to hold two control orientations, personal and collective. Because business tasks can be carried out by either a single employee or a group of employees, it would be important to foster a sense of collective control, a sense that one can control the outcome successfully in a group, as well as a sense of personal control.

PERSONAL AND COLLECTIVE CONTROL IN AN ORGANIZATIONAL SETTING ACROSS CULTURES

The previous literature suggests that the sense of personal control would be higher in the West (Weisz et al., 1984), whereas the sense of collective control is higher in East Asia (Yamaguchi et al., 2005). Weisz et al. (1984) argued that Americans tend to exert personal control, which they referred to as primary control, whereas Japanese are more prone to accommodate themselves to the realities rather than attempt to change them. When it comes to collective control, Yamaguchi et al. (2005) showed that Japanese men tend to feel safer in a situation of collective control than in a personal control situation, whereas the opposite is the case for American men. Thus, at the individual level, it appears that East Asians prefer collective control over personal control, whereas the opposite is the case with Westerners. At the cultural level, these arguments point to a negative correlation between personal control orientation and collective control orientation: Cultures characterized by higher personal control orientation tend to show lower collective control orientation and vice versa.

On the other hand, personal control orientation and collective control orientation, especially in organizational settings, would bolster each other and thus would be positively correlated. Individuals with higher sense of personal control would tend to contribute to successful achievement of a group goal and eventually hold a stronger sense of collective control. Also, individuals with a higher sense of collective control may well feel that the situation can be controlled by them to their liking within a group. Because those individuals with a high sense of collective control successfully cause the event that they desire in such situations, they may well feel competent in controlling the environment. Such feelings may lead them to hold a higher sense of personal control ability, in addition to collective control ability. Thus, there are reasons to expect that a sense of personal control and a sense of collective control are positively related. It is difficult to imagine a situation in which a higher sense of collective control leads one to hold a lower sense of personal control because by implication, successful collective control means a successful achievement of the goal that a group member has desired.

Thus, we have an interesting and apparently paradoxical expectation: The relationship between the sense of personal control and the sense of collective control at the individual level is reversed at the cultural level. In the following, we advance a set of hypotheses that embrace this challenging expectation. The following hypothesis follows from these arguments:

> *Hypothesis 1*: Individuals' sense of personal control is lower in East Asia as compared with the West, whereas individuals' sense of collective control is higher in East Asia than the West.

In a classic study, White and Lippitt (1968) examined three types of leadership: authoritarian, laissez-faire, and democratic. If we focus our discussion on the difference between laissez-faire and democratic leaderships, democratic leadership would be expected to foster a sense of collective control to a greater extent, relative to laissez-faire leadership. It is known that members work less and are more characterized by play under laissez-faire leadership; work motivation is higher under democratic leadership. This difference in work motivation and a resultant difference in performance would translate into a higher sense of collective control among members under democratic leadership, as compared with those under laissez-faire leadership:

> *Hypothesis 2*: Individuals' sense of collective control is higher in groups under democratic leadership than under laissez-faire leadership.

The simple relationship between leadership styles and sense of control would be complicated by the effect of culture, such that the facilitating effect of democratic leadership on the sense of collective control is smaller in East Asian cultural contexts, because East Asians are much more used to collective work than Westerners, regardless of the type of leadership. This reasoning would lead us to the next hypothesis:

> *Hypothesis 3*: The positive effect of democratic leadership on individuals' sense of collective control is smaller in East Asia than in the West.

Perhaps individuals with a higher sense of personal control would tend to contribute to group work more and thus hold a stronger sense of collective control. Also, individuals with a higher sense of collective control would tend to feel that they can control the situation by themselves as well, because the personal goal matches the goal of the collective control. As a result, an individual's sense of personal control would be positively related to the sense of collective control, as discussed above:

> *Hypothesis 4*: Individuals' sense of personal control is positively related to collective control.

The positive relationship between personal and collective control would be qualified by the type of culture. Perhaps in East Asia, where individuals are used to cooperating with one another to accomplish their shared goals, individuals' sense of personal control will be more efficiently generalized to their sense of collective control. Indeed, Earley (1993) has reported that performance of Chinese managers working with in-group members was much higher than those working alone. On the other hand, among American managers, their performance was better when working alone. This reasoning would lead us to the following hypothesis:

> *Hypothesis 5*: The positive relationship between the sense of personal and collective control is higher in East Asia than in the West.

More group-mindedness has been found under democratic leaders (White & Lippitt, 1968), suggesting that democratic leadership is more successful in connecting members' sense of personal control with their sense of collective control.

> *Hypothesis 6*: The positive relationship between the sense of personal control and the sense of collective control would be stronger under democratic leadership than under laissez-faire leadership.

Simulation Study

No empirical research has been conducted on the relationship between personal and collective control in organizational settings across cultures, to the best of our knowledge. Thus, we conducted a simulation study with an emphasis on the importance of multilevel analysis. In this study, we did not attempt to corroborate the hypotheses, although an empirical test of those hypotheses is highly desirable and should be done in the near future. Rather, we attempted to show that the reversed relationship at the two different levels of analysis (i.e., individual level and culture level) can coexist in a meaningful manner. In doing this, we used a multilevel random coefficient model, instead of conventional statistical analyses such as zero-order correlations or multiple regression analyses. As shown in Appendix B, the multilevel random coefficient model is superior to conventional analyses in revealing multilevel data structure.

CONCLUSION

This chapter argues that the primary–secondary control distinction proposed by Weisz et al. (1984) is based upon an assumption that individuals' repertoire of control over environment is limited to direct personal control. Although Weisz et al.'s seminal work has made a significant contribution to cross-cultural psychology by illuminating how culture affects individuals' control orientations, the simple dichotomy between primary and secondary control is not sufficient to understand individuals' repertoire of control. The conceptual framework needs to be extended to include other types of control, such as collective control and proxy control, especially when a researcher attempts to unearth how people control the environment in Asian cultural contexts. Indeed, available data indicate the importance of collective control, which has been largely neglected in the literature.

When we focus on the relationship between personal control and collective control, an interesting reversal is expected at the individual level as contrasted with the cultural level. This apparently paradoxical relationship at the two levels of analysis can be realistic and meaningful, as shown by the simulated data to which we applied multi-level analysis. Such analysis is essential for research dealing with hierarchical data structures.

Multilevel analysis is a powerful tool for cross-cultural research as well as research on organizations. It enables researchers to detect effects of variables that cannot be revealed otherwise. This chapter illustrated specifically how the simultaneous analysis of the sense of control both at the individual and group levels is made possible by multilevel analysis.

APPENDIX A

Alternative Versions of the Carcinogenic Additive Scenario (Chua, Yamaguchi, & Yates, 2001)

Note: Key differences are indicated in *bold italics* here though not in originals.

Alone-Control Condition

Scenario 1: It was recently found that a food additive usually used in the manufacturing of candy is a carcinogen. If you ingest more than one milligram of this additive over a period of two or three years, you have a good chance of developing stomach cancer. This additive has not been used on the market. *As the lone monitor of a confectionery company,* you have unfortunately already taken in more than one milligram of this additive on a daily basis for two years.

Question: How likely do you think it is that you will get stomach cancer (0– 100%): _____%

Group-Control Condition

Scenario 1: It was recently found that a food additive usually used in the manufacturing of candy is a carcinogen. If you ingest more than one milligram of this additive over a period of two or three years, you have a good chance of developing stomach cancer. This additive has not been used on the market. Unfortunately, **50 monitors of a confectionery company, including you,** have each already taken in more than one milligram of this additive on a daily basis for two years.

Question: How likely do you think it is that you will get stomach cancer (0– 100%): _____%

Group-List Condition

Scenario 1: It was recently found that a food additive often used in the manufacturing of candy is a carcinogen. If you ingest more than one milligram of this additive over a period of two or three years, you have a good chance of developing stomach cancer. This additive has not been used on the market. Unfortunately, **50 monitors of a confectionery company, including you,** have each already taken in more than one milligram of this additive on a daily basis for two years.

Question 1: Do you think that there are things that you and/or your coworkers could do that would reduce the chances that you personally will actually develop stomach cancer from your consumption of the carcinogen for the past two years (check one)?

_____No   _____Yes

If you checked "Yes," briefly list the thing(s) that you and/or your coworkers could do:

Question 2: How likely do you think it is that you will get stomach cancer (0– 100%): _____%

APPENDIX B

Data Generation

Hypothetical data were generated on the assumption that data were collected from employees of an international company with branches both in Japan and in North America. More specifically, the assumption was that 10 employees were randomly selected at 10 branches, which were also randomly selected both in Japan and in North America. Half of the branches were supposedly led by democratic managers whereas the other half were led by laissez-faire managers. Altogether 200 employees supposedly answered questoions about their senses of collective control and personal control.

The data were generated by using R, a free statistical package commonly used for statistical simulations (see Hogg, McKean, & Craig, 2005). The six hypotheses, mentioned in the main text, were assumed to be supported and the data were generated accordingly. The hypotheses had been translated into parameters in the data generation model presented below:

$$Y_{ij} = \beta_{0j} + \beta_{1j} X_{ij} + r_j, \; r_j \sim N(0, \sigma^2), \tag{1}$$

where X_j is raw score of personal control for ith person in jth company. This model is called level-1 model which expresses the relationship at individual level. The intraclass deviations of intercepts and slopes are modeled by the following level-2 model:

$$\beta_{0j} = \gamma_{00} + \gamma_{01} W_{1j} + \gamma_{02} W_{2j} + \gamma_{03} W_{1j} W_{2j} + u_{0j}$$
$$\beta_{1j} = \gamma_{10} + \gamma_{11} W_{1j} + \gamma_{12} W_{2j} + \gamma_{13} W_{1j} W_{2j} + u_{1j}$$

$$\begin{bmatrix} u_{0j} \\ u_{1j} \end{bmatrix} \sim N\left(\begin{bmatrix} 0 \\ 0 \end{bmatrix}, \begin{bmatrix} \tau_{00} & \tau_{01} \\ \tau_{10} & \tau_{11} \end{bmatrix} \right), \tag{2}$$

where W_{1j} is 1 for Japanese companies and -1 for North American companies. Similarly, W_{2j} is 1 for democratic leadership and -1 for laissez-faire leadership. The parameter values which are set to support the hypotheses are presented in Table 5. 1.

TABLE 5.1

Parameter Values to Generate the Data for the Simulation

Fixed effects				Variance components	
Intercept		Slope			
γ_{00}	20.00	γ_{10}	0.30	σ^2	2.00
γ_{01}	2.00	γ_{11}	0.10	τ_{00}	2.50
γ_{02}	1.00	γ_{12}	0.30	$\tau_{01} (= \tau_{10})$	0.00
γ_{03}	-1.00	γ_{13}	0.00	τ_{11}	0.10

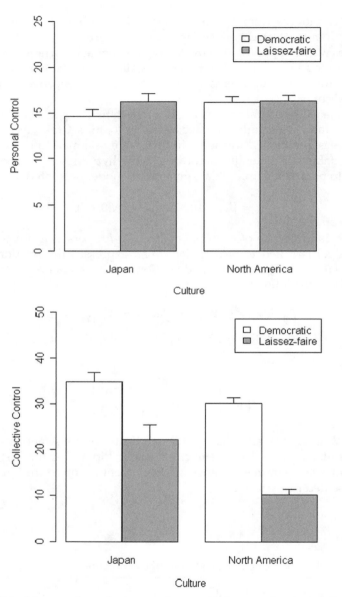

FIGURE 5.1 Means and standard errors for perceived personal control and collective control.

Data Analysis

Mean senses of personal control and collective control are shown in Figure 5.1. These figures indicate that the intended cultural differences were reproduced by descriptive statistics, although the multilevel structure (i.e.,

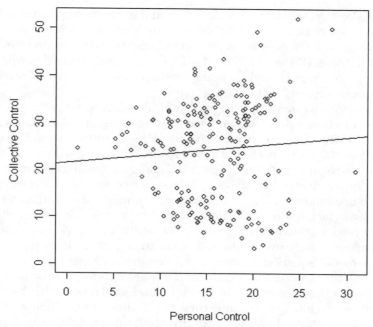

FIGURE 5.2 Scatter plot and regression line for the total sample.

the between-group effect) was not considered here. It can also be seen that the sense of collective control is higher under democratic leadership relative to laissez-faire leadership, reproducing the hypothesized relationship successfully (Hypothesis 2). However, we do not know yet at this stage if the difference in the mean sense of collective control is statistically significant. Besides, this analysis does not provide any information about the relationship between personal and collective control.

Figure 5.2 provides an overview of the relationship between the two kinds of sense of control for the total sample, without considering between-group effects. The single regression line in this figure indicates that there appears to be no significant relationship between the two senses of control if the between-group effects are ignored. In fact, the zero-order correlation coefficient for the total sample was almost null ($r = .08$, *ns*). However, this result should not be taken as indicating that there was no relationship between personal and collective control at the individual level, because the hierarchical structure of the data is completely ignored in this analysis. The lack of a significant correlation may seem unexpected, as we generated the data assuming that two senses of control are positively related. One may attempt to solve this problem by aggregating the data by branches and fit a regression model at branch level. Although the relationship between the two senses of control can be examined appropriately in this manner, the statistical power would be lowered drastically because of reduction of sample size. Furthermore, it should be noted that aggregate analyses allow us only to examine the relationship at group level, and that it is inappropriate to draw inferences about the individual-level relationship from this kind of analyses (Robinson, 1950). Also, it is important to note that what we want to know here is the individual-level relationship between personal and collective control and its cultural difference.

How should we analyze these hierarchically structured data appropriately? Let us take a closer look at the data generating equations, Equations (1) and (2). These equations have two important features. First, Equation (1) models the individual-level relationship between personal and collective control at each branch. Second, Equation (2) models not only systematic differences of intercepts and slopes for Japan and North America but also unexplained random fluctuations within these countries among branches. In fact, ordinary multiple regression analysis cannot model this kind of random fluctuations, as it cannot deal with nonindependence in observations. Furthermore, the total data structure can be expressed in a single-model equation by integrating Equations (1) and (2). These facts imply that this random-coefficient model enables us to express mean differences of collective control and the individual-level relationship between two senses of control at the same time, while allowing nonindependence among observations. In other words, by using this model we can express the multilevel structure of the data appropriately and effectively. Such models are known as multilevel models or hierarchical linear models (HLM; Raudenbush & Bryk, 2002).

Fortunately, we can fit this model to our data easily using several statistical packages. Table 5. 2 shows the result of fitting HLM to the data using the lme function in the nlme package of R. The fitted regression lines are shown in Figure 5.3, which indicates that the analysis by HLM successfully reveals the effects as produced in the data generation phase. All the coefficients were found to be significant in the predicted direction, except the three-way interaction effect (i.e., Personal control * Culture * Leadership) that was assumed to be null in the population when the data were generated.

TABLE 5.2

Summary of Multilevel Analysis

Variable	b	$SE\,b$	p
Personal control	0.262	0.069	.001
Culture	2.073	0.498	.001
Leadership	1.495	0.498	.008
Personal control * Culture	0.142	0.069	.042
Personal control * Leadership	0.434	0.069	.001
Culture * Leadership	−1.454	0.498	.010
Personal control * Culture * Leadership	0.001	0.069	.986

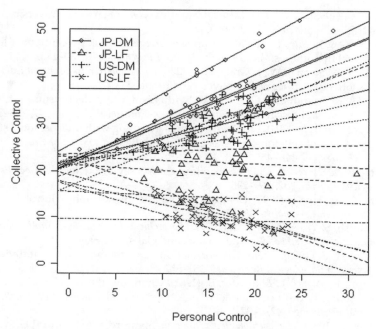

FIGURE 5.3 Scatter plot and regression lines fitted by HLM.

In conclusion, HLM enables us to examine not only the means of dependent variables but also relationships between dependent and independent variables in hierarchically structured data by fitting a single-model equation. The present hypothetical study illustrated that multilevel analysis is a useful tool for social-psychological studies across cultures.

Author Note

We thank the editors of this volume for their helpful comments on an earlier version of the manuscript.

REFERENCES

Bandura, A. (1997). *Self-efficacy: The exercise of control.* New York: Freeman.

Chua, H. F., Yamaguchi, S., & Yates, J. F. (2001, November). *Explaining the risk diffusion effect: The illusion of safety in numbers.* Paper presented at the Annual Meeting of the Society for Judgment and Decision Making, Orlando, FL.

Earley, C., P. (1993). East meets West meets Mideast: Further explorations of collectivistic and individualistic work groups. *Academy of Management Journal, 36,* 319–348.

Gilligan, C. (1993). *In a different voice.* Cambridge, MA: Harvard University Press. (Original work published 1982)

Ho, A. S. Y., & Leung, K. (1998). Group size effects on risk perception: A test of several hypotheses. *Asian Journal of Social Psychology, 1,* 133–145.

Hogg, R. V., Mckean, J. W., & Craig, A. T. (2005). *Introduction to mathematical statistics* (6th ed.). Upper Saddle River, NJ: Prentice Hall.

Hui, C. H., & Triandis, H. C. (1986). Individualism and collectivism: A study of cross-cultural researchers. *Journal of Cross-Cultural Psychology, 17,* 225–248.

Lam, A., & Zane, N. (2004). Ethnic differences in coping with interpersonal stressors: A test of self-construals as cultural mediators. *Journal of Cross-Cultural Psychology, 35,* 446–459.

Morling, B., & Evered, S. (2006). Secondary control reviewed and defined. *Psychological Bulletin, 132,* 269–296.

Morling, B., & Fiske, S. (1999). Defining and measuring harmony control. *Journal of Research in Personality, 33,* 379–414.

Raudenbush, S. W., & Bryk, A. S. (2002). *Hierarchical linear models: Applications and data analysis methods* (2nd ed.). Thousand Oaks, CA: Sage.

Robinson, W. S. (1950). Ecological correlations and the behavior of individuals. *American Sociological Review, 15,* 351–357.

Rothbaum, F., Weisz, J., & Snyder, S. (1982). Changing the world and changing the self: A two-process model of perceived control. *Journal of Personality and Social Psychology, 42,* 5–37.

Schachter, S. (1959). *The psychology of affiliation.* Stanford, CA: Stanford University Press.

Skinner, E. A. (1996). A guide to constructs of control. *Journal of Personality and Social Psychology, 71,* 549–570.

Spector, P., Sanchez, J., Siu, O., Salgado, J., & Ma, J. (2004). Eastern versus Western control beliefs at work: An investigation of secondary control, socioinstrumental control, and work locus of control in China and the U.S. *Applied Psychology: An International Review, 53,* 38–60.

Weisz, J. R., Rothbaum, F., M., & Blackburn, T. C. (1984). Standing out and standing in: The psychology of control in America and Japan. *American Psychologist, 39,* 955–969.

White, R., & Lippitt, R. (1968). Leader behavior and member reaction in three "social climates." In D. Cartwright & A. Zander (Eds.), *Group dynamics* (3rd ed., pp. 318–335). New York: Harper & Row.

Yamaguchi, S. (1998). Biased risk perception among Japanese: Illusion of interdependence among risk companions. *Asian Journal of Social Psychology, 1,* 117–131.

Yamaguchi, S. (2001). Culture and control orientations. In D. Matsumoto (Ed.), *The handbook of culture and psychology* (pp. 223–243). New York: Oxford University Press.

Yamaguchi, S., Gelfand, M., Ohashi, M. M., & Zemba, Y. (2005). The cultural psychology of control: Illusions of personal versus collective control in the United States and Japan. *Journal of Cross-Cultural Psychology, 36,* 750–761.

6

Individualism and Collectivism: Societal-Level Processes with Implications for Individual-Level and Society-Level Outcomes

Daphna Oyserman and Ayse K. Uskul

Culture can be broadly and briefly operationalized as a set of structures and institutions, values, traditions, and ways of engaging with the social and nonsocial world that are transmitted across generations in a certain time and place (e.g., Shweder & LeVine, 1984). Culture is thus temporally and geographically situated and multilevel. It is situated because it takes place in a certain time and place and is dynamically transmitted over time and across place, changing as time and place change. It is multilevel because its influence can be observed in societal-level constructs such as structures and institutions, group-level constructs such as traditions and ways of engaging in the world, and individual-level constructs such as internalized norms, personally felt values, cognitive procedures, and behaviors.

Cultural psychology focuses both on the ways that societal processes influence societal-level outcomes and on the ways that these processes influence individuals, either directly or through their effect on group-level processes.[1] Culture's situated nature has implications for each level of conceptualization. One's place within a society and the social networks within which one is embedded should influence which structural and institutional aspects of "culture" one has access to. In this way, context and changes in context that occur, for example due to immigration, may (Kitayama, Ishii, Imada, Takemura, & Ramaswamy, 2006) or may not (Atran, Medin, & Ross, 2005) carry with it cultural change depending in part on features of more proximal social networks before and after contextual change. Thus, Kitayama and his colleagues provide evidence that living in or moving to Japan's frontier areas is associated with higher individualism, in part due to the change in context. Atran and his colleagues use as their example differences in understanding of forest ecology among groups who live in somewhat different areas but importantly have differing contact with more expert groups, to show that cultural knowledge does not spread via physical moves but via social contact.

Following from this operationalization of culture, a large number of differences at the societal level, group-process level, or individual-expression level are likely due to culture. Unfortunately, such broad conceptualization can rob the term *culture* of conceptual specificity, making it all but impossible to make specific predictions about how and when culture matters. Perhaps for this reason, psychologists have sought basic organizing principles of cultures that could move the field beyond both broad generalizations and particularized description and set the stage for predictive model building. A number of potentially useful basic organizing constructs (e.g., "tight" vs. "loose" cultures, Triandis, 1995; "masculine" vs. "feminine" cultures, Hofstede, 1980; survival vs. self-expression, Inglehart 1997; honor-modesty vs. shame, Gregg, 2005; see also Cohen 2001), and frameworks (e.g., the ecocultural model, Berry, 1976, 1994; Georgas, 1988, 1993) have been proposed. To date the two constructs that most captured popular appeal are individualism and collectivism (e.g., Hofstede, 1980, 2001; Kagitcibasi, 1997; Kashima, 2001; Oyserman, Coon, & Kemmelmeier, 2002; Triandis, 1995).

Though use of individualism and collectivism as organizing constructs does provide the field with an organizing theme and focus for prediction and investigation, these organizing constructs alone do not provide a process model so that research relies on implicit process models. In this chapter we attempt to integrate these implicit models to describe both a multilevel and a societal-level process model of culture (the multilevel model focuses on individual-level consequences of culture, the societal-level model is self-explanatory). Both models begin with the same basic societal-level antecedents, but one model is multilevel in that proximal antecedents and consequences are at the individual level and the other model remains societal-level in that all antecedents and consequences are at the societal level. Most psychological research focuses on individual-level consequences, implicitly if not explicitly evoking a multilevel model.

In the following sections, we first operationalize individualism and collectivism as used both in multilevel and societal-level models, providing process models that pinpoint where research to date has concentrated and where gaps still exist. We operationalize a cultural psychological approach to the differing levels of analysis relevant to cultural psychology and ask what can and cannot be generalized from research using different levels of analysis given concerns about the ecological fallacy (see chapters 1 and 2 for a detailed discussion of levels issues in cultural research) and Simpson's paradox.

INDIVIDUALISM AND COLLECTIVISM: OPERATIONALIZATION, ASSESSMENT, AND USAGE

Modern usage of the term *individualism* is closely connected with Hofstede (1980). In the 1970s Hofstede obtained employees' ratings of workplace relevant values, averaged those into national scores, and factor analyzed them (Hofstede, 1980; see also Leung & Bond, 1989). Hofstede described one of the emerging factors as individualism (high scores on this factor were anchored at individualism, low scores at collectivism). He defined individualism as a focus on rights above duties, a concern for oneself and immediate family, an emphasis on personal autonomy and self-fulfillment, and basing identity on one's personal accomplishments. By obtaining averages across individuals, Hofstede obtained an average individual score that he used as a stand-in for a country-level score that could be correlated with other country-level variables such as Gross National Product (GNP).

A number of authors have followed Hofstede's reasoning in thinking about country-level value syndromes, arguing that individualism is associated with modernity, democracy, wealth, urbanism, higher education, and educational systems focused on positive self-regard and autonomy. Thus, for example, Inglehart (Inglehart & Baker, 2000) collected data separately as part of the World Values Survey, correlating national average value scores with national scores from other sources rating country-level attainment of education, gender equality, and other societal features. Authors using this perspective provide evidence supporting the case that collectivism as a worldview is associated with poverty, less education, hierarchical or cast-based societies, and educational systems focused on self-improvement, obedience to authority, and acceptance of social structure (e.g., Kagitcibasi, 1997).

While Hofstede was not interested in individual-level implications of cultural syndromes and attempted to obtain a country-level variable by averaging within-country individual responses, a number of researchers have developed individual-level value scales with a goal of individual-level assessment. Triandis and his colleagues have coined the terms *allocentrism* and *idiocentrism* to refer to these individual-level assessments (Triandis, 2007; Triandis, Leung, Villareal, & Clack, 1985). The consequences of individualism and collectivism at an individual level have also been described for self-concept, cognitive style, and relationality (Kitayama et al., 2006; Oyserman, Coon, & Kemmelmeier, 2002; Oyserman, Kemmelmeier, & Coon, 2002).

In their review, Oyserman, Coon, and Kemmelmeier (2002) suggest the following individual-level implications of individualism and collectivism. At the individual-level, individualism as a cultural syndrome implies that the self is permanent, separate from context, traitlike, and a causal nexus; that reasoning is a tool to separate out main points from irrelevant background or context; and that relationships and group memberships are impermanent and nonintensive, strangers may become friends or allies, and current in-group memberships may be given up for others. Conversely, at the individual-level, collectivism as a cultural syndrome implies that the self is malleable, context-dependent, and socially sensitive; that reasoning is a tool to link and make sense of the whole rather than disparate elements; and that relationships and group memberships are ascribed and fixed, "facts of life" to which people must accommodate. Strangers are not to be trusted; in- and out-group memberships are fixed.

PREDICTING INDIVIDUAL-LEVEL OUTCOME VARIABLES

Process models can help to clarify our thinking about relationships between concepts. We first address the prediction of individual-level outcome variables and thereafter discuss the strengths of these approaches.

A Process Model

An integrated process model of the individual-level effects of culture is displayed as Figure 6.1 (modified from Oyserman, Kemmelmeier, & Coon, 2002). The process model outlines the main presumed or tested links between societal and group-level antecedent factors and individual-level consequences. This simplified multilevel cultural process model draws attention to the likely influences of societal-level culture: structures, processes, systems, and artifacts; and internalized features of culture, such as values and norms, for how situations are understood—subjective construals, and the consequences of these culture-laden construals for individual action at any point in time. Internalized features of culture are subjective, heterogeneous, and nonuniform so that both within and between group differences are to be expected.

As presented from left to right in Figure 6.1, some general processes are assumed to apply. First, it is assumed that all human societies must have been influenced by evolutionary forces (e.g., natural and sexual selection and adaptation) and the ecological (e.g., climate, geographical latitude) and natural (e.g., water supply and soil conditions) features of the environments in which they developed (box 1). These basic features influence both distal culture (history, language, and religion) (box 2) and the circumstances and extent that social connection and personal autonomy

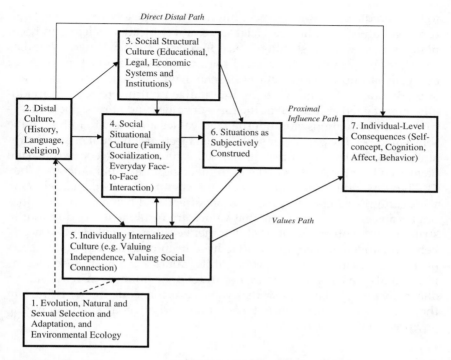

FIGURE 6.1 Culture as a multilevel process influencing individual-level outcomes. (Adapted with permission from Oyserman, Kemmelmeier, & Coon (2002). Cultural psychology, a new look: Reply to Bond (2002), Fiske (2002), Kitayama (2002), and Miller (2002). *Psychological Bulletin, 128*, 110–117. Copyright 2002 American Psychological Association)

are valued (box 5). That is, we assume that all distal cultures and value systems have some elements of individualism and some elements of collectivism. Societies established in more environmentally and ecologically resource-rich contexts would be likely to have less need for interdependent action for survival and thus likely to have fewer structures and contexts that require or cue interdependence. Conversely societies established and developed in harsher environmental and ecological niches would be likely to have more need for interdependent action for survival and so would be likely to have more structures and contexts that require or cue interdependence (for more detailed models see Cohen, 2001; Oyserman, Kemmelmeier & Coon, 2002). Between-group differences emerge due to differences in the extent that independence and interdependence patterns are embedded in distal culture and differences in the frequency of everyday contexts in which these patterns are likely to be evoked.

Though influenced by the environmental and ecological niche in which it was established, distal culture is assumed to be dynamically stable rather than static. That is, we expect distal culture to be permanent enough to have predictable consequences but not be completely fixed. Distal culture is assumed to influence social structural (educational, legal, and economic systems and institutions, box 3), social situational (what families socialize children to be like, social roles within the family, the nature of everyday face-to-face interactions in school, with age-mates, on the street, at work, box 4), and individually internalized culture (box 5). Individually internalized culture takes the form of values and norms. Social structures, social situations, and internalized values are likely to influence the sense made of any particular situation (subjective construal of social situations, box 6). Distal culture, internalized values, and subjective construal have each been posited as paths to influencing individual outcomes (box 7). These include content of self-concept, cognition, affect, and behavior. We distinguish self-concept, cognition, affect, and behavior from values not because we wish to argue that values are fundamentally different in structure from other cognitions but rather because content of self-concept, behavior, affect, and cognitive style have been described as *consequences* of individualism and collectivism while values have been described as individually internalized *markers* of individualism and collectivism. An alternative would be to posit that values are consequences of culture in the same way that self-concept, cognition, and affect are without giving any preferred status to values.

Common Approaches to Operationalization

To date, three general approaches have dominated operationalization and measurement of individualism and collectivism in multilevel models. Oyserman, Coon, and Kemmelmeier (2002) have labeled these approaches "applying Hofstede," using rating scales, and priming studies as outlined below. Each of these is presented in the process model as an explanatory path used to predict individual-level consequences of posited or assessed cultural differences. Each approach is outlined and incorporated into our multilevel model as detailed below.

Applying Hofstede

The most common approach is "applying Hofstede"; that is, citing Hofstede as the rationale for one's choices of country comparisons. Following the usage of Oyserman, Coon, and Kemmelmeier (2002), we use the term *applying* rather than *following* because this approach *does not follow* from Hofstede in the sense that he did not make the claims others make in his name. We have labeled this work as assuming a "Direct Distal Path" between distal country and individual outcomes in Figure 6.1 because that is what the researchers are doing in their empirical work.

Researchers who apply Hofstede assert that Hofstede's (1980) ranking can be used to justify the choice of countries for cross-national comparison. These researchers imply that because Hofstede (1980) defined and calculated national aggregated individualism scores, his ratings can be treated as indicators of distal culture. Reading Hofstede's initial and later work (Hofstede, 1980, 2001) makes clear that he did not intend that his ratings be assumed to be fixed, and a number of papers have criticized this method (e.g., Bond & Tedeschi, 2001; Oyserman, Coon & Kemmelmeier, 2002; Singelis, 2000).

One concern is a level of analysis issue. Researchers attempting to apply Hofstede seem to assume that individuals from countries that ranked high on individualism are highly individualistic; individuals from countries ranked low in individualism are highly collectivistic (e.g., Hui, 1988). Even if researchers refrain from making this error, a number of broader concerns have also been raised in that Hofstede's (1980) aggregated individualism scores are not really descriptive of distal culture (though studies that apply Hofstede typically assume a direct distal influence path). Aggregated individualism scores represent a nation-level aggregation of individual-level values of a certain sample of individuals at a certain place and certain point in time. Expressed values, though interesting, should not be the sole basis for cultural difference research because expressed values research requires making a number of assumptions about what culture is and how it is transmitted, as outlined below. First, using expressed values requires assuming that members of a culture can *express* their values and that standard rating scale instruments can *capture* cross-national differences in these values. Second, it requires assuming that *commonality in values* is an essential or core element of culture. Third, it requires assuming *generalizability of values across contexts*—that the values assessed in the workplace, where Hofstede collected data, generalize to values in other psychologically meaningful situations so that individuals not sampled from work but from the same country would have similar value differences. Fourth, it requires assuming that there is no meaningful *values change over time*. Thus it requires assuming that there is no meaningful developmental, temporal, or contextual change—values expressed by adults at a point in time and in one psychologically meaningful context (the workplace in the late 1970s) provide information relevant to other psychologically meaningful situations, other points in time, and other developmental or life phases.

In sum, researchers are using Hofstede's scores to study issues other than the workplace satisfaction issues on which the scores were based. This requires assuming that individualism as assessed from working adults in the domain of work is constant, not influenced by large-scale economic and political changes over time, applies to other members of the culture and in other life domains. Much of this research does not use Hofstede's scores themselves and simply alludes to Hofstede's (1980) measures as rationale for making cross-cultural comparison. This does not solve any of the problems listed previously and because any pair or small set of countries is likely to differ in many ways, documenting that responses at the individual level differ in ways one might expect given differences in individualism cannot be used to support an individualism–collectivism model of cultural difference. Other cultural syndrome models might also explain the particular differences examined or the differences may have nothing to do with cultural syndrome.

In spite of all of these well-known criticisms, a substantial body of research has focused on examination of the relationship between assumed country-level difference due to Hofstede's description of individualism (and collectivism) and individual-level outcomes. Work using this "apply Hofstede" approach has continued for more than 20 years after Hofstede's categorization and has provided a large number of studies making a link between country-level cultural constructs and individual-level effects. While problematic given the limitations of expressed values research, this work is both the most common form of cross-national research (for an extensive review, see Oyserman, Coon, and Kemmelmeier, 2002) and has provided some important cross-cultural insights. For example, participants living in countries with higher individualism scores are on average less likely to be acquiescent survey responders who simply agree with the opinions of the researcher as implied by question content (Johnson, Kulesa, Cho, & Shavitt, 2005; Smith, 2004).

Direct Assessment

The second common approach is to measure "individualism" and "collectivism" as individual-difference measures—assessing what Triandis (1995) has termed *allocentrism* and *idiocentrism* and what Markus and Kitayama (1991) have termed *independence* and *interdependence*—and to correlate this assessment with individual-level outcomes of interest. This allows the researcher to specify that difference in the dependent variable is associated with a specified set of internalized and explicitly expressed values. We have labeled this method the "Values Path" in Figure 6.1. Researchers who adopt this approach typically ask respondents to rate how much they agree with or how important they find a list of behaviors, attitudes, and value statements. Although direct assessment avoids some of the assumptions made by those who apply Hofstede, it too has many limitations. This approach assumes cross-national equivalence in how questions are understood and rating scales used. It ignores potential cross-cultural differences in the extent to which question context (such as the labels on scales) and research context (such as how the study, researcher, and other potential participants are presented) influence responses. Perhaps most importantly, it assumes that cultural values are a form of declarative knowledge that one can report on.

Just as the "applying Hofstede" approach has limitations yet provides some insights, here too, research based on an expressed value approach has provided some impressive results and some meaningful simplifying structure while it is clear that what is meant by culture is more than the direct expression of values related to individualism and collectivism. Oyserman, Coon, and Kemmelmeier's (2002) comprehensive meta-analysis of individualism and collectivism data provides evidence that in aggregate, studies based on these approaches do generally show the expected cross-national differences, with two important exceptions. Japan and to some extent Korea generally do not show the expected low valuation of individualism combined with higher valuation of collectivism. Some have argued that this anomaly invalidates the values approach; others have argued that the college student participants from whom these data were obtained no longer accept traditional Japanese and Korean values and that these societies are changing. In either case, research procedures based on direct assessment of values are vulnerable to utilizing individual-based analyses to make generalizations at the societal level as well as to overgeneralizing from findings based on college campuses to a society over time. Studying individual differences in values is not necessarily isomorphic with studying culture. In this sense, the direct values assessment approach is only relevant when used to clarify effects implied from multilevel models and does not pertain to societal-level analyses.

Priming Cultural Frame

The third, increasingly common, approach is to prime "cultural frame," focusing on cuing either individualism or collectivism and assessing the impact of this priming on individual-level cognition, affect, and behavior. While focus to date has been on a set of primes meant to evoke independence-idiocentrism-individualism or to evoke interdependence-allocentrism-collectivism, there is no necessary reason that the priming approach could not be used more broadly to study other dimensions of culture (e.g., power, face, or honor-modesty). We have labeled this method the "Proximal Influence Path" in Figure 6.1 because this approach clarifies the proximal or immediate causal path of cultural influence by making use of findings in social cognition research which consistently shows that habitually or temporarily accessible knowledge influences behavior (e.g., Bargh, Bond, Lombardi, & Tota, 1986).

Using priming as a method has a number of strengths (for a review, see Oyserman & Lee, 2007). It allows for specification of posited "active ingredients" of culture and specification that observed differences are due to these active ingredients. Because of this tighter causality, priming research has the potential to provide more clarity about the active processes that influence outcomes and allows for reasoning about culture as an aspect of situated cognition. Using priming facilitates a situated cognition approach to culture that highlights culture as dynamic process (Oyserman & Lee, 2007). How we make sense of situations, the psychological meaning of situations, is due to the sense we make of them in the moment. This sense flows from naïve theories that are cued in the moment, these naïve theories may be universal or culturally specific, cultures may also differ in the likelihood that one or another naïve theory will be cued or turned on in a particular situation.

Unlike applying Hofstede, an experimental priming approach makes it possible to study culture as a dynamic process. For example, when primed with "we" participants sit closer to confederates (Holland, Roeder, van Baaren, Brandt, & Hannover, 2004), and thus demonstrate an immediate behavioral response to a psychologically meaningful cultural situation that could not be studied without a priming manipulation. Moreover, unlike either applying Hofstede or direct value assessment an experimental approach avoids the problems associated with direct assessment such as the need to assume that respondents use the scales the same way cross-culturally and that answers provided at one time and place generalize to other times and places. By focusing on particular active ingredients of individualism and collectivism, the experimental priming approach also allows for tighter causal arguments. Thus, findings using this method can be used as part of a multimethod approach to triangulate prior correlational findings.

However, just as the other approaches have limitations, so does the priming approach. Most obviously, ecological validity is sacrificed because the primes must necessarily be narrower than the theorized underlying constructs being studied. Thus, much of the initial priming work simply had the goal of replicating prior cross-cultural findings to demonstrate that the otherwise cross-societal or cross-group effect can be turned on or cued within a society or group (see Oyserman & Lee, 2007, for a review). More generally, efficacy of this approach depends on operationalization of culture in ways relevant to presumed active ingredients of individualism and collectivism. This approach is most relevant when used to clarify effects implied from multilevel models. Relevance to societal-level analyses has not yet been explored.

As to the current state of the priming literature, a number of other limitations should also be noted. With some exceptions (e.g., Chinese participants: Lee, Aaker & Gardner, 2000; Asian and Jewish-Americans: Oyserman, Sakamoto, & Lauffer, 1998; Korean participants: Oyserman, Sorensen, Cha, & Schwarz, 2006; Nepal: Agrawal & Maheswaran, 2005), this approach has been used with European-American and Western-European participants. Much of the research focuses on effects of priming in a single country, typically the United States (e.g., Kühnen & Oyserman, 2002) or Germany (e.g., Haberstroh, Oyserman, Schwarz, Kühnen, & Ji, 2002). While clearly not as yet comprehensive, an emerging strength of the approach comes from consistent evidence that priming collectivism in European-American and Western-European samples increases subsequent collective content in self-concept, salience of collective values, and sense of closeness to others. Using this parallel between cross-national and priming study results provides some support that priming-study findings in domains that have been less extensively studied in cross-national research, such as cognitive processing, are also likely to find parallels in naturally occurring cultural settings (for a review see Oyserman & Lee, 2007).

STRENGTHS OF APPROACHES AIMED AT PREDICTING INDIVIDUAL-LEVEL OUTCOMES

Taken together, the multilevel (individual-level consequences) approaches to studying culture all focus on the extent that culture can be said to pattern or define individual-level differences in self-concept, cognition, affect, and behavior. In this sense, work in this area focuses on the extent that meaningful between-cultural group individual differences can be found over and above meaningful within-cultural group individual differences. Social psychologists have long studied the effects of social contexts, whether immediate and proximal or more distal and abstract on self-concept, cognition, affect, and behavior. Cultural psychology reminds us that contexts and their meaning may be differently organized in different societies. The question asked is whether all societies provide the same psychologically meaningful situations with the same frequency, differ in the frequency that these situations are likely to be encountered, or differ in the psychological meaning of the situations themselves. These are multilevel questions that are answerable by triangulated use of multimethod approaches, though each of the currently used approaches has limitations when used alone.

In terms of cognition, for example, research in this area asks if something about cultural contexts systematically predicts average processing speed, online perception, focus of spontaneous recall, and the like. Thus, Kitayama and his colleagues show within-Japan heterogeneity in relative ease of processing context-independent vs. context-dependent information that is associated with coming from or moving to frontier areas (Kitayama et al., 2006). Similarly, Oyserman and her colleagues show that priming "I" relative to "we" speeds processing on a color Stroop task and that this effect occurs both in the United States as well as in Korea (Oyserman et al., 2006). Taken together, studies of these types begin to provide information about what constitutes psychologically meaningful contexts and about the likely patterning of responses to these contexts.

Multilevel models provide a structured process model within which to make inferences about the psychological meaning of societal-level and group-level differences. Straightforward reverse predictions cannot be provided by these models in that knowing about individual differences does not provide prediction to group-level or society-level factors (Georgas, van de Vijver, & Berry, 2004).

PREDICTING SOCIETAL-LEVEL OUTCOME VARIABLES

While psychologists have focused on multilevel models in which societal and contextual factors are posited to predict individual-level outcomes, some researchers have focused on societal-level outcomes. Often this research involves a distal culture or values approach in that researchers seek to document meaningful correlations between an aggregated individual score (typically Hofstede's country-level aggregate scores, but also including, for example, Inglehart's World Value Survey score or Schwarz's value scores) or country-level scores assigned by Triandis (using an expert-rating technique) and nation-level variables such as GNP or language structure (e.g., is it grammatically correct to drop personal pronouns?). Some research in this vein does not attempt to directly assess individually aggregated values but rather focuses entirely on country-level variables, arguing that if certain cultural syndromes do in fact exist, then certain country-level (or region-level) patterns should exist. Vandello and Cohen (1999) have examined societal-level antecedents (population density) and consequences (e.g., divorce rates) of collectivism. Cohen (2006) also explores how cultural factors (i.e., culture of honor) moderate the relationship between societal antecedents (e.g., unequal treatment of women) and societal-level consequences (e.g., GNP). In this section, we outline a general process model that incorporates current cultural research focused on societal-level outcomes (Figure 6.2).

A Process Model

As can be seen in Figure 6.2, evolution and ecological environment (box 1) are assumed to influence both distal culture (language, religion, ideologies, histories, box 2) and the kind of values a society is likely to promulgate (box 5). As in the multilevel model, distal culture is assumed to influence social structural (box 3), social situational (box 4), and societal value (box 5) aspects of culture. Social structures (e.g., legal systems), social situations (e.g., classrooms and schooling, markets and shopping), and societal values (e.g., honor, dignity, social cohesion, stranger trust) are posited to influence societal-level consequences (box 6) such as birth rates, marriage and divorce rates, suicide rates, GNP, gender equality, and income equity.

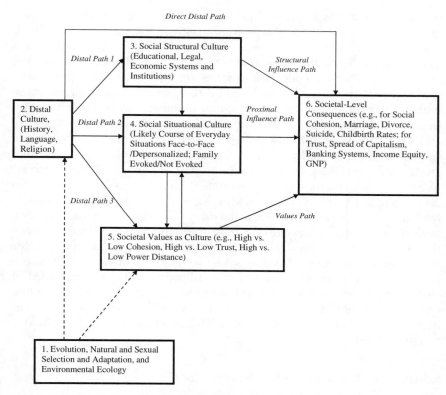

FIGURE 6.2 Culture as a societal-level process influencing societal outcomes.

Both multilevel and societal-level models assume influence of evolution and ecology on distal culture and posit an impact of distal culture on social structure, social situations and values. The process models diverge, however, in how and at what level values (box 5) and social situations (box 4) are operationalized. In the multilevel model, the values assessed are those internalized by individuals and the situations assessed are those which individuals encounter. In a societal-level model, the focus is on societal, not individual, processes and outcomes. Some researchers using a societal-level approach have obtained values via direct assessment (e.g., the World Values Survey approach); that is, aggregating across individuals to obtain national values scores. However, it is possible to infer societal-level values without resorting to direct assessment of individuals. For example, values can be obtained via coding societal artifacts such as ad campaigns, school books, children's stories, or movies.

With regard to social situations, level of analyses differences can also be discerned. Societal-level process models focus on the likely sociological meaning of everyday situations given their interest in society-level prediction, whereas multilevel process models focus on the likely psychological meaning of everyday situations given their interest in individual-level prediction. For example, to the extent that collectivism increases likelihood of distrusting out-groups and feeling obligated to in-groups, everyday situations in collective societies are more likely to be particularized rather than bureaucratized and all things being equal, situations in which interactions are with an in-group member will be preferred over those involving strangers. Take the everyday situation of shopping, a societal-level analysis would ask whether the shopping is likely to occur at small, family-run stores or chain stores, face-to-face or online, and whether credit cards are likely or unlikely to be part of the transaction. One set of everyday situations sets up personalized face-to-face interactions that do not require trust in strangers whereas the other sets up depersonalized and anonymous interactions that do require stranger trust. Although with the passing of time, cultures may adapt to changing circumstances, they will do so in culturally appropriate ways. In China for example, the American tradition of catalogue sales has not caught on, and its modern equivalent, Internet sales, requires adjustment. Thus, credit card or cash is often provided only when the product is delivered in person and examined rather than trusting that a stranger will provide the product as depicted on the Internet (Bin & Chen, 2003; Martinson, 2002; Reichheld & Schefter, 2003).

Evidence for Paths within the Process Model

Generally, research focused on societal-level outcomes has focused on either the association between distal cultural factors and social structures or social situations, or the association between social structures and societal-level outcomes. To clarify the implicit models underlying this work, in Figure 6.2 we have labeled the former "distal" path models and the latter "structural influence" path models. This work is necessarily less likely to involve experimental manipulation, providing less emphasis on empirical examination of process.

Distal Paths

Some societal-level research examines differences in features that make up distal culture (labeled "direct distal" in Figure 6.2) with the assumption that the effect of distal culture should be felt as societal-level difference in the present. This research focuses on characteristics of language as a carrier of cultural meaning with implications for societal outcomes. Some research focuses on regional difference within language. For example, Southern-Italian insults are more relational than Northern-Italian insults, which the authors associate with collectivism in the South and individualism in the North (Semin & Rubini, 1990). Other research focuses on cross-language patterns. For example, Hofstede-scored low individualism is more common in societies using languages in which it is grammatically correct to drop pronouns (Kashima & Kashima, 1998, 2003). Preferred level of abstraction also differs systematically with country-level individualism (Semin, Görts, Nandram, & Semin-Goossens, 2002)

Other societal-level research considers the effect of distal cultural features as mediated by structures, situations, and values. As can be seen in Figure 6.2, we have labeled these mediational pathways "distal path 1," "distal path 2," and "distal path 3," respectively. The association between individualism-collectivism and social structural variables has attracted considerable attention. Particular attention has been paid to the possibility that individualism (assessed as a value score), is related to societal growth and economic outcomes. Thus, Hofstede reported a negative relationship between aggregated nation-level individualism scores and a country's population, population density and demographic growth (Hofstede, 1980, 2001). Across studies affluence is associated with individualism. Thus, GNP is positively correlated with Hofstede's individualism scores (e.g., Georgas et al., 2004; Hofstede, 1980; Van Hemert, van de Vijver, Poortinga, & Georgas, 2002), GNP is positively correlated with Schwartz's autonomy versus conservation dimension (akin to individualism-collectivism; Schwartz, 1994); economic productivity is positively correlated with expert ratings of individualism (Levine, Norenzayan, & Philbrick, 2001); and economic prosperity is positively correlated with self-expression values (Inglehart, 1997).[2]

In addition to the focus on social structure, some societal-level research focuses on the association between distal culture factors and social situations. These studies typically assert that the countries or societies they are comparing differed in Hofstede's analyses and seek to examine differences in social values as expressed in social situations, such as pace of life, content of advertisements and framing of news reports. For example, Levine and Norenzayan (1999) examined the correlation between individualism as rated by Harry Triandis and pace of life as operationalized by average pace in walking and average speed of postal delivery, finding that speed is positively associated with country-level individualism. With regard to advertisements, popular Korean magazine advertisements focus primarily on conformity whereas popular American magazine advertisements focus primarily on uniqueness themes (Kim & Markus, 1999); Korean advertisements are also more likely to emphasize family well-being, in-group goals, and interdependence than U.S. advertisements (Han & Shavitt, 1994). With regard to framing of news, sports articles and editorials published in Hong Kong newspapers use situational attribution to a greater extent and dispositional attributions to a lesser frequency than those published in American newspapers (Lee, Hallahan, & Herzog, 1996).

Structural Influence Paths

Assessing a cultural syndrome is problematic. As we indicated earlier, the aggregated values or attitudes approach is limited in that it assumes that culture is a series of statements that can be made about how one engages the world. Moreover, the relationship between social structure and societal consequence variables has been studied correlationally. The difficulty in empirically assessing cultural syndrome separate from its consequences can be seen by the fact that the variables we have represented as consequences of cultural syndromes have been used by Vandello and Cohen (1999) as indicators of cultural syndrome. Their collectivism index used an array of what we have termed societal-level consequences variables (percentage of people living alone, percentage of elderly people living alone, percentage of households with grandchildren in them, divorce to marriage ratio, percentage of people with no religious affiliation, average percentage voting libertarian over the past presidential elections, ratio of people carpooling to work to people driving alone, and percentage of self-employed workers) and found a positive correlation between these factors and social-structural variables—population density, percentage of individuals engaged in herding, ratio of laborers to farmers, production of cotton, tobacco, and rice, percentage of minorities in a state, percentage of slaves per state. They also found a negative correlation between these factors and suicide rates, percentage of adults classified as binge drinkers, per capita proportion of artists and authors, gender and racial equality, as well as negative correlations with affluence and proportion of farms that were independently operated. Taken together, these results strongly suggest a cultural syndrome is operating but the syndrome itself remains a latent, not well operationalized variable to the extent that average explicit value or attitude statements have to date been the only alternate operationalization method. Other methods—such as content coding from a culture's literature, story books, newspapers, or advertisements—might provide a better latent operationalization.

The Direction of Influence

Because societal-level variables can be subjected to correlational but not experimental studies, direction of effects is open to debate. A number of authors provide evidence that wealth should be considered an antecedent rather than a consequence of individualism. Thus, Hofstede (1991), relying on his analysis over time, suggests that it is wealth that leads to individualism. He indicates that prosperity makes it possible for people to have more freedom of choice, more individual resources and to behave more selfishly. Japan provides a good example: Economic prosperity is associated with erosion of collectivism and more emphasis in individualism; Kelly (1991) argues that current Japanese cohorts are higher in hedonism and materialism, lower in commitment to societal good, and more likely to stress individual needs over community than earlier cohorts.

Similarly, Inglehart (1997; Inglehart & Baker, 2000) in his societal-level and over-time data has shown that self-expression values increase over time as economic prosperity increases. Moreover, Inglehart's data also show that large intergenerational differences exist in wealthy societies with younger birth cohorts emphasizing self-expression values more than the member of older cohorts. Inglehart and Oyserman (2004) argue that citizens in societies experiencing economic prosperity (rather than scarcity) are less likely to focus primarily on maintaining their material existence, which emancipates people from the cultural restrictions on personal choice necessary under conditions of scarcity. They further argue that economic development facilitates a shift toward the free choice aspects of individualism and away from the traditional survival aspects of collectivism, producing increasing emphasis on individual freedom-focused values and weakening the focus on traditional hierarchies. These arguments are further supported by Kagitcibasi and Ataca (2005) who documented changes in the value of children in Turkey when compared with three decades ago. The most notable change was the sharp increase in the psychological value of the child and the corresponding decrease in its utilitarian/economic value, including old-age security value. They argued that economic growth and higher education levels contributed to changes in the values people attach to their children. These perspectives suggest that societal wealth may be considered an ecological factor much like weather and social conditions rather than as a consequence of culture.

Wealth alone does not determine country-level individualism. Religion, philosophy, and historical experience interface with wealth. For example, although self-expression or individualism values increase as economic prosperity increases, rate of increase is dependent in part on religious and philosophical worldviews and historical experiences (Inglehart, 1997; Inglehart & Baker, 2000). Historically Protestant, Orthodox, Islamic, and Confucian societies cluster in cultural zones with distinctive value systems that persist even as economic development produces a shift toward individualism (Inglehart & Baker, 2000).

LEVELS ISSUES IN CULTURAL RESEARCH

We outlined both a multilevel cultural process model focused on individual-level consequences of culture and a societal-level cultural process model focused on societal-level consequences of culture. In each model, research clusters in small portions of the full model, suggesting that much research still needs to be completed if these assumed cultural processes are to be tested. Moreover, the societal-level model in particular suffers from lack of clarity about causality. Thus, it seems equally reasonable to argue that small family size increases individualism as to argue that individualism reduces desire to have large families. It is likely that both are true at some level, leading to ambiguity with regard to hypothesis testing. Equally problematic is the lack of any articulation of how cultural studies at the individual and societal levels are to be integrated to move the field forward.

Clearly, theories can focus on individuals or on groups or societies and in order for research to produce plausible evidence of the impact of cultural syndromes, the level at which a theory is articulated should match the level at which constructs are operationalized and assessed and the level of statistical analysis (Klein, Dansereau, & Hall, 1994; Rousseau, 1985). This seemingly straightforward suggestion is complicated in research domains such as cultural psychology that explicitly cross levels. Problems arise when measurement and analyses at one level are used to make inferences at other levels.

For example, cultural researchers commonly collect and compare individual-level data from two countries that Hofstede (1980) argued differ in individualism. Using country as a factor, they report any significant difference found as being a consequence of individualism. Another common approach is to collect both values responses and responses to another individual-level variable and when the two are correlated, report any significant difference in the individual-level variable as being a consequence of individualism. These common techniques may suffer from level of analyses problems to the extent that individual-level results cannot be used to draw conclusions about groups. That the individuals differ does not necessarily mean that the societies differ in cultural syndrome (see chapter 1). A number of authors have made this point; Schwartz (1992, 1994) shows some differences in how values cluster and which are correlated to one another depending on whether individual responses are aggregated at national levels and then analyzed or analyzed at the individual level (see also, Bond et al., 2004; Diener & Diener, 1995; Hui, Triandis, & Yee, 1991; Oishi, Diener, Lucas, & Suh, 1999). One reason for differences in data patterns between individuals and societies can be due to nomological networks that lead to differences in meaning of a concept at different levels of aggregation.

ECOLOGICAL FALLACY AND CROSS-CULTURAL RESEARCH

Indeed, concomitant emphasis on the individual as source of information and society as unit of generalization in cultural psychology can lead to problems described as the ecological fallacy—use of insight from one level of analyses to incorrectly draw inferences at other levels of analyses (Pedhazur, 1982; Robinson, 1950). For example, a researcher interested in whether collectivism as a cultural syndrome increases or decreases particularized treatment rather than bureaucratized treatment of individuals by public services may gather information about informal protection networks within public systems, levels of institutional corruption or institutionalized bribery of public officials. Finding patterned particularized treatment associated with differences in societies may allow for assertions about the impact of collectivism as a cultural syndrome on institutional processes. It does not allow for predictions about individual-level variables like personal honesty. As another example, a researcher interested in whether individualism and collectivism as cultural syndromes influence the intensity and closeness of interpersonal relationships may gather information about size and density of personal support networks. Finding patterned differences in density of personal relationships associated with differences in societies may allow for assertions about the impact of collectivism as a cultural frame on personal support processes. It does not allow for predictions about societal-level variables like the existence of government-sponsored safety nets such as hospitals or institutional care for the elderly or indigent.

Although processes at the individual and societal levels *may* be the same, there is no guarantee that this would necessarily be the case (e.g., because third variables may be involved). What appears to be a relationship between, for example, collectivism and public institutional corruption may not appear at the individual level, and the reverse, what appears to be a relationship between collectivism and natural support networks may not appear at the societal level (e.g., Chan, 1998; Leung, 1989). A similar phenomenon has been described as Simpson's paradox (e.g., Fiedler, 2000; Schaller, 1992; Waldmann & Hagmayer, 1995); that is, distinct relationships may appear at different levels of analysis, which, when decomposed, may not be present or may be present in opposing directions—the variables may sometimes have positive relationships, at other times negative relationships or no relationship at the separate levels (e.g., Fiedler, Walther, Freytag, & Nickel, 2003).

Take, for example, an association between willingness to care for relatives at home and Hofstede-assessed low individualism. While appearing robust, the association may be due to a third factor; for example, personal or societal wealth. Though on average country-level individualism and country-level wealth may be correlated, wealth may mediate the association of country-level individualism and willingness to care for relatives at home. For example, wealth (both personal and societal) may influence the relationship between individualism and care for relatives by influencing whether alternatives to home care are feasible or exist. Thus, those living in low individualism countries may be more willing to care for relatives at home not because they feel closer to their relatives, more obligated to them, or define themselves more in terms of social obligation than in terms of personal satisfaction; rather, they may report more willingness to care for relatives at home because on average there are no viable alternatives. Similarly, those living in high individualism countries may be less willing to care for relatives at home not because they feel less close to their relatives but because the structure of the labor market is such that no one is home to supervise care.

Indeed, cultural researchers have weighed in on this issue. Bond (2002) argues that the common ecological fallacy committed in cross-cultural psychology involves assuming that nation-level individualism or collectivism can be used to explain observed individual-level differences. Similarly, Schwartz (1994) describes the ecological fallacy as a logical fallacy and problem of construct validity in that one assumes that because a group has certain characteristics the members of the group should also have the same characteristics. As cited in Schwartz (1994), an informative example is provided by Zito (1975) who points to the discrepancy between a hung jury as a group and as individual members. As a group, a hung jury is an indecisive jury, unable to decide whether the accused is guilty or not. However, inferring that the members of that jury are also indecisive would be wrong. On the contrary, the reason the jury is hung is because its members are very decisive, and having decided, they not willing to change their minds.

Extending this issue to cultural psychology, suggests, for example, that a society may be characterized as having many stay-at-home mothers and few working mothers so that as a group, its citizens seem to value traditional family roles and centralize motherhood. Individual mothers may have little choice but to stay home, to the extent that the society also lacks structured day care and has short school days and traditional workplaces. Thus, citizens themselves may not choose traditional family roles so much as live with them. This suggests that even in multilevel models that can make individual-level predictions, care must be taken not to infer individual choice when what is observed is societal or structural patterning of choice.

Generally though, if cultural research is to make predictions about individuals, it must involve the impact of societal-level factors on individual-level variables; these cross-level models are not problematic in principle (Klein et al, 1994; Schwartz, 1994). Indeed, cross-level models can better be handled by using new-generation analytic techniques such as hierarchical linear modeling which allow individuals to be nested in social contexts rather than ignoring the potential for individuals from the same contexts to be more similar in their responses than individuals from different contexts. Because societal-level factors influence societal outcomes and the individuals that make up those societies, this is not a problem. But problems arise when individual-level meaning is drawn from societal-level data or when individual-level data and analyses are used to draw society-level conclusions. Rather than assume that individual-level correlations are associated with parallel society-level correlations, it may be more useful to broaden experimentally based enquiry into the active ingredients of culture. This entails examining social contexts and social situations in which these active ingredients may be embedded or cued, and study them separately.

CONCLUSION

We argued that generative model building and hypothesis testing in the domain of cultural psychology has benefited from narrowing focus to more specifically operationalizable constructs such as individualism and collectivism. This does not mean that future research should not begin to expand beyond this conceptualization. By operationalizing culture as a multilevel and societal-level process likely to influence individual-level and society-level phenomena, our goal was to map out what the likely processes of cultural influence are at each level and provide some feel for the kinds of research that has focused on the various posited paths in each of these models. We explored the possibility that research in cultural psychology may be vulnerable to a level of analysis problem, as formulated by the ecological fallacy or as Simpson's paradox.

The linkages between culture as society-level antecedents and culture as individual-level consequences have been tested primarily by either assuming that Hofstede's initial ratings are stable and generalizable over time and context or by obtaining individualism and collectivism value endorsement ratings and correlating them with a dependent variable of interest (all individual-level data). Both of these approaches are built on the assumption that individual-level value ratings, either aggregated, or used at the individual level, reflect an important aspect of culture which has implications for societal-level and individual-level outcomes. Alternative approaches have been sought to broaden research by increasing experimental control over the active ingredients of individualism or collectivism brought to mind in the moment, as well as to broaden research by utilizing constructs that do not depend on values ratings.

Of course the benefit of experimental studies that seek to prime active ingredients of culture and then document that these active ingredients have the hypothesized effects is the power of experimental models to provide support for causal hypotheses. The question raised by these studies is whether the effects shown at the individual level can plausibly provide evidence in support of the hypothesized societal effects of individualism and collectivism. At first pass, there clearly seems to be a level of analysis concern for authors who would argue that the results demonstrate processes occurring at the societal level. Our reading of the current literature is that authors using a priming methodology have been careful to avoid making these kinds of claims, often limiting their discussion of priming effects to evoked content of conceptual knowledge and not attempting generalizations about consequences for cultures (see Oyserman & Lee, 2007 for a review). One way for future research to utilize these findings is to begin to sample everyday face-to-face situated social contexts systematically and to begin to study the extent that these situations prime or make salient constructs that parallel those made salient in priming research. To the extent that this can be documented, then priming studies will be better linked to societal-level antecedents.

In addition to priming studies, a number of ecological models focused more directly on context, specifically attempting to make connections between physical and geographical factors, cultural syndromes, and individual differences due to culture (Berry, 1994; Triandis, 1972; Whiting, 1963, 1976). These efforts and analyses of societal-level antecedents and consequences of culture (e.g., Inglehart, 1997; Vandello & Cohen, 1999) are important because they provide a broader framework for developing testable hypotheses both about stability and change in individualism and collectivism and other cultural constructs. However, just as it is not possible to generalize back from individual differences to make the case that social groups differ, showing group-level effects does not necessarily provide predictions for individuals within the groups.

Moreover, focusing only on the societal level has a number of often overlooked problems. Clearly, it dramatically limits statistical power. If analyses are conducted only at the country level, even large-scale cross-national studies sample relatively few countries—a sample of six countries becomes an effective n of six. Other noncountry level designs leave room to examine differences by region or within country. Indeed, future research using a regional approach might increase both power and specificity of prediction by including both regions within countries and regions across countries. Appropriate statistical analysis such as hierarchical linear modeling that allows for analyses of individuals nested within countries increases power but still requires relatively large numbers of countries (e.g., six or more) for analyses. Moreover, country-level comparisons are only sensible if they compare similarly representative samples.

Typically cross-national comparisons that describe individual-level effects involve convenience samples of college students (for a review see, Oyserman, Coon, & Kemmelmeier, 2002). Those focused on societal-level effects provide exceptions; Schwartz (1994) used school teachers and, in most countries, Inglehart (1997) used random samples of adults, and both Smith (2004) and Vandello and Cohen (1999) used representative samples (albeit as secondary analyses of samples collected for other purposes). Given the expense of carrying out large multinational studies, replication of results across samples or even incremental hypotheses-testing is extremely difficult. Therefore, societal-level analyses are likely to continue to focus on individual countries as case studies. Reading across case studies can provide working hypotheses for priming studies that can at least be replicated cross-nationally.

Sensitivity to the ecological fallacy reduces the risk of concluding that characteristics of individual members of a group can be predicted by average characteristics of the group—such as concluding that country-level policies and services for the elder can be used to predict individual-level respect for the elderly. Sensitivity to Simpson's paradox reduces risk of concluding that patterns that hold at one level of aggregation are likely to predict patterns at disaggregated levels. Thus, for example, it would be inappropriate to conclude that collectivists are generally more cooperative and interdependent than individualists based on samples of these behaviors with in-group or family members because collectivists may well not be more interdependent with non-in-group and non-family members. Indeed, there is evidence that they are not (e.g., Matsumoto, 1990; Rhee, Uleman, & Lee, 1996).

Simpson's paradox reminds us that it is not possible to predict higher level relationships (in this case between collectivism and cooperation in general) from one disaggregated component relationship (in this case between collectivism and cooperation in a family or in-group situation). Indeed, a number of researchers have called for sampling of situations in which cultural practices are engaged (e.g., D'Andrade, 2001; Farr, 1991; Geertz, 1973). By sampling situations, it will be possible to see if societies do or do not differ in the situations in which a practice is engaged. It will also be possible to then use the situation as a prime and assess the extent that individuals in different countries respond uniformly to situations once presented, whether or not they are naturally occurring within a society. An example of this is work by Kitayama, Markus, Matsumoto, and Norasakknukit (1997) who had students describe self-esteem enhancing and deflating situations and found both differences between Japan and the United States in the situations generated and similarities between Japan and the United States when Japanese were presented with American situations and vice versa.

While it is important to be aware of level of analysis issues, in some ways Simpson's paradox provides an important venue for considering the level of aggregation currently being assessed in cultural research. Rather than simply assuming that the sampled relationships found can be generalized to the general universe of possible relationships, it is important to investigate. Researchers can ask whether the nature of the data collection process led to different foci for different cultural groups (e.g., participants in collective societies responding to questions in terms of how they would behave with in-group members vs. participants in individualistic cultures responding to questions in terms of how they would behave with strangers). At the societal level, culture-related variables cannot be subjected to experimentation. It is neither possible to manipulate a society's native language nor to randomly assign children to educational systems. Therefore, at the societal level, evidence must be mostly correlational and therefore open to alternate explanations or to influences by additional variables that have not yet been considered. One possible way forward is to use those natural experiments that occur—such as regime changes and economic shifts. Another possibility is to set up ecologically valid experiments; for example, Marian and Kaushanskaya's (2004) study of individual vs. collective content in memories of participants randomly assigned to recall in Russian or English. While important, neither of these solutions provides the kind of flexibility to study posited processes as do experimental manipulation, thus it seems likely that cultural psychology will continue to move between and across process models of culture that are multilevel and those that are societal-level only.

Notes

1. Of course thinking of the process of influence as unidirectional is a simplification. Just as cultures shape individual action and constitute individual psychologies, over time, individual action and psychology is likely to shape culture. In this sense, our focus is on a simplified process model since a full discussion of culture requires both a multilevel model and additional examination of the more nuanced and complex bidirectional ways in which individuals influence societies.

2. It seems reasonable to assume that the relationship between individualism and prosperity is likely to be bidirectional. On the one hand, high individualism may encourage economic activity and low individualism may encourage large families. On the other hand, it is also likely that as affluence rises, one is more able to stand separately from in-group members and as births per family increase so does the necessity of sharing both physical and social space.

REFERENCES

Agrawal, N., & Maheswaran, D. (2005). The effects of self-construal and commitment on persuasion. *Journal of Consumer Research, 31,* 841–849.

Atran, S., Medin, D. L., & Ross, N. (2005). The cultural mind: Environmental decision making and cultural modeling within and across populations. *Psychological Review, 112,* 744–776.

Bargh, J. A., Bond, R. N., Lombardi, W. J., & Tota, M. E. (1986). The additive nature of chronic and temporary sources of construct accessibility. *Journal of Personality and Social Psychology, 50,* 869–878.

Berry, J. W. (1976). *Human ecology and cognitive style: Comparative studies in cultural and psychological adaptation.* New York: Sage/Halsted/Wiley.

Berry, J. W. (1994). Ecology of individualism and collectivism. In U. Kim, H. C.Triandis, C. Kagitcibasi, S. C. Choi, & G. Yoon (Eds.), *Individualism and collectivism* (pp. 77–84). Newbury Park, CA: Sage.

Bin, Q., & Chen, S. (2003). Cultural differences in E-commerce; A comparison between the U.S. and China. *Journal of Global Information Management, 11,* 48–55.

Bond, M. H. (2002). Reclaiming the individual from Hofstede's ecological analysis—A 20-year odyssey: Comment on Oyserman et al. (2002). *Psychological Bulletin, 128,* 73–77.

Bond, M. H., Leung, K., Au, A., Tong, K., Reimel de Carrasquel, S., Murakami, F., et al. (2004). Culture-level dimensions of social axioms and their correlates across 41 cultures. *Journal of Cross-Cultural Psychology, 35,* 548–570.

Bond, M. H., & Tedeschi, J. T. (2001). Polishing the jade: A modest proposal for improving the study of social psychology across cultures. In D. Matsumoto (Ed.), *The handbook of culture and psychology* (pp. 309–324). New York: Oxford University Press.

Chan, D. (1998). Functional relations among constructs in the same content domain at different levels of analysis: A typology of composition models. *Journal of Applied Psychology, 83,* 234–246.

Cohen, D. (2001). Cultural variation: Considerations and implications. *Psychological Bulletin, 127,* 451–471.

Cohen, D. (March, 2006). Invited talk. *Culture and Cognition Symposium Series.* University of Michigan

D'Andrade, R. (2001). A cognitivist's view of the units debate in cultural anthropology. *Cross-Cultural Research, 35,* 242–257.

Diener, E., & Diener, M (1995). Cross-cultural correlates of life satisfaction and self-esteem. *Journal of Personality and Social Psychology, 68,* 653–663.

Farr, R. M. (1991). Individualism as a collective representation. In A. Aebischer, J. P. Deconchy, & M. Lipiansky (Eds.), *Ideologies et representations sociales* (pp. 129–143). Switzerland: Delval.

Fiedler, K. (2000). Beware of samples! A cognitive-ecological sampling approach to judgment biases. *Psychological Review, 107*(4), 659–676.

Fiedler, K., Walther, E., Freytag, P., & Nickel, S. (2003). Inductive reasoning and judgment interference: Experiments on the Simpson paradox. *Personality and Social Psychology Bulletin, 29,* 14–18.

Geertz, C. (1973). *The interpretation of culture: Selected essays.* New York: Basic Books.

Georgas, J. (1988). An ecological and social cross-cultural model: The case of Greece. In J. W. Berry, S. H. Irvine, & E. B. Hunt (Eds.), *Indigenous cognition: Functioning in cultural context* (pp. 105–123). Dordrecht, the Netherlands: Martinus Nijhoff.

Georgas, J. (1993). An ecological-social model for indigenous psychology: The example of Greece. In U. Kim & J. W. Berry (Eds.), *Indigenous psychologies: Theory, method & experience in cultural context* (pp. 56–78). Beverly Hills, CA: Sage.

Georgas, J., van de Vijver, F. J. R., & Berry, J. W. (2004). The ecocultural framework, ecosocial indices, and psychological variables in cross-cultural research. *Journal of Cross-Cultural Psychology, 35*, 74–96.

Gregg, G. S. (2005). *The Middle East: A cultural psychology.* Oxford: Oxford University Press.

Haberstroh, S., Oyserman, D., Schwarz, N., Kühnen, U., & Ji, L. (2002). Is the interdependent self more sensitive to question context than the independent self? Self-construal and the observation of conversational norms. *Journal of Experimental Social Psychology, 38*, 323–329.

Han, S., & Shavitt, S. (1994). Persuasion and culture: Advertising appeals in individualistic and collectivistic societies. *Journal of Experimental Social Psychology, 30*, 326–350.

Hofstede, G. (1980). *Culture's consequences: International differences in work-related values.* Beverly Hills, CA: Sage.

Hofstede, G. (1991). *Cultures and organizations: Software of the mind.* London: McGraw-Hill.

Hofstede, G. (2001). *Culture's consequences, comparing values, behaviors, institutions, and organizations across nations.* Thousand Oaks, CA: Sage.

Holland, R. W., Roeder, U. R., van Baaren, R. B., Brandt, A. C., & Hannover, B. (2004). Don't stand so close to me—The effects of self-construal on interpersonal closeness. *Psychological Science, 15*, 237–242.

Hui, C. H. (1988). Measurement of individualism-collectivism. *Journal of Research in Personality, 22*, 17–36.

Hui, C. H., Triandis, H. C., & Yee, C. (1991). Cultural-differences in reward allocation—Is collectivism the explanation? *British Journal of Social Psychology, 30*, 145–157.

Inglehart, R. (1997). *Modernization and post-modernization: Cultural, economic and political change in 43 societies.* Princeton, NJ: Princeton University Press.

Inglehart, R., & Baker, W. E. (2000). Modernization, cultural change, and the persistence of traditional values. *American Sociological Review, 65*, 19–51.

Inglehart, R., & Oyserman, D. (2004). Individualism, autonomy, self-expression and human development. In H. Vinken, J. Soeters, & P. Ester (Eds.), *Comparing cultures, dimensions of culture in a comparative perspective* (pp. 74–96). Leiden, the Netherlands: Brill.

Johnson, T., Kulesa, P., Cho, Y., & Shavitt, S. (2005). The relation between culture and response styles: Evidence from 19 countries. *Journal of Cross-Cultural Psychology, 36*, 264–277.

Kagitcibasi, C. (1997). Individualism and collectivism. In J. Berry, M. Segall, & C. Kagitcibasi (Eds.), *Handbook of cross-cultural psychology* (2nd ed., Vol. 3, pp. 1–49). Needham Heights, MA: Allyn & Bacon.

Kagitcibasi, C., & Ataca, B. (2005). Value of children and family change: A three-decade portrait from Turkey. *Applied Psychology: An International Review, 54*, 317–337.

Kashima, Y. (2001). Culture and social cognition: Toward a social psychology of cultural dynamics. In D. Matsumoto (Ed.), *The handbook of culture and psychology* (pp. 325–360). New York: Oxford University Press.

Kashima, E., & Kashima, Y. (1998). Culture and language: The case of cultural dimensions and personal pronoun use. *Journal of Cross-Cultural Psychology, 29*, 461–486.

Kashima, Y., & Kashima, E. S. (2003). Individualism, GNP, climate, and pronoun drop, is individualism determined by affluence and climate, or does language use play a role? *Journal of Cross-Cultural Psychology, 34,* 125–134.

Kelly, W. (1991). Directions in anthropology of contemporary Japan. *Annual Review of Anthropology, 20,* 395–431.

Kim, H., & Markus, H. (1999). Deviance or uniqueness, harmony or conformity? A cultural analysis. *Journal of Personality and Social Psychology, 77,* 785–800.

Kitayama, S., Ishii, K., Imada, T., Takemura, K., & Ramaswamy, J. (2006). Voluntary settlement and the spirit of independence. *Journal of Personality and Social Psychology, 91,* 369–384.

Kitayama, S., Markus, H. R., Matsumoto, H., & Norasakkunit, V. (1997). Individual and collective processes in the construction of the self: Self-enhancement in the United States and self-depreciation in Japan. *Journal of Personality and Social Psychology, 72,* 1245–1267.

Klein, K. J., Dansereau, F., & Hall, R. J. (1994). Levels issues in theory development, data collection, and analysis. *The Academy of Management Review, 19,* 195–229.

Kühnen, U., & Oyserman, D. (2002) Thinking about the self influences thinking in general: Cognitive consequences of salient self-concept. *Journal of Experimental Social Psychology, 38,* 492–499.

Lee, A., Aaker, J., & Gardner, W. (2000). The pleasures and pains of distinct self construals: The role of interdependence in regulatory focus, *Journal of Personality and Social Psychology, 78,* 1122–1134.

Lee, F., Hallahan, M, & Herzog, T. (1996). Explaining real-life events: How culture and domain shape attributions. *Personality and Social Psychology Bulletin, 22,* 732–741.

Leung, K. (1989). Cross-cultural differences: Individual-level vs. cultural level analysis. *International Journal of Psychology, 24,* 703–719.

Leung, K., & Bond, M. (1989). On the empirical identification of dimensions for cross-cultural comparisons. *Journal of Cross-Cultural Psychology, 20,* 133–151.

Levine, R., & Norenzayan, A. (1999). The pace of life in 31 countries. *Journal of Cross-Cultural Psychology, 30,* 178–205.

Levine, R., Norenzayan, A., & Philbrick, K. (2001). Cultural differences in the helping of strangers. *Journal of Cross Cultural Psychology, 32,* 543–560.

Marian, V., & Kaushanskaya, M. (2004). Self-construal and emotion in bicultural bilinguals. *Journal of Memory and Language, 51,* 190–201.

Markus, H., & Kitayama, S. (1991). Culture and the self: Implications for cognition, emotion, and motivation. *Psychological Review, 98,* 224–253.

Martinson, M. (2002). Electronic commerce in China: Emerging success stories. *Information and Management, 39,* 571–579.

Matsumoto, D. (1990). Cultural similarities and differences in display rules. *Motivation and Emotion, 14,* 195–214.

Oishi, S., Diener, E. F., Lucas, R. E., & Suh, E. M. (1999). Cross-cultural variations in predictors of life satisfaction: Perspectives from needs and values. *Personality and Social Psychology Bulletin, 25,* 980–990.

Oyserman, D., Coon, H., & Kemmelmeier, M. (2002). Rethinking individualism and collectivism: Evaluation of theoretical assumptions and meta-analyses. *Psychological Bulletin, 128,* 3–72.

Oyserman, D., Kemmelmeier, M., & Coon, H. M. (2002). Cultural psychology, a new look: Reply to Bond (2002), Fiske (2002), Kitayama (2002), and Miller (2002). *Psychological Bulletin, 128,* 110–117.

Oyserman, D., & Lee, S. (2007). Priming "culture": Culture as situated cognition. In S. Kitayama & D. Cohen (Eds.), *Handbook of cultural psychology* (pp. 255–279). New York: Guilford.

Oyserman, D., Sakamoto, I., Lauffer, A. (1998). Cultural accommodation: Hybridity and the framing of social obligation. *Journal of Personality and Social Psychology, 74,* 1606–1618.

Oyserman, D., Sorensen, N., Cha, O. & Schwarz, N. (2006). *Thinking about "Me" or "Us": Self-construal priming and fluency in east and west.* Unpublished manuscript.

Pedhazur, E. (1982). *Multiple regression in behavior research.* New York: Holt, Rinehart & Winston.

Reichheld, F., & Schefter, P. (2003). *E-loyality: Your secret weapon on the web.* Boston: Harvard Business   School Press.

Rhee, E., Uleman, J. S., & Lee, H. K. (1996). Variations in collectivism and individualism by in-group and culture: Confirmatory factor analysis. *Journal of Personality and Social Psychology, 71,* 1037–1054.

Robinson, W. S. (1950). Ecological correlations and the behavior of individuals. *American Sociological Review, 15,* 351–357.

Rousseau, D. (1985). Issues of levels in organizational research: Multi-level and cross-level perspectives. *Research in Organizational Behavior, 7,* 1–37.

Schaller, M. (1992). In-group favoritism and statistical reasoning in social inference: Implications for formation and maintenance of group stereotypes. *Journal of Personality and Social Psychology, 63,* 61–74.

Schwartz, S. (1994). Beyond individualism/collectivism: New cultural dimensions of values. In U. Kim, H. Triandis, C. Kagitcibasi, S. Choi, & G. Yoon (Eds.), *Individualism and collectivism: Theory, method and application* (pp. 85–119). Thousand Oaks, CA: Sage Publications.

Schwartz, S. (1994). The fallacy of the ecological fallacy: The potential misuse of a concept and the consequences. *American Journal of Public Health, 84,* 819–824.

Semin, G. R., Gorts, C., Nandam, S., & Semin-Goossens, A. (2002). Cultural perspectives on the linguistic representation of emotion and emotion events. *Cognition and Emotion, 16,* 11–28.

Semin G., & Rubini, M. (1990). Unfolding the category of person by verbal abuse. *European Journal of Social Psychology, 20,* 463–474.

Shweder, R., & Levine, R. (Eds.). (1984). *Culture theory; Essays on mind, self and emotion.* Cambridge: Cambridge University Press.

Singelis, P. B. (2000). Some thoughts on the future of cross-cultural social psychology. *Journal of Cross-Cultural Psychology, 31,* 76–91.

Smith, P. B. (2004). Acquiescent response bias as an aspect of cultural communication style. *Journal of Cross-Cultural Psychology, 35,* 50–61.

Triandis, H. (1972). *The analysis of subjective culture.* New York: Wiley.

Triandis, H. (1995). *Individualism and collectivism.* Boulder, CO: Westview Press.

Triandis, H. (in press). Individualism and collectivism. In S. Kitayama & D. Cohen (Eds.), *Handbook of cross-cultural psychology.* New York: Guilford.

Triandis, H. C., Leung, K., Villareal, M. J., & Clack, F. L. (1985). Allocentric vs idiocentric tendencies: Convergent and discriminant validation. *Journal of Research in Personality, 19*, 395–415.

Van Hemert, D. A., Van de Vijver, F. J. R., Poortinga, Y. H., & Georgas, J. (2002). Structural and functional equivalence of the Eysenck personality questionnaire within and between countries. *Personality and Individual Differences, 33*, 1229–1249.

Vandello, J. & Cohen, D. (1999). Patterns of individualism and collectivism across the U.S. *Journal of Personality and Social Psychology, 77*, 279–292.

Waldmann, M. R., & Hagmayer, Y. (1995). Causal paradox: When a cause simultaneously produces and prevents an effect. In J. Moore & F. Lehmann (Eds.), *Proceedings of the 17th Annual Conference of the Cognitive Science Society* (pp. 425–430). Mahwah, NJ: Lawrence Erlbaum.

Whiting, B. (Ed.). (1963). *Six cultures: Studies of child rearing.* New York: Wiley.

Whiting, B. (1976). The problem of the packaged variable. In K. Riegel & J. Meacham (Eds.), *The developing individual in a changing world* (Vol. 1, pp. 303–309). The Hague: Mouton.

Zito, G. (1975). *Methodology and meanings: Variety of sociological inquiry.* New York: Praeger.

7

Multilevel Approaches in Organizational Settings: Opportunities, Challenges, and Implications for Cross-Cultural Research

Ronald Fischer

This chapter will focus on multilevel issues in work organizations. The aim is (a) to provide a brief review of two influential areas of multilevel organizational research, namely climate and leadership and (b) to broaden the perspective of published multilevel research of organizations by including national culture as an additional level of study. Using guidelines for developing multilevel theories and research in monocultural settings (Chen, Mathieu, & Bliese, 2004; Hofmann & Jones, 2004; Klein & Kozlowski, 2000b; Kozlowski & Klein, 2000), guidelines for multilevel theories and studies incorporating national culture are presented. Cross-cultural examples are discussed where appropriate and available.

ORGANIZATIONAL CLIMATE

The concept of organizational climate has a long history that starts with research in the 1930s on the qualities of social entities as diverse as nations and groups (Peterson & Fischer, 2004). Individuals were asked to report on their perceptions of their group or leaders and these responses were thought to capture collective properties. From the 1960s, climate surveys were used to ask employees about what they experienced in their daily work life and how they perceived their surroundings within the organization. These responses were then combined to provide a description of the organization that could be used by managers to evaluate the needs for intervention or change. Climate surveys included topics like group dynamics, leadership, employee motivation, job characteristics, and management propensities to be supportive and fair.

There has been a heated debate about the meaning and function of these climate perceptions. One camp argued that these perceptions capture individuals' representations or cognitive schemata of their work environment. The focus is to understand how individuals make sense of their environment. Individuals are thought to respond to situational variables in a manner that is psychologically meaningful to them. Therefore, this perspective focuses on the individual and is concerned with the psychological description of organizational conditions (Naylor, Pritchard, & Ilgen, 1980). Climate is a reflection of the objective characteristics of the environment that individuals perceive and have to make sense of.

In contrast, a second camp focused on shared perceptions of climate that can be used to describe an entire organization or a work team. If individuals agree with each other about organizational policies, practices, or procedures that affect their well-being, these perceptions can be aggregated to the organizational level and can be used to describe the organization.

Proponents of this shared or collective climate approach have been faced with several methodological challenges. The first is the conceptualization and measurement of climate perceptions (Glick, 1985). To avoid conceptual ambiguities in the meaning of the aggregated construct, researchers phrase items so that they reflect team properties. This often means changing the referent from "I" to "we"; for example, "I am very hardworking" changes to "we (the people in this group) are very hardworking." This is what Chan (1998) has called a referent shift consensus model. The consensus in the organizational community today is to use appropriate referents (e.g., "we" instead of "I" when measuring each characteristic) when answers from individuals about the larger system are to be collected (e.g., Chen, Mathieu, & Bliese, 2004; Hofmann & Jones, 2004; Klein, Dansereau & Hall, 1994; Klein & Kozlowski, 2000b; Kozlowski & Klein, 2000; Morgeson & Hofmann, 1999). This alignment of theory with methods has been a crucial and defining step in organizational multilevel research. I review approaches to capture collective constructs, called composition models, below.

Another problem that needed to be addressed by shared climate researchers is to establish statistical methods and cut-off criteria for sufficient agreement or consensus to justify aggregation of individual-level responses (James, Joyce, & Slocum, 1988). Numerous indices and statistical procedures exist (James, 1982; James, Demaree, & Wolf, 1984, 1993; Shrout & Fleiss, 1979), but there is a continuing debate about which index or procedure is to be preferred (e.g., Bliese, 2000).

An interesting perspective emerging from this shared perception approach is that for shared perceptions to arise it is necessary that (1) individuals interact at work; (2) share a common goal or work toward an attainable outcome which predisposes them to collective action; and (3) have sufficient task interdependence so that they develop a shared understanding of behavior (Anderson & West, 1998). Since these conditions are more likely to be found in work teams than in the overall organization, researchers who have followed this perspective have argued that a shared climate is more likely to develop at a group or team level than at an organizational level, especially if the organization is large, divisionalized, and multilayered (Anderson & West, 1998).

In summary, research on climate deals with perceptions of individuals that are reflective of larger structural entities such as work groups or organizations. Researchers distinguish individual from collective and shared aspects of climate. Emphasis on the latter has led to an awareness that measures need to be aligned with the theoretical construct of interest. Second, there has also been much debate about defining sufficient levels of agreement or sharedness, with various indices and statistical tools now being available.

Leadership

Leadership as a central concept in organizational research has been extensively discussed from multilevel perspectives (e.g., Dansereau & Yammarino, 1998; Graen & Uhl-Bien, 1995; House, Hanges, Javidan, Dorfman, & Gupta, 2003; Klein & House, 1995; Waldman & Yammarino, 1999; Yammarino & Dubinsky, 1994). I focus on one specific topic, namely transformational or charismatic leadership (Bass, 1985; Conger & Kanungo, 1987), because a presentation of possible relationships between charismatic leaders and followers allows me to discuss interesting theoretical choices to be addressed in multilevel research.

Charismatic leaders are taken to influence all group members (Klein et al., 1994). These members in turn will share their perceptions of the leader as charismatic. Similar to climate, all individuals will agree with each other about the leadership characteristics and a single score can be assigned to that work group. This effect is stronger if (1) the leader's behavior is more consistent with that of all members; (2) the group members' values and beliefs about social relations are more homogeneous and in agreement with that of the leader; (3) membership is desirable for followers; (4) both followers and leader voluntarily choose to continue with their mutual relationship; and (5) task interdependence and interactions between followers are higher (Klein & House, 1995).

An alternative might be that the leader inspires only some individuals, but not others (Klein & House, 1995; Waldman & Yammarino, 1999). Charismatic leaders often emerge in situations of crisis and offer radical and novel solutions. Such leaders and their measures are sometimes seen as controversial, and hence they may alienate some members. The influence of the leader may not be uniform within a work unit and the level of inspiration of individual members can only be understood in the context of the larger group (e.g., how inspired other individuals are). Theories can also be based on a third model which holds that individuals are not influenced by their leader or the group (e.g., laissez-faire leadership; Bass, 1985). Therefore, three different models can be differentiated (Klein et al., 1994): *homogeneity, independence,* and *heterogeneity*.

Homogeneity refers to the absence of variability of subunits within higher-level units. When talking about individuals and groups, it is assumed that "group members are sufficiently similar with respect to the construct in question that they may be characterized as a whole" (Klein et al., 1994, p. 199). A single value or characteristic is sufficient to describe the group as a whole. Aggregation of responses by individuals within groups is justified if individuals within a specific unit agree about the psychological meaning of the construct that characterizes the unit as a whole (e.g., group, organization, or society). It is assumed that true variation only occurs between groups or units, but not within (James, 1982). Consequently, homogeneity in the strict sense assumes that phenomena are shared and identical within units and differences only occur between units. The homogeneity assumption of charismatic leadership (Klein & House, 1995; Waldman & Yammarino, 1999) implies that members of work teams agree with each other about the perceived characteristics of their leader and that each team can be described in terms of the overall perceived charisma by using a single score for the whole team.

The *heterogeneity* model implies the variability of subunits within higher level units. Alternative names include *frog pond, within-group,* or *parts* effect (e.g., Dansereau, Alutto, & Yammarino, 1984). Comparative or relative effects, but not absolute effects are important. A frog may be comparatively small in a big pond, but the same frog would appear large in a small pond. Therefore, the assumption is that effects are context dependent. Social comparison processes imply heterogeneity. Individuals compare themselves with others within a group in some way and their relative standing in relation to their comparison standard is important. Using our charismatic leadership example, the effect of charismatic leaders is not the same on all followers and an understanding of the leadership processes requires an examination of the relative levels of inspiration within the work group. Therefore, individual variation in relation to the group context has to be taken into account when studying group-level phenomena; still, the group itself is a meaningful entity and necessary as a contextual anchor.

The final model is *independence,* implying that subunits are independent from higher level units. It holds that individuals are free of group influence (Klein et al., 1994). This model underlies many statistical tests (e.g., individual scores are independent from each other) and this is the assumption that is most familiar to psychologists. Group membership is not considered relevant and individuals are the only source of true variation (compare individual differences on personality dimensions). It is assumed that constructs can be used to describe individuals and that these constructs represent more or less stable personality traits. Therefore, group membership or social context variables are expected to be of minor importance.

These three models of individual variation within a higher level unit have to be considered when developing theories, collecting data, and interpreting results (Klein et al., 1994). In the leadership literature the explicit use and consideration of these models has led to a clarification of theoretical boundaries (Yammarino & Dubinsky, 1994) and has helped in developing more sophisticated and differentiated theories (e.g., Graen & Uhl-Bien, 1995; Klein & House, 1995; Waldman & Yammarino, 1999).

In the remainder of the chapter, I use insights from organizational multilevel research, as described above, to specifically consider an additional level for organizational research, namely the nation level. To date, research incorporating variables at an individual, organizational, and national level is sparse. I provide a summary and an illustration of key steps and principles for multilevel cross-cultural theory development and theory testing derived from the organizational literature (Chen et al., 2004; Hofmann & Jones, 2004; Klein & Kozlowski, 2000b, Kozlowski & Klein, 2000). To illustrate crucial steps in this process, I use examples from leadership (House et al., 2003), voluntary work behavior (Fischer, Ferreira, Assmar, Redford &, Harb, 2005), and the model of culture fit (Aycan et al., 2000)

DEVELOPING CROSS-CULTURAL MULTILEVEL FRAMEWORKS FOR ORGANIZATIONAL SETTINGS

Construct Definition

The first question any researcher needs to address is this: What is the phenomenon or construct of interest? This is the question of the endogenous or dependent variable. A fundamental issue in developing useful multilevel models is the appropriate level; that is, whether the construct is best conceptualized as an individual- or collective-level construct (Morgeson & Hofmann, 1999). A failure to address this issue will have serious implications for the theory and the conceptualization, operationalization, measurement, analysis, and interpretation of resulting data (Hofmann & Jones, 2004). When discussing multilevel constructs, Morgeson and Hofmann (1999) distinguished between function and structure. The function of a construct refers to its effects or outputs and its nomological network. If two constructs show similar effects and nomological networks, they are (functionally) equivalent. One of the classical examples is individual and collective memory. The function of memory is the recollection of past events; therefore the function of the construct is similar at both levels. However, functions do not need to be identical across aggregation levels; for example, values serve different needs and functions at the individual (Schwartz & Bilsky, 1987) and national level (Schwartz, 2004).

In contrast, structure refers to processes that help these outputs and effects to come about. The structure of memory at an individual level is fundamentally different (biochemical and cognitive processes) from memory at a collective level (interpersonal and intergroup interactions). Morgeson and Hofmann (1999) highlight that: "Collective structures emerge, are transmitted and persist through the actions of members of the collective (or the collective as a whole)" (p. 253). Cross-cultural researchers are often interested in assessing cultural influence on individuals. Culture is thought to be transmitted and shared in a socialization process (Smith & Bond, 1998). Therefore, the structure of cultural constructs comes about through socialization mechanisms and the interactions between individuals within a specific cultural environment.

To give some examples of cross-cultural multilevel organizational research, Fischer et al. (2005) developed a framework for explaining levels of voluntary work behavior across different cultures. They first discussed the appropriate level of their dependent variable and conceptualized work behavior at the individual level. Variables at an organizational and nation level that might influence individuals' work behavior were also considered. Aycan et al. (2000) were interested in examining the use of human resource management (HRM) practices across cultures. Their dependent variables were perceptions of one's job (in terms of autonomy, variety of skills used, significance of task), supervisory practices (goal setting, empowerment), and reward allocation (performance–reward contingency). The authors, however, did not explicitly discuss which level they were addressing. Although they later measured items at an individual level (about individuals' beliefs about their job, see below), their explanation suggests an organizational level (as indicative of HR practices). House et al. (2003) were interested in explaining culturally endorsed leadership attributes, distinguishing specific behavioral and attribute descriptors of ideal leaders. They focused on ideal types of leadership behavior, an individual-level construct that may be shared within nations.

All three projects mentioned discussed higher-level variables that are likely to influence these lower-level perceptions. Fischer et al. (2005) focused on organizational practices as an expression of shared values and norms within an organization (organization level). Aycan et al. (2000) identified internal work culture as shared managerial beliefs about employee nature and behavior. House et al. (2003) included both practices and shared espoused values at an organization level. Finally, all three projects focused on shared values, beliefs, and practices at nation level.

All the authors used definitions of culture as a shared and complementary meaning system within an identifiable national group. Consequently, homogeneity is the most appropriate approach for both organization- and nation-level dimensions used in their research.

These examples highlight the need for researchers to start with a theoretical discussion of potential levels of their dependent and independent variables. This discussion should not only identify the appropriate level but also the mechanism of influence (direct vs. moderated) of the independent variables on the dependent variable, alternative explanations of levels and time frames for causal effects (e.g., the development of a collective construct may take a long time and require repeated interactions between key members, whereas the influence of higher level variables such as organizational structure or legal requirements on behavior of individuals is much faster). Kozlowski and Klein (2000) discuss these additional questions in more detail.

Nature of Aggregate Constructs

Multilevel theories need to address how phenomena at different levels are linked. Top-down and bottom-up processes are possible (Kozlowski & Klein, 2000). Top-down theories are about contextual influence. Individuals are embedded in groups, and groups in a society. Variables at a higher level may have a direct effect on elements at a lower level or may moderate relationships in lower-level units. In contrast, many collective phenomena have their foundation in the cognition, affect, and behavior of individuals. This creation of higher level constructs through interaction is a bottom-up process. The emergent constructs, in turn, may influence lower-level units in the form of top-down processes. Here it is important to make some distinction between emergent, collective, and aggregate constructs. Collective constructs are constructs that reside at a collective level of analysis—defined by Morgeson and Hofmann (1999), as "any interdependent and goal-directed combination of individuals, groups, departments, organizations, or institutions," or "any set [or grouping] of entities" (p. 251)—and represent descriptions of collective phenomena. An emergent construct is a collective construct that results from dynamic interactions of lower level units or their properties (Klein & Kozlowski, 2000a). Finally, aggregate constructs are made up of lower level properties, but they may not reflect collective constructs. They could just reflect the mean of individual-level variation. Collective constructs may be emergent constructs (if they are based on lower-level properties or dynamics).

For both top-down and bottom-up processes it is important that researchers answer the question as to whether they are interested in (1) describing a collection of individuals (aggregate construct) or (2) describing collective phenomena (Hofmann & Jones, 2004). Not addressing this question properly will create confusion about the aggregated and collective phenomenon. The average level of personality traits at a team level does not reflect collective personality (Hofmann & Jones, 2004). Focusing on values as expressions of culture, the aggregation of values at a collective level gives important information about what values people endorse on average, which is informative, insightful, and interesting. However, such an aggregation at a cultural level does not necessarily reflect collective values or cultural values. As discussed above in the climate section, for a shared or collective construct to emerge, agreement is necessary.

The relation of individual values that are aggregated at cultural level and culture-level values is not a trivial question. First, the aforementioned study by House et al. (2003) included questions about personal values (what society should be like) and how people perceive their current society (what society is like). Aggregations of values might be conceptualized as reflecting collections of individuals, whereas reports on practices might be seen as collective phenomena. Overall, House et al. (2003) reported acceptable levels of agreement within cultures when focusing on the dimensions overall, but not the individual items; for a critique of this approach, see Brown and Hauenstein (2005). When the values were aggregated to nation level, the average correlation across the nine nation-level dimensions was negative ($r = -.26$), indicating that specific value ratings by individuals do not coincide with cultural practices as reported by the same individuals.

Fischer (2004) asked students for value ratings using both a self-referenced value scale (important values in my life) as well as a culture-referenced value scale (important values for most people in my culture). When averaged, the former may be used to describe a collection of individuals, whereas the latter may be seen as an expression of collective phenomena. In a first study, Fischer (2004) asked two samples of New Zealand students to rate either their personal values or the values for most people in New Zealand. Significant differences for most values emerged and agreement was higher for culture-referenced rather than self-referenced values. In a second study (Fischer, 2004) students completed both self- and culture-referenced ratings. On average, the correlation between the two ratings was a mere .35. In a further study, Fischer (2006) correlated culture-referenced ratings provided by students in 10 countries with self-referenced indices provided by Schwartz (1994). The average correlation between the two ways of measuring at a culture level was .28. Focusing on other constructs rather than values, Terracciano et al. (2005) compared personality self-ratings as well as observer ratings of other individuals in 49 countries with ratings of the average individual within a country (called national character rating). Despite demonstrated reliability and validity of self, observer and national character ratings at an individual level, the median correlation between national character and self/observer ratings was not significant and virtually zero ($r = .04$). The results were not due to sample or framing effects and the authors demonstrated validity and reliability of all instruments. Although it has been reported that self-reports and observations at the individual level often show low correlations, this does not explain the discrepancy between agreement levels of constructs with specific rating instructions within nations and low correlations between the same constructs with different instructions. How shall we make sense of these divergent findings? We might find some help in interpreting these answers in the organizational multilevel literature.

Kozlowski and Klein (2000) distinguished composition models for higher level constructs into three basic types: global, shared, and configural unit properties. Global unit properties originate and are manifest at the unit level. They are relatively objective, descriptive, and easily observable characteristics of a unit. Size (e.g., number of individuals in an organization and population size), population density, and ecological climate are typical examples. In contrast, both shared and configural properties are emergent in the sense that they originate at a lower level, but are manifest at a higher level. Shared properties represent composition forms of emergence, whereas configural properties capture the variability or pattern of individual characteristics, behaviors, responses, and constructs of members within the unit. Demographic diversity is a classic example of a descriptive configural unit property; value or attitudinal diversity is an example of a latent configural unit property.

Merging the compositional models with the distinction made by Hofmann and Jones (2004) between individual versus collective constructs, we can more clearly differentiate different types of collective and aggregated constructs (see Table 7.1) as well as the information necessary to use them. The first three models in the table describe collections of individuals. The *selected score model* describes the attribute of an aggregate through the representation of a specific lower-level score. For example, in

TABLE 7.1

A Classification of Aggregate and Collective Constructs

Name of model	Level of observation	Internal consistency	Agreement within group	Aggregate reliability	Referent
Selected score model	Collection of individuals	Individual	Not necessary	NA	Individual
Summary index model	Collection of individuals	Individual	Not necessary	NA	Individual
Dispersion model	Collection of individuals	Individual	Not necessary	NA	Individual
Referent shift model	Collective	Aggregate	Necessary	Necessary	Aggregate
Aggregate model	Collective	Aggregate if applicable	NA	Necessary if applicable	Aggregate
Consensus model	Fuzzy	Aggregate	Necessary	Necessary	Individual

conjunctive tasks like assembly line work (Steiner, 1972) the capabilities of the weakest member will determine the lower limit of a potential group performance. No agreement is necessary between group members, the referent for measurement is the individual; the measure has to be reliable at individual level but aggregated reliability is not an issue.

The *summary index model* is the mere aggregate of a variable of interest. Most nation-level analyses in cross-cultural research fall into this category (e.g., Chinese Culture Connection, 1987; Hofstede, 1980; Schwartz, 1994). The summary index model captures the mean or sum of a construct for a collection of *individuals*, but need not say anything about the aggregate or collective. The only prerequisite is that there is internal consistency at an individual level; no agreement at a higher level is necessary. The interpretation of such a score from a level perspective is as the central tendency of individuals.

The *dispersion model* captures the individual-level variability or distribution of characteristics or properties rather than their central indices. Similarly to the summary index model, such models "represent descriptive statistics of individual scores within a group, but they describe the construct using a different configuration of individual-level responses in the aggregate" (Chen et al., 2004, p. 284). The most common indicator is the variance of a construct (e.g., Colquitt, Noe, & Jackson, 2002; Naumann & Bennett, 2000. Work on tightness-looseness (Gelfand, Nishii, & Raver, 2006) has focused on this variability as a dimension of cross-cultural investigation. To justify aggregation, it is necessary to show internal consistency at the individual level, no agreement is necessary and there is no need to establish reliability at an aggregate level.

When aggregated, these three composition models are most likely to capture an index about a collection of individuals. Researchers using these models have not assessed group, organizational or collective constructs. Hofmann and Jones (2004) have noted that, "it may be possible to use these compositional models to reference a true collective-level construct" (p. 309). However, they "simply suggest that researchers think critically about what they have measured and about the meaning of their aggregate variable in light of their measure and their compositional model" (p. 309). Therefore, current research on personal values aggregated to a nation level might be best interpreted as capturing average value endorsement of individuals, but it says little about the sharedness which is implied when talking about values as cultural constructs.

True collective constructs can be assessed using either referent-shift models or aggregate properties models. *Referent-shift models* have been advocated for a long time, especially in the climate literature (e.g., Glick, 1985) to avoid conceptual confusion between levels. The main distinction between a summary-index model and the referent-shift model is that for the former individuals are asked to provide a judgment of their own characteristics, attitudes, abilities, values, or norms and these judgments are aggregated. A typical item might be: "I am happy." The referent-shift model would require individuals to focus on the aggregate when answering the item; for example, "People in my group are happy." This is the cognitive schema approach in the climate literature.

Aggregation with reference-shift data is justified and indicates a true collective construct if there is internal consistency and reliability at an aggregate level and members in the group share their perceptions (in an ideal case of a collective construct all members would agree with each other; however, in reality various cut-off points for sufficient agreement have been discussed; see below). This approach was taken by Fischer, Ferreira, Assmar, Redford et al. (2006) and House et al. (2003) when measuring nation-level constructs. A referent-shift model was used, agreement was assessed and internal consistency and reliability at the aggregate level were tested. Aycan et al. (2000) used a referent-shift model to capture nation-level dimensions, but no indicators of agreement, validity, or reliability were reported.

The second model capturing collective constructs is the *aggregate properties model*. Here, the higher-level construct is directly aligned with the unit of analysis. Both central tendencies and variability can be used. In organizational research, this approach is often taken by strategic management scholars; for example, through observation of structural properties of organizations, or information obtained through key informants. House et al. (2003) and Diener, Diener, and Diener (1995) used this method (expert ratings and archival information) for validating their nation-level dimensions.

The final model is the *consensus model*. Hofmann and Jones (2004) suggested that it is fuzzy in the sense that it could be a marker for a collective construct. A consensus model refers to an individual-level variable that has been aggregated to the higher level, showing reliability at an aggregate level. Most importantly, members of the unit of interest share their perception of the construct. Using an item such as "I am happy" would form a consensus model, if there is sufficient agreement within a group and it shows reliability at aggregate level. The item "Everyone in my group is happy" would point to a referent-consensus model, if there is sufficient agreement within the group and it shows reliability at individual and aggregate level. Empirically, these two items might be similar, although Klein, Conn, Smith, and Sorra (2001) have shown that the phrasing can make a difference for organization-level constructs. Fischer, Smith et al. (2007) used self-referenced values in a working population and assessed agreement before aggregating values to a nation-level. They noted that some values showed very little agreement, especially those that may capture more personal preferences in Western societies (e.g., "devout").

However, conceptually the implied constructs are quite different. The first self-referenced variable provides an index of the shared level of individual happiness within the collective, whereas the second more directly represents the collective construct of happiness. Hofmann and Jones

(2004) suggested that the former is a marker of the second and the second is to be preferred if the construct of interest is at the collective level (Klein et al., 1994; Kozlowski & Klein, 2000; Morgeson & Hofmann, 1999). Therefore, to measure collective constructs researchers should use a referent-shift consensus model and assess agreement, reliability, and validity. Returning to the initial observation of only modest overlap between individual and collective constructs at a nation level, one might interpret aggregated scores based on self-ratings as an expression of average individual characteristics (the average personality or value within a specific group), whereas shared observations refer to higher order constructs such as collective phenomena. The relation between the aggregated self-ratings and collective phenomenon may be dependent on the construct of interest and may vary in strength. For example, Fischer (2006) found that values related to basic individual–group relationships and emotional expression (which tend to be internalized very early in one's socialization) show relatively high congruence between aggregated self-ratings and culture-ratings, whereas other values showed less congruence. Some values (like those relating to pursuit of intellectual stimulation and creativity) may not show any overlap at all, since such values might be highly dependent on individual differences in motivation and ability and reflect personal attributes rather than social norms that are internalized.

The implications for cross-cultural psychologists are potentially dramatic. What would our map of the world look like if we had used different ways of conceptualizing, operationalizing, and testing cultural dimensions? At this stage we can only speculate. It is important to emphasize that previous studies are informative and useful in that they gave us a map of the world in terms of individual preferences. However, cross-cultural psychologists are often interested in making statements about cultural processes, but have used individual-level data to gather this information. As a consequence, we (1) tend to overuse psychological constructs to explain cross-cultural differences, without paying enough attention to collective phenomena, and (2) we do not always appreciate and understand the intricate conceptual and statistical link between the two levels.

An interesting option would be to take Morgeson and Hofmann's (1999) structure perspective on collective constructs seriously. Previous cross-cultural research has focused on individual-level phenomena (Smith & Bond, 2003), but collective constructs consist and emerge out of interactions and event cycles between individuals (Morgeson & Hofmann, 1999). Smith and Bond (2003), for example, outlined the merits of a relationship-based psychology. It would be interesting to focus on the interaction patterns and events to study these ongoing event cycles and investigate collective constructs such as cultural values and dimensions. This would create the path for true multilevel theories.

The previous discussion has merged conceptual and methodological as well as interpretative issues. It needs to be stressed that first and foremost the question of the nature of constructs is a theoretical question. Are we studying a collective construct (e.g., cultural or organizational values and practices) or is the focus on average levels of individual attributes? The answer of this question should determine how researchers measure and operationalize the construct of interest. Readers of previous research should also critically question the interpretation of constructs based on the operationalization and reported information (e.g., how were constructs measured, was reliability assessed at an individual or aggregate level, were indices of agreement reported?).

Assessing Psychometric Properties of Constructs

Having discussed the various compositional models, the psychometric properties of the constructs at each level need to be assessed. An instrument that is reliable at the individual level is not necessarily reliable at the nation level. Ideally, we should assess psychometric properties at all levels, although small sample size at aggregate level may prevent adequate assessment. The assessment of the reliability and validity of multilevel constructs is slightly different from our standard practices with single-level constructs.

One of the most common ways is to study the factor structure across levels. There are sophisticated methods now available to assess the structure using both exploratory (Van de Vijver & Poortinga, 2002) and confirmatory (Muthén, 1994) factor analysis. Identification of different structures at individual and nation-level has been the strength of cross-cultural researchers (e.g., Hofstede, 1980, 2001; Kim, Triandis, Kagitcibasi, Choi, & Yoon, 1994; Schwartz, 1992; 1994; Van de Vijver & Poortinga, 2002). Fischer, Ferreira, Assmar, Redford et al. (2006) demonstrated that a theory-driven measure of individualism-collectivism norms can be replicated across levels. However, it remains a formidable challenge to demonstrate equivalence across levels (Chen et al., 2004).

Another issue is that interrater agreement needs to be assessed if the construct is supposed to be a collective construct. Various such indicators are available (see section on climate). For consensus- and referent-shift models, a sufficient level of agreement is needed to warrant aggregation. In small-group research, cut-off criteria of .6 (Brown & Hauenstein, 2005) and .7 (James et al., 1984) for interrater consistency indices have been recommended. However, at a nation level it is questionable to what extent these criteria apply since nations are much more diverse and heterogeneous (e.g., Fischer, Smith et al., 2007). This constitutes an interesting and important area for further cross-cultural research.

Reliability needs to be demonstrated. At the individual level it needs to be calculated for selected score, summary index, and dispersion models. This is straightforward and can be done using Cronbach's alpha using individual level data. Assessing the reliability of the aggregate properties model is also straightforward since the higher level unit is the level of measurement. However, consensus- and referent-shift consensus models are more complex. The indices may differ depending on whether total, average within-unit, between-unit, or separate within-unit item intercorrelation matrices are used. For the aggregate reliability, it is advisable to aggregate the individual items to the higher level and to calculate reliability at the aggregated level using the between-unit correlation matrix. In this way, the assessment of psychometric properties is adapted to the level of analysis (Klein et al., 1994). For the individual level, the average within-unit or separate within-unit intercorrelation matrices might be used.

All the analyses of psychometric properties that were presented here separately examine these properties at each level. All analyses can lead to erroneous results if all data are combined and a single index is computed. For example, the factor structure of the combined data may be different from both the structures found using the between- and within-unit correlations (Dansereau et al., 1984).

Construct Variability at Higher Level

Unless there is variation between units, there is no point in using higher level constructs. There has been some debate in the literature about whether variability between units is necessary if there is agreement within units (e.g., George & James, 1993; Yammarino & Markham, 1992). As discussed before, at least a fair agreement among members is necessary for referent shift and consensus models. George and James (1993) have argued that a shared construct exists if there are shared perceptions within a group. However, in case of agreement, individuals' perceptions of their work climate are similar in all groups. In this case we have a shared construct, but the utility of this construct for multilevel models might be limited (because there is no variability). The point is straightforward and applies to all models, without variability between nations there is nothing to model for a multilevel analysis, even if there is agreement within nations.

The Problem of the Nature and Inclusion of Higher Level Units

So far, I have been discussing the structure and function of constructs. But it is also important to pay some attention to the actual units of analysis (e.g., the groups, organizations, or societies that are the focus of our multilevel model). Two questions are of particular importance. It has been debated whether the theoretical units (e.g., groups or societies) correspond to real units and their formal or informal boundaries (Glick, 1985; Patterson, Payne, & West, 1996). For example, can a society or cultural group be described and distinguished from another society or cultural group in terms of their typical and characteristic practices? Furthermore, the strength or inclusiveness of the different levels should be discussed

(House, Rousseau, & Thomas-Hunt, 1995). For example, how strongly are individuals influenced by the national culture of the country they live in? These questions are important for specifying multilevel constructs and especially the second one poses considerable problems for cross-cultural multilevel research (Chao, 2000).

Sociopsychological Significance of Aggregates

In an investigation on work groups in a large organization, Patterson et al. (1996) found that formal units that can be defined with relative ease based on formal group boundaries (e.g., groups working together) correspond poorly to psychological group boundaries. If the focus is on collection of individuals, this variability does not provide a problem since the interest is in this area rather than the cultural collective. In addition, dispersion could be the target of investigation. Participants can be asked to identify their ethnic, cultural, and organizational identity and this can then be meaningfully incorporated in theoretical frameworks and statistical analysis. For example, it can be investigated whether minority members agree with majority members. In this case a statistic expressing the degree of agreement would be the dependent variable. Divergent views or subcultures can be integrated in model building and the effect of this variation can be tested (Colquitt et al., 2002; Lindell & Brandt, 2000).

It is crucial to assess the homogeneity of answers within a specific unit of interest before aggregating responses. In case of emerging heterogeneity of responses, this variance might provide further meaningful information and might be integrated in theory testing. Lindell and Brandt (2000) argued that within-group variance could moderate the strength of opinions within groups. Colquitt et al. (2002) found empirical evidence for this mechanism. Studying work groups in organizational settings, they found that the effect of climate was stronger if members of work groups shared a common climate perception. We might expect similar effects at a national level. If there is a strong and homogeneous cultural belief, cultural norms will be more influential than if members do not share a common culture. Preliminary research seems to indicate that some cultures show more variability across a number of constructs than others (Au, 2000). Cultural constructs such as tightness-looseness (Gelfand et al., 2006) are likely to capture some of this variation. This variability could be incorporated in research and made an explicit focus of theory. It could be expected that the effect of collective constructs is stronger if there is stronger consensus.

Inclusiveness of Levels Applied to National Cultures

The traditional approach to multilevel modeling relies on the assumption that lower level units are nested within the higher level. House et al. (1995) called this inclusiveness. They argued that effects of higher on lower levels will increase with the extent of inclusiveness. Inclusiveness is increased when members of a unit spend more time proportionally within the higher unit than with other units, when members of a lower unit are under more constant influence of the higher level unit, when members are attracted to each other, or when resources and information are shared. Applied to national culture, this implies that individuals act and operate mainly within their native sociocultural context rather than in another sociocultural context (e.g., country), are continuously exposed to the influence of their own native national culture, that members within a sociocultural environment are attracted to each other, and finally, that resources and information are shared. However, the reality is often different and this hierarchy of levels might break down (Chao, 2000). Individuals in many societies are constantly influenced by other cultural influences through mass media, Internet, international travel, increasing work group diversity due to migration, or other phenomena related to globalization.

The commonly assumed hierarchy in multilevel models of organizations is not so clear when focusing on sociocultural variables. This provides a formidable challenge and these problems need to be addressed within multilevel models. One aspect that could be modeled relatively easily in top-down models (e.g., using HLM, Raudenbush & Bryk, 2002) is to investigate whether main effects of nation-level variables become stronger in more homogeneous and tight societies (e.g., whether variability around the nation-mean or national heterogeneity moderates the impact of nation-level variables). Second, bottom-up models might investigate how and when collective constructs emerge, particularly if related to national identities or cultural constructs. For example, some countries which have a relatively young history and different subcultures tend to share a common identity and perceived culture (e.g., Brazil), whereas others do not (New Zealand). What factors would contribute to the emergence (or not) of shared collective constructs?

Construct Function across Levels: What Is the Best Model to Describe Proposed Relationships?

From the perspective of multilevel modeling, three broad types of conceptual and analytical models can be distinguished: single-level models, cross-level models, and homologous multilevel models (Kozlowski & Klein, 2000).

Single-level models deal with relationships between variables at one level of theory and analysis. Single, individual-level models are the most familiar to psychologists. Most research within psychology and management deals with and uses data at the level of individuals. However, team- or group-level models are also common (James, 1982), with climate research being the classic example. Cross-cultural research is also rich in nation-level studies (e.g., Chinese Culture Connection, 1987; Schwartz, 2004).

Single-level models do not involve variables at a higher or lower level, but they nevertheless provide a number of theoretical and analytical challenges. As discussed in previous sections, there needs to be a theoretical rationale and justification for conceptualizing a construct at a particular level (e.g., the organization or nation), the operationalization of the construct needs to be aligned with the theoretical level (using appropriate compositional models), and the construct has to be validated at the appropriate level (providing the appropriate statistical information). Once an emergent construct has been correctly identified, operationalized, and measured at a higher level, the analysis is straightforward. For example, hierarchical regression can be used to predict group-level performance on the basis of group characteristics (e.g., shared climate and leadership perceptions).

Cross-level models describe relationships among variables at different levels. Most commonly, authors use top-down approaches, assuming that higher-level variables influence lower-level variables (e.g., organizational climate influencing employee job satisfaction or performance). Three broad types of top-down models can be distinguished (Klein et al., 1994; Klein & Kozlowski, 2000b): direct effects, moderator, and frog-pond cross-level models. The first describes the theoretical relationship between a higher-level variable that has a direct effect on a variable at a lower level. For example, House et al. (2003) found that organizational practices were strongly influenced by nation-level values. Fischer and Mansell (2006) found that the nation-level in-group collectivism practices (House et al., 2003) were associated with increased levels of affective organizational commitment in samples around the world.

The second type of cross-level models, cross-level moderator models, specifies an interaction between variables, typically the higher level variable changing the relationship between two lower level variables. For example, the relationship between job satisfaction and job performance might depend on the extent to which resources are available. People might be highly satisfied, but they cannot show their performance because there is no material available for them to work on. Brodbeck, Hanges, Dickson, Gupta, and Dorfman (2004), who used data from the GLOBE project, reported analyses in which they investigated the interaction between industry and nation-level effects on organizational practices. They found that financial organizations are not strongly influenced by nation-level characteristics, suggesting low cultural influence on the operation of financial institutions and high global pressure. Fischer, Ferreira, Asmar, Omar et al. (2006) investigated the interaction between House et al.'s (2004) nation-level value dimension and perceptions of justice on self-reported work behavior at an individual level, finding that justice effects were stronger in more power distant societies.

The third category of cross-level models, cross-level frog-pond models, describes the effects of individual group members' standing within a

group on individual-level outcomes. For example, an individual's performance might predict self-esteem relative to his or her team member's performance. In a team where the average performance level is high, mediocre
performance of a single employee might lead to low self-esteem. In contrast, the same mediocre performance might lead to high self-esteem in a
team where the average performance level is low. Therefore, the relative
performance within the team is the predictor rather than the absolute
level of individual performance. Some authors may argue that frog-pond
models are not true cross-level models, but consider them as a distinct
set of multilevel models since these models do not assume that the group
average is shared and since the average is not considered as a global property of the higher level unit (Klein et al., 1994; Kozlowski & Klein, 2000).
This is a fine, but complex distinction.

Homologous multilevel models are the final group of multilevel models.
These models specify that the same relationship between variables holds
at multiple levels of analysis. The construct is operationalized at all levels
and shows the same relationship with other variables across all the levels. Therefore, the value of such models is that researchers can generalize across levels. These models are appealing because they promise to
enhance the generality and applicability of a theory. However, the challenge for most homologous models is that in order to show the same structure and function of constructs at multiple levels, the model becomes so
abstract and simplified that it is no longer of any practical value (Klein,
Tosi, & Cannella, 1999; Klein & Kozlowski, 2000b).

There have been some homologous multilevel models (e.g., Staw, Sandelands, & Dutton, 1981, as cited in Kozlowski & Klein, 2000), but these
have not been tested empirically. Despite their theoretical appeal, their
practical utility and usefulness has yet to be demonstrated. Chen, Bliese,
and Mathieu (2005) recently discussed a conceptual framework and statistical procedures for such models and it is hoped that this will help theory development and testing. Most cross-cultural models seem to imply
homology in that cultural constructs (e.g., individualism-collectivism) are
supposed to have similar relationships and functions at individual and
cultural level (Triandis, 1995). As in organizational research, there is no
convincing empirical evidence so far in support for these models.

A Final Evaluation of Multilevel Cross-Cultural Organizational Research

To the best of my knowledge, only three sets of studies explicitly tackled all three levels simultaneously. The GLOBE project focused on ideal
leadership perceptions. The authors have generally justified their conceptualization of variables at each level, used appropriate sampling methods and then measured their variables appropriately (for a critique of the
interpretation, see Peterson, 2004). Questions remain about the meaning

of the nation-level dimensions as well as the aggregation procedures used by the authors (Smith, 2006). Using these indicators in their dataset, published reports are limited to separate cross-level analyses involving two levels (nation-level on organization-level and nation-level on individual-level) and single-level analyses (validation of the nation-level variables).

Aycan et al.'s project (2000) measured variables at all three levels. However, their sampling did not allow a separation of individual and organization-level variance. Although they specified a three-level structure, they analyzed their results only at individual level. For example, Aycan et al. (2000) reported 99 regression analyses predicting their outcome variables using internal work culture as predictor in each of their samples. They found significant results supporting their hypotheses in 45 cases, significant results rejecting their hypotheses in 6 cases, and the remaining regression coefficients were nonsignificant. By conducting separate regressions in each sample between each set of variables they lost valuable information. Furthermore, their hypotheses were not supported in over half of their regressions, hardly an impressive result. However, this variation may be due to higher-level factors and can be modeled. I reanalyzed some of their reported data by using the standardized regression weights between internal work culture (organization level) and reported HR practices (individual level) per sample and correlating them with the sociocultural dimensions reported by the authors. A significant result would indicate a moderator effect, implying that their sociocultural dimensions moderate the effect of internal work culture on HR practices. Overall, I found 12 correlation coefficients larger than .5, indicating a moderate (cross-level) effect size (Cohen, 1992). For example, in paternalistic cultures, with an emphasis on mutually dependent relationships between supervisors and subordinates, supervisors used more empowerment and performance-contingent rewards, but only in organizations with a proactive internal work culture. This reanalysis of reported regression weights indicates the possibility of a cross-level moderator effect about culture-fit between national and organization characteristics (which is in line with their proposed model). The study by Aycan et al. (2000) was ground-breaking at the time it was conducted. With the progress in methodological and statistical understanding of multilevel issues, there are now greater possibilities for appropriate multilevel theories and research.

Fischer et al. (2005) provided a specific framework focusing on voluntary work behavior. They then conducted a number of pilot studies to ensure measurement equivalence across nations and levels (e.g., Fischer, Ferreira, Assmar, Redford et al., 2006). So far, they have reported analyses based on pilot studies investigating the structure and function of their instruments at nation, organization and individual level as well as cross-level analyses involving two levels (nation-level on individual level and organization-level on individual level (Assmar et al., 2006). Their main data collection is in progress. The aim is to sample 20 organizations from different sectors in each nation and then to conduct a three-level analysis investigating the interplay between nation- and organization-level variables on voluntary work behavior.

CONCLUSION

The purpose of the chapter was to briefly describe two traditional areas of multilevel research in organizational psychology and to develop an agenda for multilevel organizational research that includes culture. Guidelines developed from an organizational perspective dealing with individuals and groups can also be applied to this higher level of the nation. The main message from this past research is that a theoretical consideration of constructs at the beginning of a research process is crucial since it will determine operationalization, sampling, analysis and interpretation. Multilevel questions remain challenging and controversial, but their potential to contribute to our understanding is enormous.

Author Note

The section on "The Problem of the Nature and Inclusion of Higher Level Units" has been adapted from Fischer, R., Ferreira, M. C., Assmar, E. M. L., Redford, P., & Harb, C. (2005). Organizational behaviour across cultures: Theoretical and methodological issues for developing multilevel frameworks involving culture. *International Journal for Cross-Cultural Management, 5*, 27–48.

I would like to thank the editors and Charlotte Karam for their helpful comments on earlier versions of this manuscript.

REFERENCES

Anderson, N. R., & West, M. A. (1998). Measuring climate for work group innovation: Development and validation of the team climate inventory. *Journal of Organizational Behavior, 19*, 235–258.

Assmar, E., Fischer, R., Ferreira, M. C., Omar, A., Huynh, C. C., Dalyan, F., Baris, G., et al. (July 2006). *Extra-role behaviour across cultures: A multi-level framework and preliminary data.* Paper presented at the 18th International Congress of International Association for Cross-Cultural Psychology, Spetses, Greece.

Au, K. Y. (2000). Intra-cultural variation as another construct of international management: A study based on secondary data of 42 countries. *Journal of International Management, 6*, 217–238.

Aycan, Z., Kanungo, R. N., Mendonca, M., Yu, K., Deller, J., Stahl, G., et al. (2000). Impact of culture on human resource management practices: A 10-country comparison. *Applied Psychology: An International Review, 49*, 192–221.

Bass, B. M. (1985). *Leadership and performance beyond expectations.* New York: Free Press.

Bliese, P. D. (2000). Within-group agreement, non-independence and reliability: Implications for data aggregation and analyses. In J. K. Klein, & S. W. J. Kozlowski (Eds.), *Multilevel theory, research and methods in organizations: Foundations, extensions, and new directions* (pp. 349–381). San Francisco: Jossey-Bass.

Brodbeck, F. C., Hanges, P. J., Dickson, M. W., Gupta, V., & Dorfman, P. W. (2004). Societal culture and industrial sector influences on organizational culture. In R. J. House, P. J. Hanges, M. Javidan, P. Dorfman, & V. Gupta (Eds.), *GLOBE, cultures, leadership, and organizations: GLOBE study of 62 societies* (pp. 654–668). Newbury Park, CA: Sage.

Brown, R. D., & Hauenstein, N. A. (2005). Interrater agreement reconsidered: An alternative to the r_{wg} indices. *Organizational Research Methods, 8*, 165–184.

Chan, D. (1998). Functional relations among constructs in the same content domain at different levels of analysis: A typology of compositional models. *Journal of Applied Psychology, 83*, 234–246.

Chao, G. T. (2000). Multilevel issues and culture: An integrative view. In J. K. Klein & S. W. J. Kozlowski (Eds.), *Multilevel theory, research and methods in organizations: Foundations, extensions, and new directions* (pp. 308–348). San Francisco: Jossey-Bass.

Chen, G., Bliese, P. D., & Mathieu, J. E. (2005). Conceptual framework and statistical procedures for delineating and testing multilevel theories of homology. *Organizational Research Methods, 8*, 375–409.

Chen, G., Mathieu, J. E., & Bliese, P. D. (2004). A framework for conducting multilevel construct validation. In F. J. Yammarino & F. Dansereau (Eds.), *Research in multilevel issues: Multilevel issues in organizational behavior and processes* (Vol. 3, pp. 273–303). Oxford: Elsevier.

Chinese Culture Connection (1987). Chinese values and the search for culture-free dimensions of culture. *Journal of Cross-Cultural Psychology, 18*, 143–164.

Cohen, J. (1992). A power primer. *Psychological Bulletin, 112*, 155–159.

Colquitt, J. A., Noe, R. A., & Jackson, C. L. (2002). Justice in teams: Antecedents and consequences of procedural justice climate. *Personnel Psychology, 55*, 83–109.

Conger, J. A., & Kanungo, R. N. (1987). Toward a behavioral theory of charismatic leadership in organizational settings. *Academy of Management Review, 12*, 637–647.

Dansereau, F., Alutto, J. A., & Yammarino, F. J. (1984). *Theory-testing in organizational behavior: The "variant" approach.* Englewood Cliffs, NJ: Prentice Hall.

Dansereau, F., & Yammarino, F. J. (1998). (Eds.). *Leadership: The multiple-level approaches* (2 vols.). Westport, CT: JAI Press.

Diener, E., Diener, M., & Diener, C. (1995). Factors predicting the subjective well-being of nations. *Journal of Personality and Social Psychology, 69*, 851–864.

Fischer, R. (2004, August). *My values or my culture's values: The problem of referent choice in value measurements.* Paper presented at the 17th International Congress of International Association for Cross-Cultural Psychology in Xi'An, China.

Fischer, R. (2006). Congruence and functions of personal and cultural values: Do my values reflect my culture's values? *Personality and Social Psychology Bulletin, 32,* 1419–1431.

Fischer, R., Ferreira, M. C., Assmar, E. L. M., Redford, P., Harb, C., Glazer, S., et al. (2006). Measuring individualism-collectivism at a culture level: Development and validation of a new theory-based instrument. Paper submitted for publication.

Fischer, R., Ferreira, M. C., Assmar, E. M. L., Omar, A., Huynh, C. C., Dalyan, F. et al. (2006). Effects of justice on extra-role behaviour: A ten-culture study. Paper submitted for publication.

Fischer, R., Ferreira, M. C., Assmar, E. M. L., Redford, P., & Harb, C. (2005). Organizational behaviour across cultures: Theoretical and methodological issues for developing multilevel frameworks involving culture. *International Journal for Cross-Cultural Management, 5,* 27–48.

Fischer, R., & Mansell, A. (2006). Levels of organizational commitment across cultures: A meta-analysis. Paper submitted for publication.

Fischer, R., Smith, P. B., Richey, B. E., Ferreira, M. C., Assmar, E. M. L., Maes, J. et al. (2007). How do organizations allocate rewards? The predictive validity of national values, economic and organizational factors across six nations. *Journal of Cross-Cultural Psychology, 38,* 3–18.

Gelfand, M. J., Nishii, L. H., & Raver, J. L. (2006). On the nature and importance of cultural tightness-looseness. *Journal of Applied Psychology, 91,* 1225–1244.

George, J. M., & James, L. R. (1993). Personality, affect and behavior in groups revisited: Comment on aggregation, levels of analysis and a recent application of within and between analysis. *Journal of Applied Psychology, 78,* 798–804.

Glick, W. H. (1985). Conceptualising and measuring organizational and psychological climate: Pitfalls in multilevel research. *Academy of Management Review, 10,* 601–616.

Graen, G. B., & Uhl-Bien, M. (1995). Relationship-based approach to leadership: Development of leader-member exchange (LMX) theory of leadership over 25 years: Applying a multilevel multidomain perspective. *Leadership Quarterly, 6,* 219–247.

Hofmann, D. A., & Jones, L. M. (2004). Some foundational and guiding questions for multi-level construct validation. In F. J. Yammarino, & F. Dansereau (Eds.), *Multi-level issues in organizational behaviour and processes* (Vol 3, pp. 305–316). Amsterdam: Elsevier.

Hofstede, G. (1980). *Culture's consequences: International differences in work-related values.* Beverly Hills, CA: Sage.

Hofstede, G. H. (2001). *Culture's consequences: comparing values, behaviors, institutions and organizations across nations* (2nd ed.). Thousand Oaks, CA: Sage.

House, R. J., Hanges, P. J., Javidan, M., Dorfman, P., & Gupta, V. (Eds.). (2003). *GLOBE, cultures, leadership, and organizations: GLOBE study of 62 societies.* Newbury Park, CA: Sage.

House, R., Rousseau, D. M., & Thomas-Hunt, M. (1995). The meso paradigm: A framework for the integration of micro and macro organizational behavior.

In B. Staw & L. L. Cummings (Eds.), *Research in organisational behaviour* (Vol. 17, pp. 71–114). Greenwich, CT: JAI Press.

James, L. R. (1982). Aggregation bias in estimates of perceptual agreement. *Journal of Applied Psychology, 67,* 219–229.

James, L. R., Demaree, R. G., & Wolf, G. (1984). Estimating within-group interrater reliability with and without response bias. *Journal of Applied Psychology, 69,* 85–98.

James, L. R., Demaree, R. G., & Wolf, G. (1993). rwg: An assessment of within-group interrater agreement. *Journal of Applied Psychology, 78,* 306–309.

James, L. R., Joyce, W. F., & Slocum, J. W. (1988). Comment: Organizations do not cognize. *Academy of Management Review, 13,* 129–132.

Kim, U., Triandis, H. C., Kagitcibasi, C., Choi, S. C., & Yoon G. (Eds.). (1994). *Individualism and collectivism: Theory, method and applications.* Newbury, CA: Sage.

Klein, K. J., Conn, A. B., Smith, D. B., & Sorra, J. S. (2001). Is everyone in agreement? An exploration of within-group agreement in employee perceptions of work environment. *Journal of Applied Psychology, 86,* 3–16.

Klein, K. J., Dansereau, F., & Hall, R. J. (1994). Level issues in theory development, data collection and analysis. *Academy of Management Review, 19,* 195–229.

Klein, K. J., & House, R. J. (1995). On fire: Charismatic leadership and levels of analysis. *Leadership Quarterly, 6,* 183–198.

Klein, J. K., & Kozlowski, S. W. J. (2000a). (Eds.). *Multilevel theory, research and methods in organizations. Foundations, extensions, and new directions.* San Francisco: Jossey-Bass.

Klein, K. J., & Kozlowski, S. W. J. (2000b). From micro to macro: Critical steps in conceptualizing and conducting multilevel research. *Organizational Research Methods, 3,* 211–236.

Klein, K. J., Tosi, H., & Cannella, A. (1999). Multilevel theory building: Benefits, barriers and new developments. *Academy of Management Review, 24,* 243–248.

Kozlowski, S. W. J., & Klein, J. K. (2000). A multilevel approach to theory and research in organizations: Contextual, temporal and emergent processes. In J. K. Klein & S. W. J. Kozlowski (Eds.), *Multilevel theory, research and methods in organizations: Foundations, extensions, and new directions* (pp. 3–90). San Francisco: Jossey-Bass.

Lindell, M. K., & Brandt, C. J. (2000). Climate quality and climate consensus as mediators of the relationship between organizational antecedents and outcomes. *Journal of Applied Psychology, 85,* 331–348.

Morgeson, F. P., & Hofmann, D. A. (1999). The structure and function of collective constructs: Implications for multilevel research and theory development. *Academy of Management Review, 24,* 249–265.

Muthén, B. (1994). Multilevel covariance structure analysis. *Sociological Methods & Research, 22,* 376–398.

Naumann, S. E., & Bennett, N. (2000). A case for procedural justice climate: Development and test of a multilevel model. *Academy of Management Journal, 43,* 881–889.

Naylor, J. C., Pritchard, R. D., & Ilgen, D. R. (1980). *A theory of behavior in organizations.* New York: Academic Press.

Patterson, M., Payne, R. & West, M. (1996). Collective climates: A test of their sociopsychological significance. *Academy of Management Journal, 39,* 1675–1691.

Peterson, M. F. (2004). Culture, leadership and organizations: The GLOBE study of 62 societies. *Administrative Science Quarterly, 49,* 641–647.

Peterson, M. F., & Fischer, R. (2004). Organizational culture and climate. In C. Spielberger (Ed.), *Encyclopaedia for applied psychology* (Vol. 2, pp. 715–722). Amsterdam: Elsevier.

Raudenbush, S. W., & Bryk, A. S. (2002). *Hierarchical linear models* (2nd ed). London: Sage.

Schwartz, S. H. (1992). Universals in the content and structure of values: Theoretical advances and empirical tests in 20 countries. In M. P. Zanna (Ed.), *Advances in experimental social psychology* (Vol. 25, pp. 1–65). San Diego, CA: Academic Press.

Schwartz, S. H. (1994). Beyond individualism-collectivism: New cultural dimensions of values. In U. Kim, H. C. Triandis, C. Kagitcibasi, S. C. Choi, & G. Yoon (Eds.), *Individualism and collectivism: Theory, method and applications* (pp. 85–119). Thousand Oaks, CA: Sage.

Schwartz, S. H. (2004). Mapping and interpreting cultural differences around the world. In H. Vinken, J. Soeters, & P. Ester (Eds.), *Comparing cultures, dimensions of culture in a comparative perspective* (pp. 43–73). Leiden, the Netherlands: Brill.

Schwartz, S. H., & Bilsky, W. (1987). Toward a universal psychological structure of human values. *Journal of Personality and Social Psychology, 53,* 550–562.

Shrout, P. E., & Fleiss, J. L. (1979). Intraclass correlations: Uses in assessing rater reliability. *Psychological Bulletin, 86,* 420–428.

Smith, P. B. (2006). When elephants fight, the grass gets trampled: The GLOBE and Hofstede projects. *Journal of International Business Studies, 37,* 915–921.

Smith, P. B., & Bond, M. H. (1999). *Social psychology across cultures* (2nd ed.). Needham Heights, MA: Allyn & Bacon. (Original work published 1998)

Smith, P. B., & Bond, M. H. (2003). Honoring culture scientifically when doing social psychology. In A. Hogg & J. Cooper (Eds.), *Sage handbook of social psychology* (pp. 43–64). Thousand Oaks, CA: Sage.

Staw, B., Sandelands, L. E., & Dutton, J. E. (1981). Threat-rigidity effects in organizational behavior: A multilevel analysis. *Administrative Science Quarterly, 26,* 501–524.

Steiner, I. (1972). *Group processes and productivity.* New York: Academic Press.

Terracciano, A., Abdel-Khaled, A. M., Adam, N., Adomovava, L., Ahn, C. K., Ahn, H. N., et al. (2005). National character does not reflect mean personality trait levels in 49 cultures. *Science, 310,* 96–100.

Triandis, H. C. (1995). *Individualism and collectivism.* Boulder, CO: Westview Press.

Van de Vijver, F. J. R., & Poortinga, Y. H. (2002). Structural equivalence in multilevel research. *Journal of Cross-Cultural Psychology, 33,* 141–156.

Waldman, D. A., & Yammarino, F. J. (1999). CEO leadership: Levels-of-management and levels-of-analysis effects. *Academy of Management Review, 24,* 266–285.

Yammarino, F. J., & Dubinsky, A. J. (1994). Transformational leadership theory: Using levels of analysis to determine boundary conditions. *Personnel Psychology, 47,* 787–811

Yammarino, F. J., & Markham, S. E. (1992). On the application of within and between analysis: Are absence and affect really group-based phenomena? *Journal of Applied Psychology, 77,* 168–176.

8

Psycho-Logic and Eco-Logic: Insights from Social Axiom Dimensions

Kwok Leung and Michael Harris Bond

> By legitimation is meant socially objectivated "knowledge" that serves to explain and justify the social order...If [legitimations] are to be effective supporting the social order, however, they will have to be internalized and serve to define subjective reality as well. Legitimations, furthermore, can be both cognitive and normative in character. They do not only tell people what *ought to be*. Often they merely propose what *is*. (Berger, 1967, pp. 29–30, 32)

For most people, life is not an aimless, mindless drift; their actions and activities are conscious or unconscious manifestations of their responses to two fundamental questions: What do they want to pursue in life and how do they pursue those goals? The "what" question has been extensively researched under the rubric of values, the study of which seeks to identify general goals that people regard as important (e.g., Rokeach, 1973). In research on culture, the use of values to describe and interpret culture also has a long tradition (e.g., Kluckholn & Stodtbeck, 1961). For instance, Hofstede's (1980) now-classic work has identified four well-known cultural dimensions that are based on work values: power distance, individualism-collectivism, uncertainty avoidance, and masculinity-femininity. A fifth dimension, long-term vs. short-term orientation, was subsequently added (Hofstede, 1991), an addition to the Hofstede quartet derived from research using Chinese values (Chinese Culture Connection, 1987). A more recent research program on values has been orchestrated by Schwartz (1992), who identified 10 value types at the individual level across a wide range of cultural groups in the world. At the culture level, Schwartz (1994) identified seven value types. Other value instruments have been used at both the individual and culture levels, and it is safe to say that our discipline has mapped the world of explicit, self-reported values.

Leung et al. (2002) argue that while value-based frameworks have offered revealing insights about culture, other conceptual tools need to be explored and deployed for a comprehensive understanding of both culture and individuals. A monolithic focus on values restricts the progress of cross-cultural psychology, since individual behavior is the result of more than values, and it is behavior that we ultimately wish to understand and predict. To broaden our range of constructs-under-examination, Leung et al. proposed the construct of *social axioms*, or general social beliefs, to augment values in describing and interpreting culture and the behavior of individuals socialized into those cultures. Leung and Bond (2004) have adopted a functionalist approach to social axioms and argue that these general beliefs represent people's cognitive map of the social world they inhabit and help to guide individuals in conducting their social lives more effectively. Social axioms provide answers to the "how" question presented before; if the world operates in certain ways, then the sensible actor positions his or her behavior within that perceived set of constraints and affordances.

So what are social axioms? Beliefs vary in specificity: some are anchored in a particular social and personal context, such as "John is often forgetful when he has a heavy workload." In contrast, other beliefs are general and context-free, and may be regarded as "generalized expectancies," a concept first proposed by Rotter (1966) in describing locus of control. We use the term *social axioms* to label this type of general beliefs because, like axioms in mathematics, they are basic premises that people come to endorse and rely upon to make sense of their life space and to guide their actions. We now define these generalized beliefs about the world in this way:

> Social axioms are generalized beliefs about people, social groups, social institutions, the physical environment, or the spiritual world as well as about categories of events and phenomena in the social world. These generalized beliefs are encoded in the form of an assertion about the relationship between two entities or concepts.

Social axioms have the structure "A is related to B," and the relationship may be causal or correlational. In contrast, a value assumes the form "A is good/desirable/important." We do not deny that an evaluative dimension may underlie social axioms, because all semantic objects are characterized by an evaluative dimension (Osgood, Suci, & Tannenbaum, 1957). However, the evaluative component of a value is general, but is specific for an axiom. For instance, we classify a statement like "Wars are bad" as reflecting a pacifist value, but we regard such statements as "powerful people tend to exploit others" and "absolute power corrupts absolutely" as social axioms because they spell out a specified relationship between two entities, whether these entities are positively or negatively evaluated.

SOCIAL AXIOMS AT THE INDIVIDUAL LEVEL

The universe is real; it is happening all the time...Different men construe it in different ways. Since it owes no allegiance to any one man's construction system, it is always open to reconstruction. Some of the alternative ways of construing are better adapted to man's purposes than are others. Thus man comes to understand his world through an infinite series of successive approximations. (Kelly, 1955, p. 43)

The Initial Five-Culture Study

To identify a pancultural structure of social axioms at the individual level, Leung et al. (2002) began with the psychological literature on beliefs, which is mostly Euro-American in origin. In addition, social axioms were identified from informants and cultural sources from two distinct cultural groups: Hong Kong Chinese and Venezuelan. The beliefs generated from this culling were synthesized into a Social Axioms Survey with 182 items, which was administered to college students and adults in these two cultures. Exploratory factor analysis suggested a 5-factor solution, which showed a high degree of congruence across these two cultural groups.

Factor one is labeled *social cynicism*, because the items suggest a negative assessment of human nature, a biased view against some groups of people, a mistrust of social institutions, and a belief that people disregard ethical means in achieving their ends. The second factor is labeled *social complexity* because the items suggest a belief that there are multiple ways of achieving a given outcome and that a given person's behavior is inconsistent from situation to situation. The third factor is labeled *reward for application*, because the items suggest that effort, knowledge, careful planning, and the investment of these and other resources will lead to positive results. The fourth factor was labeled *spirituality* but subsequently renamed *religiosity*, because the items assert the existence of a supernatural being and the beneficial social functions of religious institutions and practices. The fifth factor is labeled *fate control*, because the items represent a belief that life events are predetermined by grand external forces, but that, reassuringly, there are some ways for people to influence the impact of these forces. A person may be high or low in his or her endorsement of any one of these five dimensions; the person's scores on these five constitute a comprehensive profile of his or her beliefs about the world. As these social axioms are pitched at a high level of generality, we consider these beliefs to be "valuable" beliefs (Preston & Epley, 2005), because of their broad explanatory power.

Leung et al. (2002) evaluated this five-dimensional structure of social axioms in three more cultural groups: the United States, Japan, and Germany.

Both confirmatory factor analysis and factor analysis based on Procrustes rotation suggest that the structure is reasonably equivalent across these three cultural groups. There was no plausible basis for claiming the existence of a sixth factor common across these five cultural groups.

The Global Study

As the initial study included only five cultural groups, the universality of the five-dimensional structure remained uncertain. To address this issue, Leung and Bond (2004) orchestrated a global project with the participation of over 50 colleagues from around the world and data from 40 national/cultural groups. To ensure that the final structure was not restricted by or to the five-factor structure reported by Leung et al. (2002), a meta-analytic procedure for factor analysis (Becker, 1996) was used, in which the cultural groups were treated equally, and no a priori structure was privileged by becoming the standard template against which other groups were compared. The correlation matrix of each cultural group was normalized by the Fisher transformation and these matrices were averaged to generate a combined matrix, which was then transformed back to a correlation matrix for an exploratory factor analysis. This procedure gives an equal weighting to each culture's correlation matrix, and does not assume any dimensional structure in the data.

The results suggested a five-dimensional structure, both for the 40 sets of student data as well as the 13 sets of adult data, which were analyzed separately. The final structure for the student samples is defined by 39 items that optimize equivalence across the 40 cultural groups studied (see Table 8.1 for the individual-level factor structure and composition). For evidence on the validity of this five-dimensional structure, see Leung and Bond (2004) for the etic factor structure and the Cronbach alphas factor by factor, culture by culture.

DIMENSIONS OF SOCIAL AXIOMS
AT THE CULTURE LEVEL

> Every socially constructed *nomos* must face the constant possibility of its collapse into anomie...every *nomos* is an area of meaning carved out of a vast mass of meaninglessness, a small clearing of lucidity in a formless, dark, always ominous jungle. (Berger, 1967, p. 23)

Ecological Analysis

The five-dimensional structure described before is based on the individual level, with the individual as the unit of analysis. It is well-known that

TABLE 8.1

The Structure of Social Axioms at the Individual Level Based on Student Data
from 40 Cultural Groups

Item	1 Social cynicism	2 Social complexity	3 Reward for application	4 Religiosity	5 Fate control
Powerful people tend to exploit others	.60				
Power and status make people arrogant	.59				
Kind-hearted people usually suffer losses	.57				
Kind-hearted people are easily bullied	.53				
People will stop working hard after they secure a comfortable life	.45				
Old people are usually stubborn and biased	.45				
The various social institutions are biased towards the rich	.44				
It is rare to see a happy ending in real life	.44				
To care about societal affairs only brings trouble for yourself	.42				
People deeply in love are usually blind	.39				
Young people are impulsive and unreliable	.38				
People may have opposite behaviors on different occasions		.60			
Human behavior changes with the social context		.54			
One's behaviors may be contrary to his or her true feelings		.54			
One has to deal with matters according to the specific circumstances		.48			
Current losses are not necessarily bad for one's long-term future		.40			
There is usually only one way to solve a problem (reversed)		.39			

(continued)

TABLE 8.1

Continued

Item	1 Social cynicism	2 Social complexity	3 Reward for application	4 Religiosity	5 Fate control
Hard working people will achieve more in the end			.59		
Adversity can be overcome by effort			.56		
Every problem has a solution			.50		
Knowledge is necessary for success			.49		
One who does not know how to plan his or her future will eventually fail			.45		
Competition brings about progress			.42		
Failure is the beginning of success			.40		
Caution helps avoid mistakes			.36		
Belief in a religion helps one understand the meaning of life				.75	
Religious faith contributes to good mental health				.72	
There is a supreme being controlling the universe				.62	
Belief in a religion makes people good citizens				.61	
Religion makes people escape from reality (reversed)				.59	
Religious beliefs lead to unscientific thinking (reversed)				.54	
Religious people are more likely to maintain moral standards				.51	

(continued)

TABLE 8.1

Continued

Item	1 Social cynicism	2 Social complexity	3 Reward for application	4 Religiosity	5 Fate control
Individual characteristics, such as appearance and birthday, affect one's fate					.60
There are many ways for people to predict what will happen in the future					.60
There are certain ways to help us improve our luck and avoid unlucky things					.52
Most disasters can be predicted					.51
Fate determines one's successes and failures					.48
Good luck follows if one survives a disaster					.48

dimensions at the individual level may, and often do, deviate in number and composition from dimensions at the culture level (e.g., Leung & Bond, 1989). To evaluate this possibility, Bond et al. (2004) analyzed the dimensionality of social axioms at the culture level, using item means from each of the now 41 cultural groups of college students as the input data. This input enables us to perform an "ecological factor analysis," as Hofstede (1980) labeled the procedure and then demonstrated for his work-related values.

Factor analysis of these culture averages rather than individual scores revealed a 2-dimensional structure. Factor 1 is labeled *dynamic externality*, because it contains items from four of the individual-level axiom dimensions: Reward for application, religiosity, fate control, and social complexity, although the dimension is primarily defined by items from reward for application and religiosity. The items in this factor tapping religiosity and fate control involve the assertion of outside forces at play and give rise to the label *externality*, but the emphasis on effort and cognitive engagement gives a dynamic quality to this construct. Factor 2 is labeled *societal cynicism*, because all the items are from the individual-level factor of social cynicism, but derived from a cultural group's average scores, thus representing "citizen" endorsements. The adjective *societal* is used to signal that this factor is derived from these culture-level inputs. These two factors are correlated at a low level, $r(39) = .21$, *ns*, and share little common variance.

TABLE 8.2

Axiom Dimensions at the Culture Level Based on Student Data from 41 Cultural
Groups

Item	Dynamic externality	Societal cynicism
Belief in a religion helps one understand the meaning of life	.92	
Good deeds will be rewarded, and bad deeds will be punished	.92	
Religious faith contributes to good mental health	.90	
There is a supreme being controlling the universe	.90	
All things in the universe have been determined	.90	
Belief in a religion makes people good citizens	.89	
The just will eventually defeat the wicked	.82	
Religion makes people escape from reality	−.82	
One will succeed if he/she really tries	.81	
Hard working people will achieve more in the end	.74	
Every problem has a solution	.72	
Religious people are more likely to maintain moral standards	.71	
Religious beliefs lead to unscientific thinking	−.70	
Knowledge is necessary for success	.67	
Failure is the beginning of success	.65	
There are many ways for people to predict what will happen in the future	.62	
Ghosts or spirits are people's fantasy	−.60	
Human behavior changes with the social context	−.58	
Competition brings about progress	.58	
Caution helps avoid mistakes	.55	
Adversity can be overcome by effort	.51	
To care about societal affairs only brings trouble for yourself		.81
Kind-hearted people usually suffer losses		.76
Old people are usually stubborn and biased		.73
It is rare to see a happy ending in real life		.69
People will stop working hard after they secure a comfortable life		.63
Old people are a heavy burden on society		.61
Kind-hearted people are easily bullied		.55
People deeply in love are usually blind		.54
Humility is dishonesty		.53
Power and status make people arrogant		.52
Powerful people tend to exploit others		.46

To establish the robustness of this two-factor structure, an ecological
factor analysis was conducted on the adult data from 13 cultural groups
as well. Even with such a small sample, the congruence between the structures based on student and adult data was reasonable, supporting the

generality of the structure (see Table 8.2 for the ecological factor structure and composition).

To establish the meaning of these two culture-level dimensions of social axioms, they were correlated with other well-known dimensions of culture (Hofstede, 2001; House, Hanges, Javidan, Dorfman, & Gupta, 2004; Inglehart & Baker, 2000; Schwartz, 1994; Smith, Dugan, & Trompenaars, 1996). To illustrate our procedure, we use Hofstede's individualism–collectivism dimension as an example. We correlated the scores of our two axiom dimensions with Hofstede's individualism–collectivism scores for cultures that are included in both our and his research. The correlations obtained are thus at the level of national culture.

Dynamic externality was correlated significantly with: both dimensions of Inglehart and Baker (2000), traditional orientation and survival values; two dimensions of Hofstede (1980), power distance and individualism (negatively); four dimensions of Schwartz (1994), conservatism, intellectual autonomy (negatively), egalitarian commitment (negatively), and harmony (negatively); one dimension of Smith et al. (1996), loyal involvement; two dimensions of House et al. (2004) that describe the current status of a culture, viz., humane orientation and in-group collectivism; and three dimensions of House et al. that describe the ideal state of a culture, viz., uncertainty avoidance, future orientation, and gender egalitarianism (negatively).

These correlations suggest that dynamic externality is generally related to power distance, collectivism, and conservatism. In addition, because of the association of dynamic externality with lower levels of socioeconomic development, which will be elaborated later, its correlation with high uncertainty avoidance and high future orientation perhaps suggests that hard labor and difficult living have engendered beliefs in the predictability of external forces and in the hope for a better future. The lower preference for gender egalitarianism in these cultures may reflect the continuous influence of conservatism. In sum, dynamic externality seems to overlap considerably with value-based cultural dimensions, although it does contain some novel, distinctive features not captured in previous culture-level studies.

Societal cynicism was only correlated with one value dimension of Inglehart and Baker (2000), survival; with two Hofstede (2001) dimensions, individualism (negatively) and long-/short-term orientation; and with three dimensions of House et al. (2004) that describe the ideal state of a culture, uncertainty avoidance, performance orientation (negatively), and gender egalitarianism (negatively). These correlations tend to be fewer and weaker than those for dynamic externality, with the exception of the survival dimension of Inglehart and Baker (2000). We conclude that the belief dimension of societal cynicism represents a feature of culture that is not captured well by extant and well established culture-level dimensions of value.

Multilevel Analysis of Axiom Dimensions

The individual- and culture-level dimensions of social axioms described above are derived independently from the same dataset. Recent advances in multilevel structural equation modeling permit the estimation of the two types of dimension simultaneously (e.g., Cheung & Au, 2005; Goldstein, 2003; Muthén, 1994), and multilevel analysis has indeed been eagerly applied in cross-cultural research (e.g., Van Hemert, Van de Vijver, & Poortinga, 2002; Van de Vijver & Poortinga, 2002) where it has obvious applications.

Cheung, Leung, and Au (2006) have adopted such a multilevel approach to evaluate the individual and culture-level structures of social axioms. The generality of the five-dimensional structure of social axioms at the individual level was first confirmed with meta-analytic structural equation modeling, a more stringent test than the exploratory factor analysis undertaken by Leung and Bond (2004). In this step, the homogeneity of the correlation matrices across cultures was first assessed; the RMSEA index for the homogeneity model was high, suggesting a good fit. In other words, the correlation matrices are reasonably similar across cultures, supporting the previous and somewhat arbitrary pooling of the correlation matrices across cultures. The fit of the five-factor model as defined by Leung and Bond (2004) was then evaluated with this pooled correlation matrix. Both RMSEA and SRMR, two fit indexes that are appropriate for large samples, pointed to a good fit.

In the second step, three multilevel models were tested with the pooled correlation matrix: (1) a five-factor model at both levels; (2) a five-factor model at the individual level and a two-factor model (i.e., dynamic externality and societal cynicism) at the culture level, a model based on the previous exploratory analyses described before; and (3) a five-factor model at the individual level, and a five-factor model at the culture level, which is further grouped into two second-order factors (i.e., dynamic externality and societal cynicism). In essence, the third model attempts to reconcile the first and the second models.

Results do not support the first model, but both the second and the third models were supported by favorable RMSEA and SRMR (Cheung et al., 2006). In summary, the original structures proposed by Leung and Bond are compatible with the results of this statistically more stringent analysis. However, we cannot rule out the model in which the five factors are equivalent across the two levels, but at the culture level, the five factors further group into two second-order factors. Nonetheless, even for this model, the more complex structure at the second level is clearly different from the relatively orthogonal five-factor model at the individual level. At this point, there are insufficient statistical grounds for differentiating the second and third models, and future work is needed to identify the better model.

LINKING INDIVIDUAL- AND CULTURE-LEVEL DIMENSIONS OF SOCIAL AXIOMS

...society now functions as the formulative agency of individual consciousness. (Berger, 1967, p. 15)

Meaning of Axiom Dimensions at the Individual Level

It is clear that social axioms exhibit different structures across the two levels, and in this section, we explore theoretically meaningful ways to link the dimensions across the two levels. The functionalist view of Leung and Bond (2004) assumes that at the individual level, the five axiom dimensions provide a framework for individuals to make effective choices in their actions and activities. Evolutionary psychologists suggest that people need to develop competence in two broad domains: social interaction and problem solving (Keller, 1997). In the social domain, an important ability is concerned with deceiving others and detecting deception so as to protect or expand one's own gains and not have them appropriated by others, phenomena which have been documented extensively among primates and humans (e.g., Humphrey, 1983; Whiten & Byrne, 1997). Varying degrees of social cynicism represent a cognitive response to these fundamental needs for survival and adaptation, as each person's position has been formulated in the rough-and-tumble of social living to date. However, social cynicism responds to broader concerns than deception, and includes a heightened concern with exploitation, oppression, and other negative elements of social life that threaten the well-being of a person negotiating a social system.

In the problem-solving domain, Leung and Bond (2004) propose three fundamental issues that must be resolved for effective management of daily challenges: First, individuals need to determine whether problems encountered are generally solvable, and what are the causes of these problems. Fate control represents a general judgment that fate controls the difficulties encountered in the social world, but *pari passu* that people are able to predict and alter the decree of fate so that they can mitigate or overcome these difficulties. Second, individuals need to have a general assessment of how likely problem-solving activities are to lead to success, and reward for application represents a general assessment of the cost-benefit features of individual actions and activities in response to environmental demands. Third, individuals need to have a general assessment of whether a contingent approach is required, or a "one-size-fits-all" strategy is adequate in problem solving. Persons who believe in a "complex" world accept inconsistency across different domains of social life and subscribe to contingent approaches that take into account situational and individual variations as causes of events. Such an assessment of how the world works suggests multiple solutions to any given problem and has significant consequences for the problem-solving styles adopted in a person's problem-solving activities.

Finally, humans differ in the degree of their need to seek meaning in their existence (e.g., Williams, 1997), and spiritual activities are an important and universal way of providing a sense of order and meaning to human existence. As Berger (1967) analyzes its functions, "Religion legitimates social institutions by bestowing upon them an ultimately valid ontological status, that is, by locating them within a sacred and cosmic frame of reference" (p. 33). Individuals within a given society endorse this belief in the function of religious institutions more or less strongly for themselves, making religiosity a variable individual belief. We argue that religiosity represents both a general response to the spiritual need of humans and a solution to many social problems. In fact, the items defining this dimension are mainly concerned with the perceived functionality of religious activities and institutions. As we read the content of the items defining this dimension, religiosity seems to be more concerned with solutions to the challenges of creating social order and encouraging civility than with the satisfaction of spiritual needs, which can of course be met outside the institutional framework of organized religious practice.

Meaning of the Axiom Dimensions at the Culture Level

While we propose that the five individual-level axiom dimensions provide a guide to individual behavior, this logic obviously does not apply to the culture level because culture does not have a consciousness of its own for making choices. Instead, researchers generally view culture-level dimensions as characterizations of cultural groups (e.g., Hofstede, 1980). Only two dimensions are identified at the societal level, suggesting that societies are less differentiated than are individuals in terms of their axiom profiles. Dynamic externality encompasses items from four individual-level axiom dimensions, and is primarily defined by items from reward for application and religiosity. We note that Bond et al. (2004) reported that dynamic externality is negatively correlated with national wealth, and we speculate that this conflation of items from different individual-level dimensions is primarily a response to poverty, and arises from the cultural press channeled through socialization agencies to overcome difficulties in survival.

Even after controlling for wealth, however, countries higher in dynamic externality are more likely to report a lower quality of life, a higher average number of people per room, a lower life expectancy, a higher adult illiteracy rate, a lower level of human development, lower human rights observance, lower political rights and civil liberties, a lower percentage of GDP spent on education and on health, a lower capacity for reducing human vulnerability by means of human sustenance and environmental health, a lower social and institutional capacity for environmental sustainability, and fewer TV receivers per capita. This profile suggests that even after differences in economic development have been controlled for, societies higher in dynamic externality are generally characterized by conservative educational, social, and political development. However, these aversive conditions result in cultural socialization of citizens for average belief profiles high in reward for application and religiosity, both orientations conducing toward entrepreneurialism and prosociality.

If a society constantly faces hardship associated with low living standards, social customs, structures, and institutions are likely to evolve into a configuration that is adaptive in the face of such hardship. Belief of its citizens in effort and hard work sustains the struggle against the hardship, and beliefs associated with religiosity conduce toward social order and civility. Fatalism reflects some degree of helplessness in the face of the hardship, but the belief that fate can be altered offers some control over the future. Finally, low social complexity focuses citizen attention and effort on subduing the hardships faced in a unified way. Viewed from this perspective, the covariation of these four axiom dimensions across societies seems interpretable as a consequence of the need to cope with difficult circumstances in living. An interesting observation is that individuals seem to be more varied than societies in how they react to hostile environments. For instance, it is easy to find both rich and poor individuals who are either religious or fatalistic, and that is why the four individual-level axiom dimensions do not cluster together. At the level of societies or nations, however, these four dimensions are not distinguishable.

Societal cynicism exhibits what Cheung et al. (2006) describe as "cross-level equivalence," or what Leung and Bond (1989) labeled a "strong etic" dimension, in that its content is similar across the two levels. This convergence implies that the individual belief system characterized by mistrust toward and disengagement from people and social systems corresponds to a cultural dimension of the same nature. For instance, Bond et al. (2004) reported that after controlling for economic development, societal cynicism is associated with lesser voter turnout in a nation, a lower average satisfaction with one's company or work organization, citizens' lower life satisfaction, a lower average level of conscientiousness (a factor in the big-five personality model), a general rejection of the view that leadership is based on charisma and values, generally more disagreement within in-groups, and a stronger belief among the citizenry in exerting an amount of effort that is proportional to the pay received. This pattern of national characteristics suggests a disengagement of a nation's citizenry, its human capital, from investment of their resources into their own society.

Individual- and culture-level dimensions are sometimes consequences of different dynamics and processes (Leung & Bond, 1989), but cynicism happens to be equivalent across levels. As described before, social cynicism has survival value because it helps individuals avoid social traps and scams. At the societal level, we argue that social and political turmoil along with instability in a nation may have moved its citizenry toward a cynical belief system troubled by such disintegrating and dangerous events. Consistent with this logic, those societies highest in societal cynicism tend to have experienced political or economic turmoil triggered by disruptive social changes in the past 20 years, such as those in Eastern Europe (Bond et al., 2004). Our functionalist perspective would argue that cynicism may be an adaptive belief constellation in societies marked by such unsettling events.

We note that both dynamic externality and societal cynicism are associated with hardship, but the source of that hardship appears to be different. Dynamic externality is primarily driven by poverty, and its correlation with GDP per capita is high ($r(39) = -.65$) (Bond et al., 2004). In contrast, societal cynicism is more driven by disruptive social, political, and economic changes that impinge on institutions and the lives of individuals. Such changes obviously affect the economic well-being of societies, but the correlation between societal cynicism and GDP per capita ($r(39) = -.40$) is lower than the $r(39) = -.65$ for dynamic externality (Bond et al., 2004).

Psycho-Logic and Eco-Logic: Insight from the Dimensions of Social Axioms

It is well-documented but underappreciated that the meaning of constructs may shift when moving between the individual level and the group level (e.g., Leung & Bond, 1989; Chan, 1998). Hofstede (1980, 2001) describes this phenomenon vividly by suggesting that individual-level dimensions are driven by psycho-logic, whereas culture-level dimensions are driven by eco-logic. These two types of logic are fundamentally different, and as psychologists, we are prone to err in applying psycho-logic to interpret culture-level phenomena, thus committing the "reverse ecological fallacy" (Hofstede, 1980, chap. 1). Unfortunately, we are thus far unable to articulate clearly what are the defining characteristics of these two types of logic. We propose that the social axioms project provides some insight for helping us to differentiate these two types of logic.

Different Theoretical Bases of Psycho-Logic and Eco-Logic

It is possible to develop different bases for psycho-logic and eco-logic, and then contrast their differences. We assume a functionalist perspective in interpreting axiom dimensions at the individual level, and this psycho-logic derives from concerns for individual survival, adaptation to social groups and self-extension. Each of the five axiom dimensions offers a unique approach for coping with the various demands of an individual's social living.

At the culture level, however, this psycho-logic cannot be directly applied. Instead, the eco-logic we adopt is derived from the basic premise that the membership in the same society is confronted with a shared set of problems, although the perceived intensity of the problems obviously varies to some degree across individual members. We argue that the intensity of this common set of problems confronting a given society shapes the characterization of that society in terms of its social customs, norms and laws, its social structures, and the goals of its institutions.

The case of dynamic externality provides a good illustration of this approach. We argue above that it delineates the belief constellation of societies that are confronted with a difficult external social and physical environment and have to bear the brunt of toil and hardship. Bond et al. (2004) reported some society-level correlations that are consistent with the two core definers of this dimension; namely, reward for application and religiosity. Societies high in dynamic externality are associated with less unemployment, more work hours per week, and a stronger competitive motive, echoing their endorsement of effort and hard work. Societies high in dynamic externality are indeed set up in a way that rewards application. As described before, the social welfare system of these societies is underdeveloped, and citizens of these societies have to count on their own efforts to make ends meet and cope with crises. The simple rule of survival seems to be the harder they work, the more they get.

In a similar vein, the positive association of dynamic externality with higher church attendance, more frequent praying, and a higher importance attached to religion and God is consistent with the endorsement of items from the belief dimension of religiosity. Difficult living seems to be associated with more involvement in religious institutions and practices. Religion is an integrative social force, and promotes the cooperation and spirit of self-sacrifice necessary to maximize societal development, whether that religious tradition is Weberian Protestantism, Bhakti Hinduism, or any other transcendent "ism." In summary, this reasoning suggests that the emphasis on investing one's resources into the struggle of life, religiosity, and to a smaller extent fate control and low social complexity, by societies high in dynamic externality is a collective response to the challenges posed for a group's survival by difficult circumstances and low living standards.

It is possible for psycho-logic and eco-logic to converge, and a case in point is societal cynicism, whose content is similar to that of social cynicism. Cross-level equivalence is evident, and some empirical results support this convergence. As mentioned before, societies higher in societal cynicism are likely to report a lower level of job satisfaction. Leung, Ip, and Leung (2007) further showed that in a longitudinal design, social cynicism is correlated negatively with job satisfaction at the individual level. In other words, cynicism is related to job satisfaction in a similar manner at the culture as well as the individual levels. In this case, a society may be viewed as a collection of people acting in unison, and what can be observed across individuals can be observed across societies.

As mentioned before, social cynicism has survival value for the individual. At the culture level, societies higher in societal cynicism are usually associated with political or economic turmoil triggered by rapid social changes over the past decades. Perhaps cynicism is also adaptive in a society marked by a history of disruptive events, working to demobilize citizens, to focus their attention onto personal matters, and to resist personal investment in social institutions. The survival value of cynicism at both levels seems to be able to account for the cross-level invariance of this axiom dimension.

Guidelines for Developing Theoretical Bases for Eco-logic

Our experience with the social axioms research has suggested three major guidelines for formulating theoretical bases characterizing eco-logic. The first guideline is concerned with the common experience of a cultural group. The theoretical basis for psycho-logic is necessarily oriented toward the individual, and psychology has a long history of developing such frameworks. For eco-logic, however, the focus is to explain why a society exhibits a certain profile, and the common puzzle is that the elements of this profile do not cluster together in a *psychologically* meaningful way. Take reward for application and fate control as examples. It is hard to understand psychologically why items reflecting a belief in hard work cluster with items emphasizing predetermination. While such a clustering does not occur across individuals, their covariation at the societal level is sensible if we assume that they are both responses of a cultural group confronted with hardship. As explained before, in a demanding context, many people subscribe to the functionality of hard work, and many people also see fate as an important force shaping social outcomes, because it is societally defocusing and disintegrating for citizens to see their society's hardships as caused by their own doing. This analysis suggests that the theoretical basis for an eco-logic should be tied to the common experience of a cultural group, and it is this common experience that provides a framework to account for psychologically puzzling patterns found at the culture level.

The second guideline involves a *contextual approach* to the interpretation of a culture-level construct. In individual-level research, an important way to determine the meaning of a construct is for the researcher to "phenomenologize" the items defining this construct; that is, to ponder what this constellation of items means for an individual person. However, for culture-level constructs, this approach usually does not work because, as pointed out before, the clustering of items often defies a psychological interpretation. For instance, the meanings of Hofstede's (2001) now-famous five cultural dimensions are not always readily apparent from an inspection of their constituent items, even though we often try to invest them with psychological interpretations they cannot logically bear. Those who work with constructs derived from an ecological analysis of averages from individual ratings must struggle carefully against psychologizing the labels they use to describe their constructs (Bond, 1994). The resulting "ecological" labels (e.g., Confucian work dynamism; Chinese Culture Connection, 1987), often sound bizarre to those trained as psychologists; those that fit our psychological traditions, like Hofstede's (1980) masculinity-femininity, generate no end of unnecessary controversy. Other labels that capture the societal-level features of the construct, like hierarchy (Schwartz, 1994) or integration (Chinese Culture Connection, 1987), are logically much more appropriate. It is often difficult for psychologists to name these constructs as systemic variables, since their composition derives from averages of psychological items. But, we must shift our labeling to correspond with our procedures!

In summary, to decipher the meaning of culture-level constructs, a contextual approach is needed, in which the constructs are assessed in light of socioeconomic-political dimensions as well as other societal features that may endow these constructs with meaning. In the case of dynamic externality, for example, our conjecture about its meaning is based on its correlations with low national wealth and a host of socioeconomic-political indicators (Bond et al., 2004).

The third guideline is concerned with the use of a *culture-level nomological network* to substantiate the interpretation of a culture-level construct. An advantage of society-level research is that a wide variety of country-level indexes are available for validating the meaning of a culture-level construct. As described before, dynamic externality is hypothesized to be related to poverty, and consistent with this argument, it is indeed related to a wide range of relevant, society-level indicators, as hypothesized. These relationships provide evidence for the association of dynamic externality with less favorable social, economic, and political development, and support the hardship argument advanced for interpreting the meaning of this dimension.

In fact, Hofstede (1980) employed a similar strategy to substantiate the interpretation of his dimensions of culture. Eco-logic can be evaluated with society-level indicators in the same way as a psychological construct is validated by means of a nomological network of relationships with other psychological-level variables. At this level of theorizing, we psychologists are doing sociology, a foreign discipline for most of us, and one requiring constructs and dynamics of its own. For most of us, this represents a paradigm shift, and, as Kuhn (1962) persuasively argues, such shifts are difficult to undertake personally or orchestrate in one's discipline.

REMAINING ISSUES AND DIRECTIONS FOR FUTURE RESEARCH

> When we add up all these factors—social definitions of reality, social relations that take these [definitions of reality] for granted, as well as the supporting therapies and legitimations—we have the total plausibility structure of the conception in question. (Berger, 1969, p. 52)

Linking Social Systems and Psychological Processes

A social system may be regarded as an integrated constellation of plausibility structures, a totality of social institutions, an ecological niche, an economic-political-legal-historical confluence that conduces toward a national-societal-cultural profile of beliefs defined by the two dimensions we have identified, societal cynicism and dynamic externality. Each national system will then generate a "plausibility press" resulting in its two scores on these dimensions.

We have already discussed some of the characteristics of social systems high or low on these two dimensions. To date, this work has been rather piecemeal, lacking a comprehensive model of social systems that lead to greater or lesser levels of societal cynicism or dynamic externality. It is also incomplete in that we cannot at present state how much of the explainable variance in these dimensions can be accounted for by antecedent variables, though it appears to be only moderate. Other unmeasured aspects of social systems probably contribute toward the plausibility press in one direction or the other. So, Bond et al. (2004) wrote,

> A cultural system, in both its objective and subjective manifestations, is responsive and adaptive (Berger & Luckman, 1966). Such subjective manifestations as beliefs will shift in response to changes in objective circumstances, both in terms of newly available resources and emerging constraints. Mapping of these subjective shifts will be potentiated by the availability of national indicators more likely to be connected to these subjective outcomes. (p. 567)

The availability of such indicators is, however, only a start to the creative theorizing needed. Just how do a social system and its characteristics function to shape any aspect of its citizens' psychological software, including beliefs? Addressing this question entails developing a model of how social systems operate with respect to psychological outcomes, exactly the question that will be later assessed by our multilevel modeling of psychological outcomes.

We psychologists are not well equipped by our disciplinary training to consider distal, systemic variables and their interrelationships. To be fair, we have attempted to examine national systems empirically, using available national indices in a bottom-up, data-driven way to discover the basic features of national systems. Cattell's initiative in factor analyzing these national indices led to the ambitious project called the "dimensions of nations" (Rummel, 1972). Sporadic attempts to characterize national systems have continued, most recently in the project spearheaded by Georgas, using Berry's eco-social framework as an orienting model (Georgas & Berry, 1995; Georgas, Van de Vijver, & Berry, 2004). These endeavors are intellectual stimuli, grist for our theoretical mill, that provide us with tools to conjure with, as we push ourselves towards a psychologically relevant theory about how a national system functions to shape psychological processes. In this essential work, we psychologists can learn from the work of other "big-picture" thinkers about the key drivers of social systems (e.g., Diamond, 1999) and about the ways that systems may function (e.g., Ball, 2004). We are just beginning to undertake this type of contextual thinking, but it is essential if we ever are to link distal variables like culture, to proximal outcomes, like individual behavior, in scientifically credible ways.

But theorizing about social systems is only a part of the intellectual challenge ahead. How does the psychologically relevant press of a given social system become internalized in the psychological structure of the individuals who function within that system? Each person is a genetically variable filtration system through whom that particular press must be drawn. This individual likewise occupies a particular culture-gender-age-class niche in that social system that we know will shape his or her belief profile (Singelis et al., 2003). In conjunction with one another, this cornucopia of influences acts in concert to produce the more microscopic outcomes we typically study as psychologists.

Additionally, and depending on the society an individual populates, he or she will enjoy some latitude of choice in the specific microsocial systems he or she joins. In discussing beliefs, Berger (1969) argues that, "One of the fundamental propositions of the sociology of knowledge is that the plausibility, in the sense of what people find credible, of views of reality depends on the social support these receive" (p. 50). Depending on the coherence of a society's subsystems with respect to the plausibility press of the overarching social system, an individual freer to choose will be able to join various microsocial support systems and develop an individual profile of beliefs different from that of his or her fellow citizen. At present we have little evidence on this process in general and none with respect to the socialization of social axioms.

This issue of socializing the psychological is central to the challenge posed by this edited collection of essays: How do we flesh out the intermediary steps between the societal and the individual levels of analysis? Each topic of psychological investigation (beliefs in the present case, dialectical

thinking, values, motivations, self-construals, relationship types, interpersonal norms), whatever psychological outcome is of interest, faces this
explanatory conundrum. How can we chart the translation of the cultural
or the national context into individual lives? As psychologists, this is our
task. Its successful accomplishment will require us to identify the levels
of influence on our psychological outcomes, and to explicate how these
levels interpenetrate.

CONCLUSION

In this chapter, we have explored the different meanings of axiom dimensions at the individual and culture levels, thus opening up several directions for future research. First, axiom dimensions at the culture level may
provide explanations for cultural similarities and differences that are not
readily accounted for by well-known value-based dimensions of cultural
variation. Second, individual-level axiom dimensions add to the repertoire of individual differences variables and provide a new framework for
understanding and predicting behavioral variations across individuals.

These two types of research involve a single level only, and are well-
known in cross-cultural research. A third, novel direction is made possible
by recent advances in multilevel theorizing and data-analytic techniques,
which permit the cross-level analysis of axiom dimensions. Take societal cynicism as an example. Societies vary in societal cynicism, and so
do individuals within a single society. A question arises as to whether
individuals high in cynicism would behave similarly across societies that
vary in societal cynicism. To answer this question, it is possible to set up a
two-level model and test whether societal (culture-level) and social (individual level) cynicism exert their effects on behaviors independently or
interactively. To complicate matters, contextual variables may moderate
the relationships between societal and social cynicism. That is, the effects
of societal and social cynicism may be independent in one societal context,
but their effects may interact in another societal context. At this point, it
is hard to speculate what kind of contextual variables may moderate the
effects of cynicism at the two levels, but it is clear that this line of enquiry
will take cross-cultural research to totally uncharted waters. Cross-level
analysis is nascent, but we believe that it will lead to many exciting dis-
coveries, providing the impetus for revolutionizing our thinking in many
domains of research. Social axioms provide an excellent content area to
demonstrate what cross-level analytic techniques are able to illuminate
and where they can take us in terms of theoretical advancement.

> The open question for man is not whether reality exists or not, but what he can make of it. Thus a man come to understand for himself what is happening— within and without—...as the impact of his own actions demonstrates what is possible. (Kelly, 1966, p. 26)

Author Note

This chapter was prepared with the support of a grant from the Hong Kong Research Grants Council (CityU 1466/05H).

REFERENCES

Ball, P. (2004). *Critical mass: How one thing leads to another.* London: Arrow.

Becker, G. (1996). The meta-analysis of factor analyses: An illustration based on the cumulation of correlation matrices. *Psychological Methods, 1,* 341–353.

Berger, P. L. (1967). *The sacred canopy: Elements of a sociological theory of religion.* Garden City, NY: Doubleday.

Berger, P. L. (1969). *A rumor of angels: Modern society and the rediscovery of the super-natural.* Harmondsworth: Penguin.

Berger, P. L., & Luckman, T. (1966). *The social construction of reality: A treatise in the sociology of knowledge.* Garden City, NY: Doubleday.

Bond, M. H. (1994). Into the heart of collectivism: A personal and scientific journey. In U. Kim, H. C. Triandis, C. Kagitcibasi, S. C. Choi, & G. Yoon (Eds.), *Individualism and collectivism: Theory, method, and applications* (pp. 66–76). Thousand Oaks, CA: Sage.

Bond, M. H., Leung, K., Au, A., Tong, K. K., Reimel de Carrasquel, S., Murakami, F. et al. (2004). Culture-level dimensions of social axioms and their societal correlates across 41 cultures. *Journal of Cross-Cultural Psychology, 35,* 548–570.

Chan, D. (1998). Functional relations among constructs in the same content domain at different levels of analysis: A typology of composition models. *Journal of Applied Psychology, 83,* 234–246.

Cheung, M. W. L., & Au, K. (2005). Applications of multilevel structural equation modeling to cross-cultural research. *Structural Equation Modeling, 12,* 598–619.

Cheung, M. W. L., Leung, K., & Au, K. (2006). Evaluating multilevel models in cross-cultural research: An illustration with social axioms. *Journal of Cross-Cultural Psychology, 37,* 522–541

Chinese Culture Connection (1987). Chinese values and the search for culture-free dimensions of culture. *Journal of Cross-Cultural Psychology, 18,* 143–164.

Diamond, J. (1999). *Guns, germs, and steel: The fate of human societies.* New York: Norton.

Georgas, J., & Berry, J. W. (1995). An ecocultural taxonomy for cross-cultural psychology. *Cross-Cultural Research, 29,* 121–57.

Georgas, J., van de Vijver, F., & Berry, J. W. (2004). The ecocultural framework, eco-social indices and psychological variables in cross-cultural research. *Journal of Cross-Cultural Psychology, 35*, 74–96.

Goldstein, H. (2003). *Multilevel statistical models* (3rd ed.). London: Arnold.

Hofstede, G. (1980). *Culture's consequences: International differences in work-related values*. Beverly Hills, CA: Sage.

Hofstede, G. (1991). *Cultures and organizations: Software of the mind*. London: McGraw-Hill.

Hofstede, G. (2001). *Culture's consequences: Comparing values, behaviors, institutions and organizations across nations* (2nd ed.). Thousand Oaks, CA: Sage.

House R. J, Hanges, P. J, Javidan, M., Dorfman, P., & Gupta, V. (Eds.). (2004). *Cultures, leadership, and organizations: GLOBE study of 62 societies*. Newbury Park, CA: Sage.

Humphrey, N. K. (1983). The adaptiveness of mentalism. *Behavioral and Brain Sciences, 6*, 343–390.

Inglehart, R., & Baker, W. E. (2000). Modernization, cultural change and the persistence of traditional values. *American Sociological Review, 65*, 19–51.

Keller, H. (1997). Evolutional approaches. In J. W. Berry, Y. H. Poortinga, & J. Pandey (Eds.), *Handbook of cross-cultural psychology* (Vol. 1, pp. 215–255). Boston, MA: Allyn & Bacon.

Kelly, G. A. (1955). *The psychology of personal constructs* (Vol. 1). New York: Norton.

Kelly, G. A. (1966). Ontological acceleration. In B. Maher (Ed.), *Clinical psychology and personality* (pp. 7–45). New York: Wiley.

Kluckhohn, F. R., & Strodtbeck, F. L. (1961). *Variations in value orientations*. Evanston, IL: Row, Peterson.

Kuhn, T. S. (1962). *The structure of scientific revolutions*. Chicago: University of Chicago Press.

Leung, K., & Bond, M. H. (1989). On the empirical identification of dimensions for cross-cultural comparisons. *Journal of Cross-Cultural Psychology, 20*, 133–151.

Leung, K., Bond, M. H., Reimel de Carrasquel, S., Muñoz, C., Hernández, M., Murakami, F. et al. (2002). Social axioms: The search for universal dimensions of general beliefs about how the world functions. *Journal of Cross-Cultural Psychology, 33*, 286–302.

Leung, K., & Bond, M. H. (2004). Social axioms: A model for social beliefs in multi-cultural perspective. *Advances in Experimental Social Psychology, 36*, 119–197.

Leung, K., Ip, O., & Leung, K. K. (2007). Longitudinal analysis of effects of social cynicism and well-being on job satisfaction. Paper submitted for publication.

Muthén, B. O. (1994). Multilevel covariance structure analysis. *Sociological Methods and Research, 22*, 376–398.

Osgood, C. E., Suci, G. J., & Tannenbaum, P. H. (1957). *The measurement of meaning*. Urbana: University of Illinois Press.

Preston, J., & Epley, N. (2005). Explanations versus applications: The explanatory power of valuable beliefs. *Psychological Science, 16*, 826–832.

Rokeach, M. (1973). *The nature of human values*. Glencoe, IL: Free Press.

Rotter, J. B. (1966). Generalized expectancies for internal versus external control of reinforcement. *Psychological Monographs, 80*, 1–28.

Rummel, R. J. (1972). *The dimensions of nations*. Beverly Hills, CA: Sage.

Schwartz, S. H. (1992). The universal content and structure of values: Theoretical advances and empirical tests in 20 countries. *Advances in Experimental Social Psychology, 25*, 1–65.

Schwartz, S. H. (1994). Beyond individualism and collectivism: New cultural dimensions of values. In U. Kim, H. C. Triandis, C. Kagitcibasi, S. C. Choi, & G. Yoon (Eds.), *Individualism and collectivism: Theory, method and applications* (pp. 85–119). Thousand Oaks, CA: Sage.

Singelis, T. M, Her, P., Aaker, J., Bhawuk, D. P. S., Gabrenya, W., Gleaned, M. et al. (2003). *Ethnic and regional differences in social axioms.* Unpublished manuscript, California State University.

Smith, P. B., Dugan, S., & Trompenaars, F. (1996). National culture and managerial values: A dimensional analysis across 43 nations. *Journal of Cross-Cultural Psychology, 27*, 231–264.

Van de Vijver, F. J. R., & Poortinga, Y. H. (2002). Structural equivalence in multi-level research. *Journal of Cross-Cultural Psychology, 33*, 141–156.

Van Hemert, D. A., Van de Vijver, F. J. R., & Poortinga, Y. H. (2002). The Beck Depression Inventory as a measure of subjective well-being: A cross-national study. *Journal of Happiness Studies, 3*, 257–286.

Whiten, A., & Byrne, R. W. (Eds.) (1997). *Machiavellian intelligence II: Extensions and evaluations.* Cambridge: Cambridge University Press.

Williams, K. D. (1997). Social ostracism. In R. M. Kowalski (Ed.), *Aversive interpersonal behaviors* (pp. 133–170). New York: Plenum.

9

Can We Learn about National Differences in Happiness from Individual Responses? A Multilevel Approach

---

Richard E. Lucas and Ed Diener

Psychologists have been interested in subjective well-being (SWB) for a number of reasons. For one thing, researchers pursue an understanding of SWB because they believe such an understanding could lead to the identification of the fundamental nature of human beings. According to this reasoning, it should be possible to identify basic needs by studying hedonic reactions to various life circumstances (Veenhoven, 1995; Wilson, 1967). For instance, if strong social relationships reliably lead to higher well-being and the lack of such bonds reliably lead to lowered well-being, then one could argue that human beings have a *basic need* for belonging-ness (Baumeister & Leary, 1995). Similarly, if factors such as income and material possessions are uncorrelated with well-being, one might argue that humans are not inherently materialistic beings.

Yet SWB is not simply a tool that psychologists use to develop theories about human nature. Psychologists also realize that SWB is a valued end in itself. Most people desire high levels of happiness. In fact, when asked to evaluate the life outcomes they would find most desirable, people report that being happy is more valued than almost any other outcome. Diener and Oishi (2004) showed that participants from 28 nations consistently ranked happiness as more important than wealth, attractiveness, health, love and affection, and even going to heaven! Therefore, psychologists study well-being because they hope to identify factors that will allow people to achieve a permanent increase in their feelings of happiness.

To accomplish these goals, researchers often begin by using cross-sectional, between-person designs to identify robust correlates of well-being. More sophisticated experimental or longitudinal designs can then be used to follow up these initial findings and to identify the processes that are responsible for these effects. For instance, researchers have noted that in between-person analyses, marital status exhibits robust associations with SWB variables (Haring-Hidore, Stock, Okun, & Witter, 1985; Wood, Rhodes, & Whelan, 1989). After identifying this association, researchers turned to more sophisticated designs to clarify the processes underlying this effect. Within-person analyses show that at least some of the differences between marital groups are due to lasting changes that occur following marital events like widowhood and divorce (Lucas, 2005; Lucas, Clark, Georgellis, & Diener, 2003).

After decades of research, social scientists have turned to an additional level of analysis to understand the processes that underlie SWB—the analysis of national differences. Initially, these studies were conducted because they provided a convenient way to test basic theories about well-being. Oftentimes, participants in single-nation psychological studies of SWB vary little on the variables of interest. In contrast, participants from different nations often exhibit greater variability in these predictor variables. For instance, most of the college students who typically participate in psychological studies have their basic needs met. Therefore, it is impossible to determine whether basic needs have an influence on well-being without finding populations where such needs are left unmet. When nationally representative surveys are available, they provide a convenient source of data for testing hypotheses using samples with greater variability (e.g., Diener, Diener, & Diener, 1995).

In addition, recent developments in the way that SWB measures are used have led to a more intense focus on national differences by a wider group of researchers. For instance, economists have argued that in addition to being a desired goal, SWB may be an indicator of experienced utility (Frey & Stutzer, 2002; Kahneman, 1994). Thus, SWB might be used by individuals to guide economic decisions, and thus, the construct should be studied by economists. Extending this idea, economists, psychologists, and public policy makers have suggested that well-being measures can be used to guide policy decisions. Diener and Seligman (2004) argued that many policy decisions are geared toward increasing the economic or physical health of a population. However, these outcomes are desired because they are thought to lead to greater happiness. Because each is only imperfectly (and often only weakly) correlated with the ultimate outcome of happiness, policy makers may want to focus on developing policies that have the explicit goal of increasing well-being. To accomplish this goal, it will be necessary to measure and track SWB levels of large populations.

Yet the extension of research on SWB to national level requires a shift in levels of analysis. Of course, such shifts can often lead to ambiguities in interpretation, and drawing conclusions about phenomena at one level using data that are measured at another level may not always be appropriate. In this chapter, we first discuss some concerns that have been raised about between-nation analyses of SWB constructs. We then review research on the within- and between-nation correlates of well-being. Finally, we present new research that investigates the comparability of the well-being construct at different levels of analysis.

CONCERNS ABOUT BETWEEN-NATION ANALYSES

As Van de Vijver and Poortinga (2002) have noted, shifting levels of analysis can lead to a number of errors in interpretation, and these various errors fall along two underlying dimensions. The first dimension reflects structure errors versus level errors. According to Van de Vijver and Poortinga, "a *structure error* refers to the use of a concept at a level to which it does not apply, whereas a *level error* refers to the incorrect attribution of a score value from one aggregation level to another" (p. 142). The second dimension reflects aggregation errors versus disaggregation errors. Aggregation errors occur when "characteristics of a lower hierarchical level of aggregation (e.g., a person) are incorrectly attributed to some higher level (e.g., an organization or country)" (Van de Vijver & Poortinga, 2002, p. 142). Disaggregation errors occur "when a higher order characteristic is incorrectly attributed to a lower order" (p. 142).

Four broad errors can result from the combination of these two underlying dimensions. For instance, a disaggregation/structure error occurs when one assumes that a construct that is measured at a higher level has a similar meaning at a lower level. In contrast, an aggregation/structure error would occur when one assumes that a construct that is measured at a lower level has a similar meaning at a higher level. This latter type of error is particularly relevant to discussions of SWB because happiness (which is measured at the individual level) may have a completely different meaning when aggregated at the national level. As we discuss below, once individual differences are averaged out, the remaining nation-level variance may simply reflect response styles or a general tendency to respond with greater positivity.

It is important to note that cross-level interpretational errors do not only occur when conducting nation-level analyses. SWB researchers often work at the level of the individual, yet they often apply their research findings to theories about within-person processes. For example, as we review below, social activity and social relationships are reliably associated with SWB in between-person studies. This fact may lead psychologists to suggest that an individual could increase his or her happiness by participating in more social activities. However, the cross-level parallelism that is implied by such advice may not always exist. In fact, Lucas, Le, and Dyrenforth (2005) showed that for some types of social activity, between-person analyses lead to different conclusions than do within-person analyses. Although within-person analyses show that spending time at parties and in bars is fun (i.e., people report more positive affect when at parties or bars than when they are not at parties or bars), between-person analyses show that people who spend more time at parties and bars are no happier than those who spend less time in these activities. This lack of cross-level parallelism is likely due to a shift in the meaning of "time spent in parties and bars" as one moves from the within- to the between-person level. Although parties are fun, the extent to which an individual spends time at parties is a variable that may index personality characteristics that are unrelated or negatively associated with happiness. In this case, within- and between-person analyses provide different information.

Although issues of cross-level comparisons arise when examining within- and between-person data, these issues are often more salient when national differences (or other cross-cultural comparisons) are discussed (Hui & Triandis, 1985). This is because there are often prominent differences among cultural groups, and any number of plausible explanations could be developed to account for national differences in reports of well-being. For instance, Kahneman and Riis (2005) raised the concern that when aggregated within nations, SWB scores may reflect nothing more than "culturally determined positivity" (p. 10). In other words, national levels of happiness may not reflect the true happiness of the population. Instead, between-nation variance may simply reflect something akin to a response set. In support of this idea, Kahneman and Riis made two arguments.

First, when examining national levels, the differences between nations are often too large, at least when considered in light of what we know about the within-nation effects of important life circumstances. For example, Kahneman and Riis (2005) pointed out that the French tend to be less happy than Americans. In the 1981, 1990, and 1999 World Values surveys, participants from France reported average life satisfaction scores of 6.71 (SD = 2.08), 6.78 (SD = 1.98), and 7.01 (SD = 1.99). By comparison, participants from the United States reported much higher average life satisfaction scores: 7.66 (SD = 1.96), 7.73 (SD = 2.01), and 7.66 (SD = 1.82).[1] Kahneman and Riis noted that the difference between the two nations is consistently as large as the within-nation difference between employed and unemployed individuals. Thus, an employed French person is as happy as an unemployed American, a finding that they considered to be implausible.

In addition, Kahneman and Riis (2005) suggested that aggregated levels of life satisfaction correlate too strongly with other suspect self-report ratings. Specifically, they showed that among a select group of 18 wealthy Western nations, life satisfaction and self-reports of health correlate .85.

Although this could be interpreted as evidence for the importance of health in determining one's life satisfaction, Kahneman and Riis (2005) suggested that self-reports of health were themselves "reality free." Specifically, they showed that among these 18 wealthy nations, self-reports of health were completely unrelated to "the most widely used objective measure of national health, adult life expectancy" (p. 10). Thus, if aggregated levels of self-reported health are unrelated to an objective measure of national health and aggregated levels of self-reported health are strongly correlated with aggregated levels of life satisfaction, then this suggests that aggregated levels of life satisfaction may also be "reality free."

Yet both of these arguments rely on potentially inappropriate cross-level comparisons. For instance, when Kahneman and Riis (2005) suggested that the difference between the United States and France is too large, they relied on their knowledge of the size of within-nation effects to make this judgment. However, within-nation effects often provide inappropriate comparison standards against which to compare the size of between-nation effects. Intuition may not serve researchers well when comparing findings across levels.

In addition, the claim that national levels of self-reported health are reality free may be too strong. Although it is true that one would hope these measures would correlate with objective measures of health, the fact that they do not correlate with one particular indicator does not necessarily suggest a problem. For one thing, by restricting their analysis to relatively wealthy nations of the Organisation for Economic Co-operation and Development (OECD), Kahneman and Riis (2005) limited the amount of variance that exists in their criterion measure. This range restriction naturally reduces correlations. Repeating the analyses using the full set of OECD nations (which are themselves fairly select) results in a much higher (though still far from perfect) correlation between self-reported health and adult life expectancy: $r = .55$, $p < .01$.

Furthermore, there may be other factors that legitimately affect one's health that are independent of life expectancy (particularly in a set of nations with particularly high life expectancy). For instance, the OECD provides reports about a variety of health outcomes and health predictors. These additional health measures can help establish the validity of both self-reports and national life expectancy as indicators of global national health. Even in the fairly select group of 18 wealthy OECD nations, self-reports of health correlate moderately with other health-related variables including the number of cavities and missing teeth the nations' citizens have by age 12 ($r = -.59$, $p < .05$), the amount of fat calories that the average person eats ($r = -.59$, $p < .05$), and the average amount of alcohol that the average person drinks ($r = -.51$, $p < .05$). Importantly, national life expectancy is uncorrelated with theoretically relevant variables such as per capita health expenditures ($r = .15$, *ns*), rates of injuries due to car accidents ($r = .04$, *ns*), or the amount of fat ($r = -.04$, *ns*) and alcohol ($r = .23$, *ns*) in the average citizen's diet.[2] Although life expectancy may be the most widely cited health statistic *for some purposes*, the weak correlations between this statistic and other relevant variables show that it does not provide a comprehensive index of a unified national health construct.

Finally, other research directly addresses concerns about the association between national character and reports of well-being, and results from these studies do not always support a culturally based positivity explanation. For instance, both Steel and Ones (2002) and Van Hemert, Van de Vijver, and Poortinga (2002) examined the correlations between two well-being measures and various self-reported nation-level predictors. Both studies found that national levels of happiness correlated negatively with national levels of social desirability (as measured by the Eysenck Personality Lie Scale).

The point that we are trying to make is that it may be tempting to use knowledge about within-nation effects to evaluate cross-national differences; yet such comparisons may be inappropriate and misleading. One must be cautious when making the leap from the individual level to the national level, and methodologies designed for multilevel analysis should ideally be used. In the remainder of this chapter, we discuss what we can learn about national differences in well-being from individual responses. Then we use techniques that are appropriate for multilevel data to investigate the psychometric properties of national measures of well-being.

RESEARCH ON THE CORRELATES OF HAPPINESS

Researchers have been studying SWB for decades, and there now exists a large database of findings. This literature shows that many external life circumstances that were once expected to strongly predict well-being are often only weakly related to happiness (Diener, Suh, Lucas, & Smith, 1999, for a review). In contrast, certain personality characteristics consistently exhibit moderate to strong correlations (Diener & Lucas, 1999). Below we review the literature on the individual-level correlates of SWB, focusing specifically on those variables that could potentially translate into important cross-national differences. We then discuss the extent to which these correlations replicate at the national level. Because this chapter focuses on the issue of multilevel data in cross-cultural research, we do not have enough space to provide a complete review. Thus, what follows is just a brief sketch of some of the most robust findings.

Income

Perhaps the most surprising finding reported in the literature is that at the individual level, money does not seem to matter much for happiness (Myers, 2000). Lucas and Dyrenforth (2006) recently reviewed the conclusions from two meta-analyses (Haring, Stock, & Okun, 1984; Pinquart & Sörensen, 2000), a narrative review of cross-national results (Diener & Biswas-Diener, 2002), and many waves of a yearly nationally representative survey (the General Social Survey; Davis, Smith, & Marsden, 2003). Their review showed that the correlation between income and happiness tends to fall between .17 and .21. Although this correlation is robust, it is small by traditional standards, accounting for at most 4% of the variance in SWB measures. This appears to support the counterintuitive finding that money does not buy happiness.

We must caution, however, that such correlations must be interpreted carefully. If income and happiness correlate .20, then this means that for each standard deviation increase in income, there is a corresponding increase of about one fifth of a standard deviation in happiness. It is unclear whether an effect of this size would contradict people's intuition. Because income standard deviations tend to be fairly small, people may not expect a one standard deviation increase to have a strong effect on their happiness. Instead, when they say that they believe money will increase happiness, they may mean that they believe winning a million dollars (which is many standard deviations above the mean income) will increase their happiness several points. In this case, the empirical evidence might support their intuition.

It is also true that most people would probably agree that money is not the *only* factor that influences happiness. Because happiness is multiply determined, there may be a fairly low upper limit to the size of the correlation between any one factor and happiness (Ahadi & Diener, 1989). Thus, the low correlation may actually be quite consistent with people's intuition. Finally, research consistently shows that most people are happy most of the time (Diener & Diener, 1996). This may be the most surprising aspect of the income/happiness relation—even people with the lowest incomes report happiness scores that are in the positive range. However, even this fact may not be as counterintuitive as it may first seem. People may report very low income for many reasons, not all of which would be expected to lead to low levels of SWB. In addition, those individuals who have very low incomes but who are available to participate in national surveys may not be the most destitute, even if they have low incomes. In support of this idea, Veenhoven (1995) showed that the size of the association between income and happiness is stronger in poorer nations than in richer nations, and Biswas-Diener and Diener (2001) showed even among two very poor groups, resources made a difference in happiness. Slum dwellers in Calcutta were significantly more satisfied with their life than were pavement dwellers. Thus, although it is true that income exhibits relatively weak associations with SWB variables, this finding does not necessarily mean that money does not matter for individuals' happiness.

Because of these concerns, researchers have turned to nation-level studies as a way to resolve questions about the role of income in happiness. Virtually every study that has looked at cross-national differences in happiness has examined the role of income (e.g., Arrindell et al., 1997; Diener et al., 1995; Easterlin, 1995; Economist Intelligence Unit, 2005; Inglehart & Klingemann, 2000; Kirkcaldy, Furnham, & Martin, 1998; Schyns, 1998; Steel & Ones, 2002; Van Hemert, Van de Vijver, & Poortinga, 2002). Diener and Biswas-Diener (2002) reported that the correlations between per capita income (or other similar variables) and national happiness tend to fall between .50 and .70. Consistent with individual-level data, there appear to be diminishing returns for national levels of income (Diener & Seligman, 2004). Once a nation reaches about U.S.$10,000 in per capita income, there are only small increases in happiness with increasing wealth (Frey & Stutzer, 2002; Helliwell, 2003a; Schyns, 2003). This finding suggests that wealth matters only until a set of basic needs are met. In an analysis that addressed this hypothesis directly, Diener et al. (1995) predicted national SWB from income after controlling for basic needs. They showed that per capita income still predicted national SWB, even after controlling for the extent to which basic needs were being met.

Different researchers have arrived at different conclusions about the effect of income change on national levels of well-being. For instance, among wealthy nations, dramatic changes in per capita income have led to few if any lasting increases in happiness over time (Diener & Biswas-Diener, 2002; Easterlin, 1995). However, Hagerty and Veenhoven (2003) found that in a sample of 21 nations examined over time, there were significant correlations between income and happiness in six nations and nonsignificant correlations in all others. Importantly, there were no significant negative correlations. Hagerty and Veenhoven also found evidence that increases in income are associated with the biggest increases in happiness among poorer nations.

These results show that at both the individual and national level, income is associated with happiness. The associations tend to be weaker at the individual level than at the national level (as might be expected based on the principles of aggregation; see Diener & Biswas-Diener, 2002, for a review). In addition, the associations tend to be weaker among wealthier individuals and wealthy populations. However, this may be due to the fact that moderately wealthy individuals and nations get very close to the theoretical maximum score on well-being measures. Diener and Seligman (2004), for example, presented a figure plotting per capita Gross Domestic Product against national life satisfaction. They showed that the wealthiest nations had average life satisfaction scores between 7 and 8 on a zero to 10 scale. Unless we expect every individual in a wealthy nation to be happy (even those with poor health, poor relationships, and unhappy personalities), it it may be unreasonable to expect average happiness scores for any group to exceed 8.

Health

A second individual difference that has relevance for between-nation comparisons is health. As with income, intuition might suggest that health should be strongly correlated with happiness, particularly since people tend to say that health is the most highly valued life domain in their lives (Campbell, Converse, & Rodgers, 1976). A great deal of research confirms that health and well-being are correlated, at least when subjective measures of health are assessed. For instance, Okun, Stock, Haring, and Witter (1984) conducted a meta-analysis of over 200 effect sizes, and they found correlations around .30. Similarly, in our own analysis of the most recent World Values Survey (World Values Survey, 2006), the unweighted average within-nation correlation between single-item measures of self-reported health and global life satisfaction was .23. Thus, perceptions of health are associated with self-reported levels of happiness.

Yet other studies suggest that the association weakens considerably or even disappears when more objective measures of health are examined. Okun and George (1984), for instance, found that in most of the studies they reviewed, physician ratings of health were not significantly correlated with well-being. Similarly, Brief, Butcher, George, and Link (1993) found that although subjective reports of health tended to correlate around .30 to .40 with life satisfaction, more objective reports of health (in the form of self-reported doctor and hospital visits) only correlated about .10 with life satisfaction. Thus, the discrepancy across measures raises questions about the nature of this association. Are unhealthy people less happy than healthy people, or do unhappy people simply perceive their health as being bad? If the latter is true, why do people believe that health will have such a large impact on their happiness?

As with income, correlations between health and happiness are complicated, and a number of issues have not fully been resolved. First, it is not clear whether objective measures such as doctors' ratings, symptom checklists, or records of hospital visits are more valid than participants' own global evaluations. Although doctors' ratings and other such measures are less subjective than self-reports of global health, they may not capture all aspects of health. Thus, individuals who visit the doctor infrequently or who have similar numbers of symptoms may exhibit wide variability in actual health.

In addition, it is possible that typical objective measures are simply wrong. In support of this idea, Nelson et al. (1983) showed that when doctors were asked about the reasons for the discrepancies between physician and patient ratings of health, the doctors admitted that 44% of the disagreements were due to clinician error. An additional 12% were due to insufficient knowledge of the patients. This study demonstrates that objective reports can be flawed and that patients' subjective ratings may actually be more valid than physician ratings. In fact, a number of studies have now shown that subjective reports of health can predict outcomes such as longevity, even after controlling for objective reports of health (Ganz, Lee, & Siau, 1991; McClellan, Anson, Birkeli, & Tuttle, 1991; Mossey & Shapiro, 1982; Rumsfeld et al., 1999). Thus, it is unclear whether researchers should dismiss the moderate correlations between subjective health and SWB simply because the correlations weaken when objective measures are used.

Finally, it is possible that people who tend to be included in psychological research studies are in relatively good health. One way to address this concern would be to conduct research on individuals with relatively extreme health conditions. And although psychologists initially believed that people adapt to a wide variety of health conditions, Diener, Lucas, and Scollon (2006) have shown that many of these findings have been misinterpreted. For instance, researchers often cite Brickman, Coates, and Janoff-Bulman's (1978) classic study of lottery winners and spinal-cord-injured patients as evidence that people have a remarkable ability to adapt to just about any life circumstance. Brickman et al. concluded that the spinal-cord-injured patients were not as unhappy as one might expect. Diener et al., however, pointed out that this small group of patients was, in fact, significantly less happy than a control group, and this difference was large by traditional standards ($d = .78$). A number of reviews have confirmed that the spinal-cord-injured people report happiness levels that are considerably lower than those of control groups (Dijkers, 1997; Hammell, 2004). And furthermore, Lucas (2007) used two large-scale, nationally representative panel studies to show that the onset of a permanent disability leads to drops in life satisfaction varying from moderate to large, and very little adaptation occurs over time. Thus, these studies suggest that major health problems can have large effects on happiness.

Fewer studies have directly linked national levels of SWB to national levels of health than studies that have linked SWB with income; however, those that do, suggest that health plays a role. As Kahneman and Riis (2005) noted, self-reports of health correlate strongly with self-reports of life satisfaction. For example, in the 47 nations from the most recent World Values Survey that have both life satisfaction and self-reported health data, the correlation across all nations is .52, $p < .001$. In addition, life satisfaction also correlates with objective measures of health. For instance, life expectancy at birth correlates .62, $p < .001$ with average life satisfaction in the 77 nations that participated in one of the two most recent World Values Surveys. The Economist Intelligence Unit (2005) showed that this effect held even after controlling for income and a variety of other nation-level characteristics. Finally, Diener et al. (1995) examined a composite "basic needs" variable that consisted of four separate health-related statistics: the percent of a population with access to safe drinking water, the rate of infant mortality, the mean life expectancy, and the percent of a population with sanitary toilet facilities. This composite measure correlated between .37 and .60 with four separate measures that consistently show that national differences in health play a role in national well-being.

Social Relationships

Psychologists have long recognized the benefits of social relationships for a wide variety of important outcomes in people's lives. Decades worth of research shows that social relationships seem to have a protective effect when it comes to risk for mental illness, poor physical health, and even risk of death (e.g., Berkman & Syme, 1979; House, Landis, & Umberson, 1988; House, Robbins, & Metzner, 1982). Thus, it is not a surprise that relationships have also been linked with SWB. In his broad review of the external correlates of happiness, Argyle stated that "social relationships have a powerful effect on happiness and other aspects of well-being, and are perhaps its greatest single cause" (2001, p. 71). Similarly, Myers suggested that although "age, gender, and income...give little clue to someone's happiness...better clues come from knowing...whether [people] enjoy a supportive network of close relationships" (2000, p. 65). These statements suggest that social relationships are probably the most important factor in determining one's level of happiness.

We agree that social relationships matter, but the story is, again, not so simple. As argued elsewhere (Lucas & Dyrenforth, 2006), most of the major reviews that have been cited in support of the strong effects of social relationships have two limitations. First, they rarely review evidence about the existence of social relationships or the amount of time spent with relationship partners. Instead, the studies that are reviewed often focus on the extent to which individuals *value* relationships or report being *satisfied* with their relationships. These more subjective variables are likely to correlate with happiness for reasons other than the effects of relationships on happiness. For instance, it is difficult to determine whether a relationship satisfaction measure reflects the quality of that relationship or a general tendency to be satisfied with domains in one's life. The strong correlations between relationship satisfaction and satisfaction with other domains (including satisfaction with one's environment, with one's housing, and with one's income) suggest that the latter is at least partially true.

Second, many major reviews fail to report effect sizes for the variables that they examine. Because of this limitation, Lucas and Dyrenforth (2006) collected evidence from a series of meta-analyses along with a number of nationally representative surveys. They found that social relationship variables are significantly associated with happiness, but the effect sizes tend to be quite small—smaller even than the effect of income. Variables such as the size of one's social network, the number of close friends that one can name, and the amount of time spent with various friends and acquaintances all tend to correlate less than .20 with a variety of SWB variables. Thus, social relationship variables represent a robust correlate of happiness, but their effects are similar to the size of other predictors including income and health.

Existing research also shows that one particularly important relationship—marriage—tends to be weakly, though consistently related to happiness (Haring-Hidore et al., 1985; Mastekaasa, 1994; Wood et al., 1989). Married people are happier than single people, who in turn are happier than those who are widowed or divorced. Again, however, the effect sizes tend to be small. Haring-Hidore et al. reported an average correlation of just .14 between marital status and well-being. In addition, Lucas et al. (2003) and Lucas (2005) showed that only widowhood and divorce were associated with lasting changes in happiness over time. People who got married quickly adapted back to their baseline levels of happiness and reported no lasting change in happiness.

It is possible that the effects of social relationship also influence happiness at the national level. For instance, the Economist Intelligence Unit (2005) attempted to predict national life satisfaction ratings from nine specific factors including family life (operationalized as divorce rate) and community life (operationalized as church attendance and trade-union membership). Although they did not report raw correlations, both factors significantly predicted life satisfaction, even after controlling for all the other variables. Using a different database of national happiness scores, Diener et al. (1995) found that divorce rates correlated .31 with an aggregate of four national happiness measures (though correlations ranged from .04 to .57). Interestingly, van Hemert et al. (2002) found that the percent of men and women who were married was negatively correlated with SWB and positively correlated with national levels of depression. However, this study included a relatively small sample of nations.

The implications of the association between social relationships and SWB at the national level are, at this point, unclear. On the one hand, Putnam (2001) suggested that social capital can lead to increases in many dimensions of quality of life, and Helliwell (2003b) showed that happiness levels are high (and suicide rates are low) where trust in others is high. This has led some to suggest that increasing individualism leads to declines in social capital and a lessened importance of social relationships. In turn, this should lead to reduced happiness over time. However, Veenhoven (1999) argued against such an interpretation and showed that more individualistic nations tend to be happier than less individualistic nations. Diener et al. (1995) even showed that this effect is significant and strong even after controlling for a variety of related variables including income. Furthermore, Allik and Realo (2004) showed that individualistic nations had higher levels of social capital. Of course, the links between individualism, social capital, and social relationships may not be straightforward. Therefore, nation-level research on all three variables will be required before this question can be resolved.

Personality

One of the most surprising things about happiness is the extent to which it appears, at least in part, to be built in to the person. Researchers know that happiness is heritable—twin and adoption studies show that at least 40 to 50% of the variance in happiness can be explained by genes (e.g., Lykken & Tellegen, 1996). In addition, research shows that happiness is at least moderately stable over time (Fujita & Diener, 2005). Thus, it is not surprising that some of the strongest predictors of happiness are stable personality traits. For instance, a great deal of research shows that the personality trait of neuroticism is strongly related to negative affect and the personality trait of extraversion is strongly related to positive affect (Costa & McCrae, 1980; see Diener & Lucas, 1999, for a review). It is important to note that these associations are not simply due to the fact that both are assessed using self-report methods. Even when a variety of methods of assessing personality or happiness are used, the correlations are moderate to strong.

One possible explanation of these associations is that personality affects other external factors, and these external factors then influence happiness. For instance, extraverts may have more friends or their increased sociability may make them more successful at work. However, the fact that the effects of personality tend to be much larger than the effects of these potentially mediating factors reduces the likelihood of such explanations. Furthermore, studies that have directly tested these effects tend to find that personality is still related to well-being even after controlling for a number of potential mediators. For instance, Lucas et al. (in press) showed that even after controlling for a variety of measures of social contact, extraverts were still happier than introverts. Because of this literature, many personality researchers believe that there is a direct, physiological link between the personality traits of extraversion and neuroticism and the emotional traits of positive and negative affect.

The strong correlation between personality and happiness has an important implication for research on national levels of well-being. If much of the variance that exists among individuals is due to differences in personality, then researchers must be careful when using individual-level data to interpret between-nation effects. At the individual level, temperament effects may swamp any environmental effects, which in turn may lead to the impression that very little matters for well-being. However, once responses are aggregated within an entire nation, individual differences should be eliminated, and much of the remaining variance may be due to the effects of external circumstances. Of course, it is possible that there are valid national differences in personality (Steel & Ones, 2002), but theoretical and empirical work on the existence of such differences is quite limited at this point.

Additional Predictors

Although researchers have looked at a variety of additional demographic characteristics and their associations with happiness, few of these investigations have identified strong correlations. And of the additional correlates that have emerged, few have relevance for between-nation analyses. For instance, there are few sex differences in well-being, and those that are found tend to be quite small (Haring et al., 1984; Lucas & Gohm, 2000). Similarly, although questions about the effect of age on well-being have not completely been resolved, most research suggests that changes over much of the lifespan are not large (though there is a steeper drop-off in late life, particularly as one approaches death; Mroczek & Spiro, 2005). Education and intelligence also have positive, but very weak associations with happiness.

Yet one other individual difference variable that could play a role in national differences in well-being is religion or religiosity. Individual-level research consistently shows that religious people tend to be happier than the nonreligious (Diener et al., 1999; Ferriss, 2002). The mechanisms behind this effect are not clear, though it could be due to the greater social support that one receives from being involved in a group or to the sense of meaning that belief in something larger than oneself provides. In any case, the effect also seems to exist at the national level. For instance, Helliwell (2003a) found that at the national level, belief in a god and attendance at religious services are associated with average happiness.

There are also additional nation-level characteristics that have no individual-level counterpart. For instance, a number of researchers have shown that characteristics of government predict national happiness or even differences in regional happiness within nations. Diener et al. (1995) showed that human rights correlate with happiness, and both Donovan and Halpern (2003) and Inglehart and Klingemann (2000) showed that the extent of democracy within a nation predicts national SWB. Frey and Stutzer (2000, 2002) were even able to show that within a single nation (Switzerland), an index of direct democracy was associated with regional well-being. Unfortunately, many of these characteristics are highly correlated with one another, and disentangling their effects is difficult. Many of the studies that we have reviewed use the same or overlapping datasets. And because national measures of well-being are often hard to acquire, sample sizes tend to be small. Thus, regression analyses that attempt to identify the unique contribution of various variables are often unstable across studies. As a result, different researchers sometimes come to different conclusions about which factors have unique effects on national well-being. It is likely that these questions will begin to be resolved as more and more nations track the well-being of their citizens.

MULTILEVEL FACTOR ANALYSIS OF WELL-BEING MEASURES

As Van de Vijver and Poortinga (2002) noted, one way to avoid aggregation and disaggregation errors is to restrict interpretation to the level at which data have been collected. However, such a strategy is extremely restrictive, and they suggested that a better approach would be to use statistical techniques that can empirically address the nature of the association between individual- and nation-level characteristics. Thus, in the following section, we use multilevel techniques to examine the structural equivalence of SWB measures at multiple levels of analysis. Cross-level structural equivalence refers to a similarity in meaning across levels. Tools that are often used to examine the nature of constructs at the individual-level analyses can also be used to examine multilevel data. Specifically, multilevel factor analysis (Muthén, 1991) has been proposed as a technique that could be used to examine structural equivalence in multilevel data. If a similar factor structure emerges among a set of items at multiple levels of analysis, then this suggests that the construct has similar psychological meaning at each level.

Muthén (1991, 1994) proposed a series of steps that could be used to examine the underlying structure of a set of items or scales. Although his procedure ultimately relies on confirmatory factor analytic techniques, Van de Vijver and Poortinga (2002) modified the procedures for use with exploratory factor analysis in cross-cultural research.[3] First, exploratory factor analysis is conducted on the items or scales using the full data-set, ignoring the multilevel structure. Second, estimates of cross-cultural differences (usually in the form of intraclass correlations) are computed. If these are sufficiently large, then the nested nature of the data may affect results and multilevel techniques should be used (Muthén and Van de Vijver and Poortinga recommend that at least 5% of the variance should be due to nations). In the third step, between-nation and pooled-within-nation correlation or covariation matrices are computed. Next, an exploratory factor analysis is conducted using the pooled-within-nation correlation matrix. The factor structure is then compared to the structure obtained in each individual nation using congruence coefficients following targeted rotation. Exploratory factor analysis is then conducted with the between-nation correlation matrix. Again, the resulting factor structure is compared to that obtained from the pooled-within-nation matrix and congruence coefficients are calculated to assess similarity in structure across levels.

To demonstrate this process, Van de Vijver and Poortinga (2002) examined the structure of a postmaterialism scale in 39 regions using data from the 1990–1991 World Values Survey. Using the procedures outlined above, they showed that region accounted for a substantial amount of variance in the postmaterialism scale, and thus, multilevel techniques were called for. They then showed that the within-region structure represented in the pooled-within-region correlation matrix was replicated quite well across most nations. Most importantly, however, they showed that the factor structure at the region level was similar to the factor structure at the individual level. Specifically, they showed that there was a single factor underlying the postmaterialism items, and the items loaded on this factor in a similar way within and between regions. This suggests that the construct has a similar meaning at the two levels.

We can also use similar analyses to examine the structure of well-being measures. However, if we were to find that a unidimensional measure such as the Satisfaction with Life Scale (SWLS; Diener, Emmons, Larsen, & Griffin, 1985) had a similar structure at the within- and between-nation levels, these results might still be somewhat ambiguous. If a single factor emerged, one could argue that the single factor meant different things at different levels. The SWLS could validly assess life satisfaction at the individual level, whereas it might still tap "culturally determined positivity" (Kahneman & Riis, 2005, p. 10) at the national level. Thus, stronger evidence for the validity of aggregated SWB measures would be found if distinct well-being constructs loaded on separate factors in both within- and between-nation analyses.

To test this possibility, we turned to the International College Student (ICS) data, a large-scale study of college students from 40 nations collected by colleagues of Ed Diener (see Suh, Diener, Oishi, & Triandis, 1998, for a description of this sample). As part of this project, participants were asked to complete the five-item SWLS, along with a measure assessing the frequency with which they experienced each of eight specific emotions: fear, affection, anger, joy, sadness, guilt, contentment, and pride. Typically, in within-nation analyses, life satisfaction, positive affect, and negative affect items load on three distinct factors (Lucas et al., 1996). Thus, at the individual level, life satisfaction, positive affect, and negative affect reflect separable (though related) constructs. If these constructs are meaningful at the national level, a similar three-factor structure should emerge. If, on the other hand, aggregated SWB reflect national differences in positivity, only one factor should emerge in nation-level factor analyses.

Following the recommendation of Muthén (1991, 1994) and Van de Vijver and Poortinga (2002), we first conducted an exploratory analysis on the 13 well-being items using the full sample, ignoring the nested structure of the data. Three factors emerged with eigenvalues greater than one, and

TABLE 9.1

Factor Loadings for the Full Sample (Ignoring Nested Structure), within-Nation, and between-Nation Correlation Matrices

Variable	Life satisfaction			Negative affect			Positive affect		
	F	W	B	F	W	B	F	W	B
SWLS1	0.69	0.69	0.76						
SWLS2	0.65	0.64	0.68						0.36
SWLS3	0.74	0.72	0.93						
SWLS4	0.61	0.60	0.79						
SWLS5	0.56	0.55	0.62						0.41
Fear				−0.54	−0.54	−0.74			
Affection			0.44			−0.44	0.52	0.49	0.36
Anger				−0.60	−0.55	−0.89			
Joy							0.65	0.66	0.77
Sadness				−0.70	−0.67	−0.88			
Guilt				−0.49	−0.48	−0.73			
Content	0.30		0.33				0.66	0.62	0.78
Pride						−0.58	0.51	0.47	0.67

Note. F = Full sample, ignoring nested structure; W = Within; B = Between (before Procrustes rotation). Loadings printed in bold are those that are should theoretically be linked with the underlying factor. Loadings less than .30 are not shown.

the scree plot also suggested that a three-factor solution was appropriate. Varimax rotated factor loadings for the three-factor solution are presented in the first, fourth, and seventh columns of Table 9.1. As can be seen, each item had its strongest loading on the hypothesized factor. In addition, with only one exception (for contentment loading on the life satisfaction factor), each factor loading for nonhypothesized factors was less than .30.

We next computed intraclass correlations for all 13 variables in order to determine whether between-nation variance was likely to affect these results. These values ranged from .06 to .13, with an average intraclass correlation of .09 ($SD = .03$). Because between-nation differences account for a substantial proportion of the variance, multilevel analyses should be conducted. Therefore, we computed between-nation and pooled-within-nation correlation matrices for the 13 variables using M*plus* (Muthén & Muthén, 2004). We then conducted exploratory factor analyses on each of the two matrices. We also conducted separate factor analyses on the 13 items within each of the 40 nations. Finally, we calculated Tucker's phi congruence coefficients comparing each set of loadings to those obtained from the pooled-within-nation matrix after Procrustes rotation. Following the recommendation of Barrett (2005), we also calculated double-scaled Euclidian distance values for each comparison. Procrustes rotations, congruence values, and double-scaled distances were computed using Orthosim 2.01 (Barrett, 2005).

As with the analysis that ignored the nested nature of these data, an exploratory factor analysis of the pooled-within-nation correlation matrix showed that there were three factors with eigenvalues greater than one. In addition, the scree plot suggested that a three-factor solution would be most appropriate. Varimax-rotated factor loadings for this solution are presented in the second, fifth, and eighth columns of Table 9.1. Results are almost identical to those estimated using the full sample. Again, each item loads on the hypothesized factor, and in this case, no item had a loading greater than .30 on any nonhypothesized factor. Thus, looking just at the within-nation variance, it appears that separable life satisfaction, positive affect, and negative affect factors exist in these data.

Table 9.2 shows congruence coefficients and double-scaled Euclidian distances and compares solutions in each of the 40 nations with the solution from the pooled-within-nation matrix (after Procrustes rotation). Recommendations for minimal acceptable coefficients vary (e.g., Barrett, 1986; Eysenck & Eysenck, 1982; Mulaik, 1972; Ten Berge, 1996; Van de Vijver & Leung, 1997), with guidelines ranging from .80 to .95. In general, the values reported in Table 9.2 tend to fall above the most frequently recommended cutoff of .90, though there are a few nations (highlighted in bold) where congruence coefficients, double-scaled Euclidian distance measures, or both, fall below .85.

Perhaps the most important part of this analysis is the comparison of the between-nation and pooled-within-nation analyses. As with the full-sample and pooled-within-nation analyses, there were three eigenvalues greater than one, and the scree plot suggested that a three-factor solution was appropriate. Columns 3, 6, and 9 of Table 9.1 show the varimax-rotated factor loadings from the between-nation analysis. In addition, the first row of Table 9.2 shows the congruence and double-scaled Euclidian distance coefficients when comparing the between-nation solution to the pooled-within-nation solution after Procrustes rotation. As in the previous two analyses, the items tend to load strongly on their hypothesized factors. However, in one case, an item loads more strongly on a nonhypothesized factor than on the hypothesized factor—affection loads more strongly (.44) on the life satisfaction factor than on the positive affect factor (.36). In addition, a greater number of items show secondary loadings that are higher than .30 in the between-nation analysis than in either of the individual-level analyses. However, after Procrustes rotation, the similarity coefficients show that the factor structure is quite comparable across the two levels. Thus, although there may be a bit more overlap among items at the between-nation level, there are three recognizable factors that closely mirror those found at the within-nation level. This is strong evidence that these variables have similar psychological meaning at the individual and

TABLE 9.2

Congruence and Double-Scaled Euclidian Distance Coefficients for Procrustes Rotations

Within Versus:	N	Congruence	DSES
Between		.94	.90
Argentina	90	.93	.90
Australia	292	.98	.95
Austria	164	.96.	.92
Bahrain	124	.78	.81
Brazil	112	.97	.94
China	558	.96	.92
Columbia	100	.97	.93
Denmark	91	.94	.90
Egypt	120	.97	.93
Estonia	119	.82	.83
Finland	91	.92	.89
Germany	108	.95	.91
Ghana	118	.93	.90
Greece	129	.96	.92
Guam	186	.85	.84
Hong Kong	142	.89	.87
Hungary	74	.96	.92
India	93	.93	.89
Indonesia	90	.97	.93
Italy	289	.97	.93
Japan	200	.95	.91
Korea	277	.98	.95
Lithuania	101	.95	.92
Nepal	99	.65	.92
Nigeria	244	.87	.76
Norway	99	.96	.86
Pakistan	155	.95	.91
Peru	129	.96	.92
Portugal	139	.97	.93
Puerto Rico	87	.97	.93
Singapore	131	.96	.92
Slovenia	50	.97	.92
South Africa	134	.98	.95
Spain	373	.99	.96
Taiwan	327	.99	.95
Tanzania	533	.89	.86
Thailand	92	.82	.83
Turkey	100	.95	.91
US	443	.98	.95
Zimbabwe	109	.97	.93

national level. The fact that more than one factor emerged suggests that between-nation variance in SWB measures does not simply reflect cultural differences in positivity. At least at the structural level, there is some degree of equivalence across the between- and within-nation levels. It is important to note that this evidence applies only to comparisons regarding the structural aspects, and researchers must still be careful to avoid level errors (Van de Vijver & Poortinga, 2002).

Of course, it is possible that college student samples are select groups that are not representative of the populations from which they come. For instance, with increased education may come increased exposure to Western culture. However, this would lead to a reduction in between-nation variance, making it more difficult to find structural equivalence across the two levels. In addition, average SWLS scores from the ICS data correspond well with national levels of life satisfaction from other more representative sources. For instance, we took the 32 nations that were represented in both the ICS study and in one of the two most recent waves of the World Values Survey and compared average satisfaction scores across the two studies. Average satisfaction scores in the ICS correlated .68 ($p < .001$) with average satisfaction in the World Values Survey. In addition, we compared the ICS values to aggregate nation-level well-being scores reported in Diener et al., 1995). Again, the correlation for the 27 overlapping nations was a strong .64 ($p < .001$). Thus, there is no reason to believe that these college student samples are substantially different from the wider population from which they were drawn.

CONCLUSION

For decades, researchers have been interested in understanding the determinants of individual levels of SWB. These researchers have used increasingly sophisticated methods to identify robust correlates of happiness and to clarify the processes that are responsible for individual differences in happiness. Because nation-level variables can often affect individual happiness, and because aggregated measures of a population's happiness can inform policy decisions, it is no surprise that studies of national differences are becoming increasingly common. Yet before these studies can provide unambiguous information about the process that underlie happiness or the policies that governments should pursue, it is important that researchers have a clear idea about how the construct of SWB varies when measured at different levels.

At the individual level, SWB reflects an individual's subjective evaluation of the quality of his or her life as a whole. The research reviewed in this chapter suggests that at a national level, SWB measures may have a similar meaning—they appear to tap between-nation differences in the quality of life as a whole. This conclusion is supported by a number of different pieces of evidence. First, national measures are related to predictor variables in theoretically meaningful ways. For example, the Economist Intelligence Unit was able to predict 85% of the variance in national levels of happiness from just 12 variables (all of which were measured using non-self-report techniques). Many of the variables that correlate with SWB at the national level also correlate at the individual level. This correspondence provides evidence that SWB has similar meanings across levels (van Hemert et al., 2002).

In addition, between-nation variance in well-being measures exhibits a meaningful structure, and this structure corresponds well to that found at the individual level. Clear life satisfaction, positive affect, and negative affect factors emerge from a multilevel analysis. These results suggest that the between-nation variance does not simply reflect positivity. Instead, it appears that aggregated measures of positive affect, negative affect, and life satisfaction reflect distinct, but theoretically meaningful aspects of the nations' quality of life as a whole. Although it was beyond the scope of the current chapter to do this, future research could determine whether national levels of these distinguishable facets correlate in predictable ways with distinct sets of predictors. Such analyses would further knowledge about the nature of nation-level SWB.

Together these results suggest that measures of well-being can provide useful information about the quality of life of a nation. Although these measures must be interpreted carefully, and although research on the psychometric properties of aggregated measures must continue, the initial evidence regarding the use of these measures is encouraging. With the appropriate use of multilevel techniques, further progress can be made.

Notes

1. Between-nation standard deviations ranged from .68 to 1.20 across years.
2. Because health data were not reported for all nations in all years, any available data from 1990 to 1995 were aggregated across years to provide an average value for each nation. Correlations were calculated among those nations with data. These criterion variables were chosen somewhat haphazardly to demonstrate that correlations with any single criterion variable provide only partial evidence about validity. We do not mean to suggest that self-reports of health provide a *better* measure of national health than life expectancy. Other theoretically relevant variables also show weak correlations (or even correlations in the opposite direction) with these aggregated self-reports. Furthermore, because these correlations are calculated using a small number of nations, they are subject to the influence of outliers and are not very stable. However, this is also true of the initial correlations published in Kahneman and Riis (2005).

3. Confirmatory factor analytic techniques could not be used in this case: even the simplest three-factor multilevel model with 13 observed variables had more estimated parameters than nation-level units; thus, the model could not be estimated.

REFERENCES

Ahadi, S., & Diener, E. (1989). Multiple determinants and effect size. *Journal of Personality and Social Psychology, 56,* 398–406.

Allik, J., & Realo, A. (2004). Individualism-collectivism and social capital. *Journal of Cross-Cultural Psychology, 35,* 29–49.

Argyle, M. (2001). *The psychology of happiness* (2nd ed.). New York: Routledge.

Arrindell, W. A., Hatzichristou, C., Wensink, J., Rosenberg, E., van Twillert, B. R., Stedema, J. et al. (1997). Dimensions of national culture as predictors of cross-national differences in subjective well-being. *Personality and Individual Differences, 23,* 37–53.

Barrett, P. (1986) Factor comparison: An examination of three methods. *Personality and Individual Differences, 7,* 327–340.

Barrett, P. (2005). *Orthosim 2.01* [Statistical Software]. Retrieved February 1, 2006 from http://www.pbarrett.net/factor_similarity.htm

Baumeister, R. F., & Leary, M. R. (1995). The need to belong: Desire for interpersonal attachments as a fundamental human motivation. *Psychological Bulletin, 117,* 497–529.

Berkman, L. F., & Syme, S. L. (1979). Social networks, host resistance, and mortality: A nine-year follow-up study of Alameda county residents. *American Journal of Epidemiology, 109,* 186–204.

Biswas-Diener, R., & Diener, E. (2001). Making the best of a bad situation: Satisfaction in the slums of Calcutta. *Social Indicators Research, 55,* 329–352.

Brickman, P., Coates, D., & Janoff-Bulman, R. (1978). Lottery winners and accident victims: Is happiness relative? *Journal of Personality and Social Psychology, 36,* 917–927.

Brief, A. P., Butcher, A. H., George, J. M., & Link, K. E. (1993). Integrating bottom-up and top-down theories of subjective well-being: The case of health. *Journal of Personality and Social Psychology, 64,* 646–653.

Campbell, A., Converse, P. E., & Rodgers, W. L. (1976). *The quality of American life: Perceptions, evaluations, and satisfactions.* New York: Russell Sage Foundation.

Costa, P. T., & McCrae, R. R. (1980). Influence of extraversion and neuroticism on subjective well-being: Happy and unhappy people. *Journal of Personality and Social Psychology, 38,* 668–678.

Davis, J. A., Smith, T. W., & Marsden, P. V. (2003). *General social surveys, 1972–2002* [Computer File]. Ann Arbor, MI: Inter-University Consortium for Political and Social Research. Available at: http://webapp.icpsr.umich.edu/GSS/

Diener, E., & Biswas-Diener, R. (2002). Will money increase subjective well-being? *Social Indicators Research, 57,* 119–169.

Diener, E., & Diener, C. (1996). Most people are happy. *Psychological Science, 7,* 181–185.

Diener, E., Diener, M., & Diener, C. (1995). Factors predicting the subjective well-being of nations. *Journal of Personality and Social Psychology, 69,* 851–864.

Diener, E., Emmons, R. A., Larsen, R. J., & Griffin, S. (1985). The Satisfaction with Life scale. *Journal of Personality Assessment, 49,* 71–75.

Diener, E., & Lucas, R. E. (1999). Personality and subjective well-being. In D. Kahneman, E. Diener, & N. Schwarz (Eds.), *Well-being: The foundations of hedonic psychology* (pp. 213–229). New York: Russell Sage Foundation.

Diener, E., Lucas, R. E., & Scollon, C. N. (2006). Beyond the hedonic treadmill: Revisions to the adaptation theory of well-being. *American Psychologist, 61,* 305–314.

Diener, E., & Oishi, S. (2004). Are Scandinavians happier than Asians? Issues in comparing nations on subjective well-being. In F. Columbus (Ed.), *Asian economic and political issues* (Vol. 10, pp. 1–25). Hauppauge, NY: Nova Science.

Diener, E., & Seligman, M. E. P. (2004). Beyond money: Toward an economy of well-being. *Psychological Science in the Public Interest, 5,* 1–31.

Diener, E., Suh, E. M., Lucas, R. E., & Smith, H. L. (1999). Subjective well-being: Three decades of progress. *Psychological Bulletin, 125,* 276–302.

Dijkers, M. (1997). Quality of life after spinal cord injury: A meta analysis of the effects of disablement components. *Spinal Cord, 35,* 829–840.

Donovan, N., & Halpern, D. (2003, November). *Life satisfaction: The state of knowledge and implications for government.* Paper presented at the conference on well-being and social-capital, Harvard University, Cambridge, MA.

Easterlin, R. A. (1995). Will raising the incomes of all increase the happiness of all? *Journal of Economic Behavior and Organization, 27,* 35–47.

Easterlin, R. A. (2003). Explaining happiness. *Proceedings of the National Academy of Sciences, 100,* 11176–11183.

Economist Intelligence Unit (2005). *The Economist Intelligence Unit's Quality-of-Life Index.* Retrieved July 17, 2005 from http://www.economist.com/media/pdf/QUALITY_OF_LIFE.pdf

Eysenck, H. J., & Eysenck, S. B. G. (1982) Recent advances in the cross-cultural study of personality. In C. D. Spielberger & J. N. Butcher (Eds.) *Advances in personality assessment.* Hillsdale, NJ: Lawrence Erlbaum.

Ferriss, A. L. (2002). Religion and the quality of life. *Journal of Happiness Studies, 3,* 199–215.

Frey, B. S., & Stutzer, A. (2000). Happiness prospers in democracy. *Journal of Happiness Studies, 1,* 79–102.

Frey, B. S., & Stutzer, A. (2002). *Happiness and economics: How the economy and institutions affect human well-being.* Princeton, NJ: Princeton University Press.

Fujita, F., & Diener, E. (2005). Life satisfaction set point: Stability and change. *Journal of Personality and Social Psychology, 88,* 158–164.

Ganz, P. A., Lee, J. J., & Siau, J. (1991). Quality of life assessment: An independent prognostic variable for survival in lung cancer. *Cancer, 67,* 3131–3135.

Hagerty, M. R., & Veenhoven, R. (2003). Wealth and happiness revisited—Growing national income does go with greater happiness. *Social Indicators Research, 64,* 1–27.

Hammell, K. W. (2004). Exploring quality of life following high spinal cord injury: A review and critique. *Spinal Cord, 42,* 491–502.

Haring, M., Stock, W. A., & Okun, M. A. (1984). A research synthesis of gender and social class as correlates of subjective well-being. *Human Relations, 37,* 645–657.

Haring-Hidore, M., Stock, W. A., Okun, M. A., & Witter, R. A. (1985). Marital status and subjective well-being: A research synthesis. *Journal of Marriage and the Family, 47,* 947–953.

Helliwell, J. F. (2003a). How's life? Combining individual and national variables to explain subjective well-being. *Economic Modelling, 20,* 331–360.

Helliwell, J. F. (2003b). *Well-being and social capital: Does suicide pose a puzzle?* Unpublished manuscript, University of British Columbia, Vancouver, British Columbia, Canada.

House, J. S., Landis, K. R., & Umberson, D. (1988). Social relationships and health. *Science, 241,* 540–545.

House, J. S., Robbins, C., & Metzner, H. L. (1982). The association of social relationships and activities with mortality: Prospective evidence from the Tecumseh Community Health Study. *American Journal of Epidemiology, 116,* 123–140.

Hui, C. H., & Triandis, H. C. (1985). Measurement in cross-cultural psychology: A review and comparison of strategies. *Journal of Cross-Cultural Psychology, 16,* 131–152.

Inglehart, R., & Klingemann, H.-D. (2000). Genes, culture, democracy, and happiness. In E. Diener & E. M. Suh (Eds.), *Culture and subjective well-being* (pp. 165–183). Cambridge, MA: MIT Press.

Kahneman, D. (1994). New challenges to the rationality assumption. *Journal of Institutional and Theoretical Economics, 150,* 18–36.

Kahneman, D., & Riis, J. (2005). Living and thinking about it: Two perspectives on life. In F. A. Huppert, N. Baylis, & B. Keverne (Eds.), *The science of well-being.* (pp. 285–304). New York: Oxford University Press.

Kirkcaldy, B. D., Furnham, A., & Martin, T. (1998). National differences in personality, socio-ecomonic, and work-related attitudinal variables. *European Psychologist, 3,* 255–262.

Lucas, R. E. (2005). Time does not heal all wounds: A longitudinal study of reaction and adaptation to divorce. *Psychological Science, 16,* 945–950.

Lucas, R. E. (2007). Long-term disability is associated with lasting changes in subjective well-being: Evidence from two nationally representative longitudinal studies. *Journal of Personality and Social Psychology, 92,* 711–730.

Lucas, R. E., Clark, A. E., Georgellis, Y., & Diener, E. (2003). Reexamining adaptation and the set point model of happiness: Reactions to changes in marital status. *Journal of Personality and Social Psychology, 84,* 527–539.

Lucas, R. E., Diener, E., & Suh, E. (1996). Discriminant validity of well-being measures. *Journal of Personality and Social Psychology, 71,* 616–628.

Lucas, R. E., & Dyrenforth, P. (2006). Does the existence of social relationships matter for subjective well-being? In K. D. Vohs & E. J. Finkel (Eds.), *Self and relationships: Connecting intrapersonal and interpersonal processes* (pp. 254–273). New York: Guilford.

Lucas, R. E., & Gohm, C. L. (2000). Age and sex differences in subjective well-being across cultures. In E. Diener & E. M. Suh (Eds.), *Culture and subjective well-being* (pp. 291–317). Cambridge, MA: MIT Press.

Lucas, R. E., Le, K., & Dyrenforth, P. S. (in press). Explaining the extraversion/ positive affect relation: Sociability cannot account for extraverts' greater happiness. *Journal of Personality.*

Lykken, D., & Tellegen, A. (1996). Happiness is a stochastic phenomenon. *Psychological Science, 7,* 186–189.

Mastekaasa, A. (1994). Marital status, distress, and well-being: An international comparison. *Journal of Comparative Family Studies, 25,* 183–205.

McClellan, W. M., Anson, C., Birkeli, K., & Tuttle, E. (1991). Functional status and quality of life: Predictors of early mortality among patients entering treatment for end stage renal disease. *Journal of Clinical Epidemiology, 44,* 83–89.

Mossey, J. M., & Shapiro, E. (1982). Self-rated health: A predictor of mortality among the elderly. *American Journal of Public Health, 72,* 800–808.

Mroczek, D. K., & Spiro, A. I. (2005). Change in life satisfaction during adulthood: Findings from the veterans affairs normative aging study. *Journal of Personality and Social Psychology, 88,* 189–202.

Mulaik, S. (1972). *The foundations of factor analysis.* New York: McGraw-Hill.

Muthén, B. O. (1991). Multilevel factor analysis of class and student achievement components. *Journal of Educational Measurement, 28,* 338–354.

Muthén, B. O. (1994). Multilevel covariance structure analysis. *Sociological Methods & Research, 22,* 376–398.

Muthén, B. O., & Muthén, L. (2004). *Mplus 3.01* [Statistical Software]. Los Angeles, CA: Muthén & Muthén.

Myers, D. G. (2000). The funds, friends, and faith of happy people. *American Psychologist, 55,* 56–67.

Nelson, E., Conger, B., Douglass, R., Gephart, D., Kirk, J., Page, R. et al. (1983). Functional health status levels of primary care patients. *JAMA: Journal of the American Medical Association, 249,* 3331–3338.

Okun, M. A., & George, L. K. (1984). Physician- and self-ratings of health, neuroticism and subjective well-being among men and women. *Personality and Individual Differences, 5,* 533–539.

Okun, M. A., Stock, W. A., Haring, M. J., & Witter, R. A. (1984). Health and subjective well-being: A meta-analysis. *International Journal of Aging and Human Development, 19,* 111–132.

Pinquart, M., & Sörensen, S. (2000). Influences of socioeconomic status, social network, and competence on subjective well-being in later life: A meta-analysis. *Psychology and Aging, 15,* 187–224.

Putnam, R. (2001). *Bowling alone: The collapse and revival of American community.* New York: Simon & Schuster.

Rumsfeld, J. S., MacWhinney, S., McCarthy, M., Jr., Shroyer, A. L. W., VillaNueva, C. B., O'Brien, M. et al. (1999). Health-related quality of life as a predictor of mortality following coronary artery bypass graft surgery. *JAMA: Journal of the American Medical Association, 281,* 1298–1303.

Schyns, P. (1998). Cross-national differences in happiness: Economic and cultural factors explored. *Social Indicators Research, 43,* 3–26.

Schyns, P. (2003). *Income and life satisfaction: A cross-national and longitudinal study.* Delft, the Netherlands: Eburon.

Steel, P., & Ones, D. S. (2002). Personality and happiness: A national-level analysis. *Journal of Personality and Social Psychology, 83,* 767–781.

Suh, E., Diener, E., Oishi, S., & Triandis, H. C. (1998). The shifting basis of life satisfaction judgments across cultures: Emotions versus norms. *Journal of Personality and Social Psychology, 74,* 482–493.

Ten Berge, J. M. F. (1996). The Kaiser, Hunka and Bianchini factor similarity coefficients: A cautionary note. *Multivariate Behavioral Research, 31,* 1–6.

Van de Vijver, F. J. R., & Leung, K. (1997) *Methods and data analysis for cross-cultural research.* Newbury Park, CA: Sage

Van de Vijver, F. J. R., & Poortinga, Y. H. (2002). Structural equivalence in multilevel research. *Journal of Cross-Cultural Psychology, 33,* 141–156.

Van Hemert, D. A., Van de Vijver, F. J. R., & Poortinga, Y. H. (2002). The Beck Depression Inventory as a measure of subjective well-being: A cross-national study. *Journal of Happiness Studies, 3,* 257–286.

Veenhoven, R. (1995). The cross-national pattern of happiness: Test of predictions implied in three theories of happiness. *Social Indicators Research, 34,* 33–68.

Veenhoven, R. (1999). Quality-of-life in individualistic society. *Social Indicators Research, 48,* 157–186.

Wilson, W. R. (1967). Correlates of avowed happiness. *Psychological Bulletin, 67,* 294–306.

Wood, W., Rhodes, N., & Whelan, M. (1989). Sex differences in positive well-being: A consideration of emotional style and marital status. *Psychological Bulletin, 106,* 249–264.

World Values Survey. (2006). Available from http://www.worldvaluessurvey.org.

10

The Five-Factor Model and Its Correlates in Individuals and Cultures

Robert R. McCrae and Antonio Terracciano

Personality traits are among the most familiar of individual difference variables, both to laypersons, who use them incessantly in daily life, and to psychologists, who have studied them throughout the history of their discipline. Major advances in trait psychology have occurred in recent years, chiefly fostered by an emerging consensus that personality traits can be described in terms of five basic dimensions. In this chapter we will summarize what is known about the Five-Factor Model (FFM) at the individual level and, more tentatively, at the culture level; report new data on the culture-level correlates of factors and their facets; address some issues in data analysis and interpretation at two levels; and discuss some implications for public policy.

This chapter is based chiefly on the results of two projects. In the first, McCrae (2001, 2002) reported secondary analyses of self-report personality data from volunteer samples collected by other researchers in 36 cultures around the world. In the second study (McCrae, Terracciano et al., 2005a, 2005b), McCrae and Terracciano invited collaborators from 51 cultures to gather observer-rating data from college students who rated college-age or adult men and women. Appendices to this chapter give mean values for 30 personality traits from that Personality Profiles of Cultures (PPOC) Project, which other researchers may find useful.

THE FIVE-FACTOR MODEL (FFM) AT TWO LEVELS

The Individual-Level FFM

The dimensional structure of personality traits has been a contentious issue for generations (Eysenck, 1947). Some lexical researchers believe that only three factors are universal (De Raad & Peabody, 2005), and some cross-cultural psychologists believe there are personality factors unique to particular cultures (Cheung & Leung, 1998). But the most widely accepted view today is that personality traits are adequately summarized by five factors.

The dimensions, or factors, of the FFM were originally identified by Tupes and Christal (1961/1992) in analyses of observer ratings of personality, and they have subsequently been replicated in self-report measures using dozens of instruments (Markon, Krueger, & Watson, 2005). Most commonly they are designated by the names Neuroticism vs. Emotional Stability (N), Extraversion vs. Introversion (E), Openness vs. Closedness to Experience (O), Agreeableness vs. Antagonism (A), and high vs. low Conscientiousness (C). Many personality questionnaires have been developed to assess these factors (De Raad & Perugini, 2002), of which the most widely used is the Revised NEO Personality Inventory (NEO-PI-R; Costa & McCrae, 1992). The NEO-PI-R assesses 30 specific traits, six for each of the five factors. (They are listed in Table 10.1; the scale labels may give a better idea of the nature and scope of the factors.)

Studies using the NEO-PI-R and other measures have established that all five traits (1) show high rank-order stability over periods of many years; (2) can be assessed by self-reports or the ratings of knowledgeable informants, with modest to moderate agreement across these different sources; (3) are strongly heritable; and (4) are useful in the prediction of a variety of behaviors and outcomes, from vocational interests to longevity (McCrae & Costa, 2003). Because of these properties, traits of the FFM have assumed an increasingly prominent role in clinical, developmental, health, and industrial/organizational psychology. If aggregate personality traits function in the same way, they have great promise as culture-level variables.

Early research established that the FFM was replicable across subgroups: men and women, old and young adults, black and white Americans. Research in the past decade has also established that the FFM is universal (McCrae, Terracciano et al., 2005a; Paunonen et al., 1996). The NEO-PI-R has been translated into over 40 languages, and the factor structure has been more-or-less clearly replicated in all of them. This means that the 30 NEO-PI-R facets retain some measure of convergent and discriminant validity in translation. Further evidence for the validity of these trait constructs comes from the many validation studies that have been reported: N predicts unpleasant moods in China (Yik, Russell, Ahn, Fernández Dols, & Suzuki, 2002); O is inversely related to HIV stigmatization in Russia (McCrae, Costa et al., 2007); C predicts job performance in Europe (Salgado, 1997).

Researchers who have followed this literature have become blasé; McCrae, Terracciano et al. (2005a) reported 50 cross-cultural replications of the NEO-PI-R structure in a single paper. Yet the fact that any two cultures should show the same personality structure is remarkable, given the profound differences that may be found in religious beliefs, language, political systems, and other features of culture. Contemporary psychological anthropologists sometimes give the impression that it is hopelessly difficult to understand someone from another culture (Spiro, 1999), and yet the same trait constructs that Americans employ are readily used by Thais, Turks, and Taiwanese to describe themselves.

Five-factor theory (FFT; McCrae & Costa, 1999) explains this by asserting that personality traits are based in biology, not culture. They are latent constructs that underlie but are not equivalent to observable behaviors. Although expressed in patterns of thoughts, feelings, and behaviors that are influenced by cultural variables, traits themselves are not caused by culture. Instead, these latent psychological constructs—the Basic Tendencies of FFT—are directly linked to biological bases. There is one human species and one human genome, so from the perspective of FFT it should be no more surprising that the FFM is found everywhere than it is that people everywhere have two eyes, two ears, and a nose.

The Culture-Level FFM

Because the FFM can be found in individual-level analyses in all cultures, one can score culture members on the five factors and calculate an average score for each factor. Assuming scalar equivalence—that is, that the raw scores have the same interpretation in all cultures—we can compare cultures and conclude, for example, that the members of one culture have, on average, higher levels of E than the members of another. It is tempting to translate this observation to the culture level and say that the first is an *extraverted culture*, but it is premature to do so (Van de Vijver & Poortinga, 2002). E is defined by the covariation of traits such as gregariousness, activity, and assertiveness, but it is not necessarily true that these variables covary when assessed at the culture level. That hypothesis can be tested by using aggregate or average personality traits as the variables in what Hofstede (2001) called an *ecological factor analysis*. Few such analyses have been reported, and they remain mysterious to most psychologists, so a recent article (McCrae, Terracciano et al., 2005b) in which NEO-PI-R observer rating data from 51 cultures were analyzed prefaced its ecological factor analyses by some simulations.

Jüri Allik (personal communication, August 10, 2004) pointed out that, other things being equal,[1] ecological factor analyses ought to parallel individual-level factor analyses on purely statistical grounds (for more formal statistical treatments of these issues, consult Muthén, 1991, 1994; Van de Vijver & Poortinga, 2002). If Trait X is correlated with Trait Y at the individual level, then any group that happens to have many individuals high on Trait X will also tend to have many who are high on Trait Y. Our simulations confirmed this observation: When we randomly reassigned individuals from 51 cultures to 202 groups (thereby eliminating effects of culture), factor analysis of the group means reproduced the individual-level structure as Allik predicted (Tucker's ϕs = .93 to .96; values above .85 are considered a replication, Haven & Ten Berge, 1977). Thus, replication of the individual-level structure on the culture level is not remarkable evidence that the superorganic (Kroeber, 1917) somehow follows the same psychological laws as the organic; replication means simply that cultures do not actively interfere with the operation of statistics. Such interference could occur in at least two ways, and we studied both through simulations.

First, we examined the effects of randomly altering means of the NEO-PI-R facets in each of the 202 groups by adding or subtracting a few points. These changes were intended to mimic the effects of error introduced by poor translations or cultural variations in response styles. These changes seriously degraded the factor structure (ϕs = .47 to .77 after targeted rotation). If such problems were in fact widespread in cross-cultural comparisons of NEO-PI-R scales, the individual-level structure would not be found at the culture level, and conversely, if the structure is replicable at the culture level, it would imply that there is relatively little such error in cross-cultural comparisons.

Second, we considered the possibility that there were systematic cultural effects superimposed on the individual-level structure. We contrasted hypothetical "thinking" and "feeling" groups, adding a constant to the Openness to Ideas facet in the thinking groups and to the Openness to Feelings facet in the feeling groups. Note that this procedure would not affect the individual-level factor structure within any culture, because linear transformations (such as adding a constant) do not affect correlations. In this culture-level simulation, after targeted rotation the individual-level factor structure was replicated (ϕs = .86 to .97), except for the O factor (ϕ = .14), which contrasted Openness to Ideas and Feelings. Thus, if there are genuine and systematic cultural effects, they can be detected in ecological factor analyses.

What did the real culture-level factor analysis show? Four of the factors, N, O, A, and C, replicated the individual-level structure (ϕs = .86 to .94), and the fifth, E, approximated it (ϕ = .81). Overall, these results imply, first, that the NEO-PI-R scales at the culture level are not seriously compromised by random error such as that introduced by poor translations; and second, that the constructs represented by the five factors are applicable to cultures as well as people. It is meaningful to say that some cultures are conscientious, and others are agreeable, because the traits that define these factors covary at the culture level. There is a culture-level FFM.

But it is not identical to the individual-level FFM. The culture-level E factor (see Table 10.1, fourth data column) was defined by five of the six E facets and by Openness to Feelings and Altruism, which usually have

TABLE 10.1

Factor Loadings on the Extraversion Factor at the Individual and Culture Level for Self-Reports and Observer Ratings, and a Simulation

NEO-PI-R Facet Scale	Individual level		Culture level		
	Form S[a]	Form R[b]	Form S[c]	Form R[d]	Simulation
N1: Anxiety	.02	−.07	−.05	.08	.04
N2: Angry hostility	−.03	−.05	−.03	−.09	−.04
N3: Depression	−.10	−.18	−.21	−.21	−.23
N4: Self-consciousness	−.18	−.23	−.42	−.40	−.16
N5: Impulsiveness	.35	.33	.66	.50	.43
N6: Vulnerability	−.15	−.08	−.33	−.40	−.05
E1: Warmth	.66	.72	.64	.68	.74
E2: Gregariousness	.66	.76	.75	.64	.64
E3: Assertiveness	.44	.40	.61	.32	.39
E4: Activity	.54	.58	.70	.45	.53
E5: Excitement seeking	.58	.54	.65	.41	.45
E6: Positive emotions	.74	.70	.71	.72	.66
O1: Fantasy	.18	.27	.45	.55	.53
O2: Aesthetics	.04	.14	−.23	−.26	.08
O3: Feelings	.41	.46	.58	.50	.41
O4: Actions	.22	.24	.09	−.16	.04
O5: Ideas	−.01	−.05	−.09	−.02	−.02
O6: Values	.08	.11	.60	.52	.53
A1: Trust	.22	.38	.10	.41	.49
A2: Straightforwardness	−.15	−.08	−.11	.45	−.06
A3: Altruism	.52	.38	.66	.63	.41
A4: Compliance	−.08	−.05	−.43	−.24	−.06
A5: Modesty	−.12	−.11	.36	.34	−.11
A6: Tender-eindedness	.27	.27	.07	.16	.31
C1: Competence	.17	.07	.51	.45	.19
C2: Order	.06	−.07	−.22	−.28	−.11
C3: Dutifulness	−.04	−.01	.13	.21	−.02
C4: Achievement striving	.23	.14	−.26	.11	.22
C5: Self-discipline	.17	.03	.11	.17	.12
C6: Deliberation	−.28	−.26	−.33	−.44	−.30

Note. These are principal components targeted to the American normative factor structure. Loadings greater than .40 in absolute magnitude are given in italics. [a]Self-reports from the American normative sample ($N = 1,000$; Costa & McCrae, 1992). [b]Observer ratings from 50 cultures from the PPOC Project ($N = 11,985$; McCrae et al., 2005a). [c]Self-reports from 36 cultures ($N = 27,965$; McCrae, 2002). [d]Observer ratings from 51 cultures from the PPOC Project ($N = 12,156$; McCrae et al., 2005b).

secondary loadings on individual-level E (Table 10.1, first and second data columns). However, it was also defined by several other traits, including Impulsiveness, Openness to Fantasy and Values, and Competence, which are not related to E on the individual level. Further, as shown in the third data column of Table 10.1, the pattern of results closely resembled that from an earlier ecological factor analysis of self-report data. This suggests that there are systematic culture-level effects on personality trait scores above and beyond the effects of aggregating individual scores.

The interpretation of this finding is speculative at this point, but one possibility is that it is driven by economic development. Inglehart (1997) has argued that nations with long histories of prosperity move from modern, materialist values to postmaterialist values, which include imagination and tolerance—values related to Openness to Fantasy and Values. Western cultures were the first to experience this shift in values, and Western countries are distinguished from the rest of the world chiefly by high levels of E (McCrae, Terracciano et al., 2005b). Perhaps O1: Fantasy and O6: Values are correlated with E at the culture level simply because they were encouraged among cultures that happen to be extraverted. (By this argument, if Asian countries had had longer histories of economic prosperity than European countries, O1 and O6 would have had negative loadings on the culture-level E factor.)

To test the feasibility of this hypothesized mechanism, we conducted a new simulation. We used data from 12,156 observer ratings (McCrae, Terracciano et al., 2005b). Data were first standardized within culture and randomly reassigned to 202 groups. Factor analysis of these group-level data clearly replicated the FFM. We then simulated the postmaterialist scenario by adding two T-score points to O1 and O6 in groups that scored above average on the E factor (the "Western" groups). This lowered the factor congruence of E from .97 to .92, and produced the factor loadings shown in the last column of Table 10.1. Note that O1 and O6 now show loadings comparable to those found in real culture-level data. Thus, a fairly subtle effect of culture on personality trait scores could produce the culture-level structures that have been observed. This is one of the first pieces of evidence that cultures can influence the level of personality traits—a proposition that would have seemed self-evident to earlier students of culture-and-personality, but which is currently a matter of debate (Hofstede & McCrae, 2004).

The Scalar Equivalence of Culture-Level FFM Scales

The knowledgeable reader may feel some uneasiness in discussing the culture-level FFM: Is it, after all, legitimate to factor aggregate scores from different cultures before it has been established that they show scalar equivalence? Cross-cultural research clearly establishes the validity of the NEO-PI-R within different cultures, but that does not ensure the validity of NEO-PI-R comparisons across cultures. In order to compare two or more different cultures on the level of a trait, it is necessary to demonstrate scalar equivalence (Van de Vijver & Leung, 1997), that is, to show that the same raw score represents the same trait level in all the cultures. This is in fact a prerequisite to comparisons of any two groups: When men are compared to women, or depressed patients to controls, or liberals to conservatives, it is presumed that the measures used work the same in both groups. In the case of cross-cultural comparisons, however, that assumption has frequently been questioned. Translating an instrument may introduce changes in the "difficulty," or likelihood of endorsing, the items. Cultures may differ in response styles such as acquiescence or self-enhancement (Smith & Fischer, this volume). Members of different cultures may use different standards of comparison. Observed differences thus may be artifacts, and must be interpreted in light of the available evidence for scalar equivalence.

McCrae, Terracciano et al. (2005b) have argued that scalar equivalence, like construct validity, is something that must be established through a pattern of evidence, and that there are two ways to approach this task. The bottom-up approach uses analyses of individual-level data, chiefly through differential item functioning analyses (DIF; Huang, Church, & Katigbak, 1997) or through bilingual retest studies (Piedmont, Bain, McCrae, & Costa, 2002). In the former, the properties of individual items are assessed relative to the scale as a whole; marked differences of item properties in two groups suggest inequivalence. However, DIF analyses are ambiguous: A measure may have scalar equivalence even if all its items are biased, provided that the biases are random and cancel each other out (a likely possibility with item translations). Further, the finding of no DIF provides only weak evidence of equivalence, because artifacts may mask real differences. Consider the case in which two distributions of item responses are identical: For every person in culture A with a certain pattern of responses, a single person can be identified in culture B with the same pattern. Means, standard deviations, and all other statistical properties of the items and scales will, of course, be identical across cultures, and DIF analyses would conclude that there is no bias present. But suppose that in fact every single response in culture B (but none in culture A) had been inflated by one point through the operation of acquiescent responding. Item bias analyses could not detect that massive but systematic bias.

In bilingual retest studies, the same respondents, with presumably the same personalities (but see Ramírez-Esparza, Gosling, Benet-Martínez, Potter, & Pennebaker, 2006), complete the measure twice, in two different languages. If the translations are equivalent, means from the two administrations should be the same. Six such studies have compared translations of the NEO-PI-R, and found only small and scattered differences (McCrae, Terracciano et al., 2005b). But bilingual studies address only issues of translation; biases introduced by response styles would presumably affect both administrations, and thus not be detectable by comparing them.

Ultimately, researchers using a bottom-up approach would need to adopt multiple methods (Van de Vijver & Leung, 1997). If the same differences between two cultures are found when different instruments or different sources of data (e.g., self-reports vs. ratings) are used, if questionnaire results parallel behavior counts or daily diary findings, then the difference is probably real, and the original instrument possessed scalar equivalence. Although effective, this approach is slow and arduous, especially when multiplied across many cultural comparisons.

The top-down approach proceeds directly to the culture level and assesses the validity of aggregate scores. After all, if comparisons of cultures were meaningless because of pervasive artifacts, then aggregate scores could not show construct validity for the intended constructs. But demonstration of validity for culture-level scores requires data from a fairly large number of cultures (which are the cases in culture-level analyses), and it requires the availability of appropriate criteria. Both of these were difficult to find until quite recently. New studies (McCrae, 2001; McCrae, Terracciano et al., 2005b), however, provide encouraging results. Aggregate measures of the factors and facets of the NEO-PI-R show substantial correlations across methods (self-reports vs. observer ratings), are related to national values and Hofstede's (2001) dimensions of culture, and show a meaningful geographic distribution (Allik & McCrae, 2004). None of these findings would have been possible if the scales wholly lacked scalar equivalence, so some degree of scalar equivalence can be asserted at the culture level. The fact that at least rough scalar equivalence was found across a range of cultures and a range of traits suggests that personality assessment is more robust than had been feared, and bodes well for the cross-cultural use of well-constructed personality measures in general.

Thus, the culture-level factor analyses reported in McCrae, Terracciano et al. (2005a, 2005b) are legitimate, and are in fact further evidence of scalar equivalence. As mentioned, introducing random error by adding to or subtracting from group facet scores sharply degraded the FFM structure; that is what should happen if there are pervasive violations of scalar equivalence. Because the FFM structure was replicated at the culture level, scalar inequivalence cannot be a major problem. This does not mean that all scales in all cultures are fully equivalent, any more than all scores for all individuals are accurate when a validated measure is used. Assertions about the levels of traits in any given culture need to be tentative and evaluated in the light of other available knowledge, but we need not be nihilistic about cross-cultural comparisons.

The top-down approach to scalar equivalence has one limitation: It is directly applicable only to the culture-level aggregate scores. Elsewhere McCrae (2002) argued that scalar equivalence would also generalize to individuals, so that NEO-PI-R scores from anyone in the world could meaningfully be interpreted in terms of American norms (or, for that matter, any other set of norms). This is a matter of practical importance, because counselors and clinicians sometimes deal with multiethnic populations (Rossier, 2005) for whom local norms are not available. McCrae's proposed solution requires full scalar equivalence, which includes the requirement that the measurement units be equivalent across cultures:

A difference of 10 raw-score points in Peru should mean the same as a 10-point difference in Estonia. But culture-level correlations that establish top-down scalar equivalence deal only with means, and do not take into account the dispersion of scores around the mean.

It is now well established that there are cultural differences in the standard deviations of NEO-PI-R scales, with systematically lower variances in non-Western cultures (McCrae, Terracciano et al., 2005b). The interpretation of that phenomenon is uncertain. One possibility is that the scales really do possess measurement unit equivalence; in that case, personality is simply more homogeneous in non-Western countries (just as eye color is more homogeneous in Asia than in Europe). In this case, one could legitimately use a single set of norms to describe anyone in the world. But another possibility is that lower variances in non-Western cultures are due to acquiescence and other forms of measurement error (McCrae, Terracciano et al., 2005b).[2] If that is true, deviations around the mean are attenuated, and the scores of high- (or low-) scoring members of non-Western cultures would be under- (or over-) estimated by the use of Western norms. Whether this distortion is large enough to make any practical difference remains to be seen.

CULTURE-LEVEL CORRELATES OF FACTORS AND FACETS

At the individual level, personality traits are well known predictors of outcomes of behavioral, social, and clinical importance (Ozer & Benet-Martínez, 2006; Paunonen, 2003). Such associations are usually similar across cultures (e.g., McCrae, Costa et al., 2007), but there are other instances in which they are not, and culture-level variables might explain such cross-cultural differences. Also of interest are the culture-level correlates of aggregate personality traits. Allik's principle should apply here as well: Other things being equal, correlations seen on the individual level should also be found on the culture level. For example, extraverts are generally happy (Costa & McCrae, 1980), so nations with high aggregate levels of E should also show high levels of subjective well-being. Research is needed, however, to establish whether or not other things really are equal. In this section, we will explore the role of culture-level variables of interest from clinical and social perspectives. In part, our findings are of substantive interest; in part, they are illustrative of the possibilities and problems of this relatively new kind of analysis.

Culture-level correlates of aggregate personality traits have rarely been studied, mostly because of the paucity of large cross-cultural datasets that are required for such analyses. Among the few studies, Lynn and

Martin (1995) related Eysenck Personality Questionnaire (EPQ) data from 37 nations to social indicators. Despite a nonuniform sampling strategy across nations for personality traits, culture-level E was positively related to homicide rate and negatively related to suicide. Diener, Diener, and Diener (1995) found that high income, individualism, human rights, and societal equality correlated strongly with nation-level subjective well-being (SWB), and Steel and Ones (2002) examined whether the SWB data were related to EPQ and NEO-PI-R self-report data across 39 and 24 matching cultures, respectively. Consistent with the associations at the individual level, aggregate N and E were associated with SWB, particularly with the NEO-PI-R self-report data.

In the PPOC Project (McCrae, Terracciano et al., 2005b), we extended previous studies by using observer ratings of both adults and college students collected through a uniform sampling strategy across cultures. Although the data were not from representative samples, several indicators, such as geographical clustering and correlations with aggregate self-report data (McCrae, Terracciano et al., 2005b), suggested that cross-cultural comparisons with these aggregate values are meaningful. McCrae and colleagues found a strong pattern of culture-level correlates for E, which was related to individualism, self-expression, and subjective well-being, and for O, which was related to low power distance, valuing affective and intellectual autonomy, and secular-rational values. As expected, N was related to uncertainty avoidance; E, O, and A were all related to Gross Domestic Product per capita (GDP).[3]

McCrae and colleagues did not systematically examine culture-level correlates of NEO-PI-R facet scores. Six facets define each of the broad factors; they are redundant with the overall factor to the extent that they share common variance. But there is also evidence of discriminant validity for the facet scales at the individual level (McCrae & Costa, 1992), and one study (McCrae, Costa et al., 2007) suggests differential validity at the aggregate level. Therefore, in this chapter we present new culture-level correlational analyses of several clinical, demographic, and social indicators at both factor and facet levels.

The main personality dataset for these analyses uses aggregate scores based on observer ratings from the 51 cultures of the PPOC Project (McCrae, Terracciano et al., 2005b). These aggregate values are provided in appendixes 10.A and 10.B to facilitate culture-level analyses by other investigators. The international norms used in McCrae, Terracciano et al. (2005b) are available from the first author. Researchers who gather observer-rated NEO-PI-R data in new cultures can standardize them using these norms and add them to the database. Aggregate self-report data from 38 cultures (McCrae, 2002; see also appendix 10.C) were used to replicate the observer rating associations (at $p < .05$, one-tailed). Note that this is a very conservative replication strategy, because the two sets of cultures are distinct (only 28 overlap).

Country-level criteria were obtained from Internet sources, mostly from World Health Organization (WHO) and United Nations (UN) databases or reports.[4] For most cultures the matching between aggregate personality data and culture-level variables was straightforward. English and Northern Irish aggregate personality scores were matched with UK national data. Similarly, French- and German-speaking Swiss personality scores were matched with Swiss data. Hong Kong personality scores were matched with Hong Kong data when available, otherwise with Chinese national data.

It is relatively easy to find national data summaries on the Internet and relate them to aggregate personality traits. Particularly when facets are examined as well as factors, the sheer number of correlations can grow very large, and the likelihood of chance findings is high. Bonferroni correction is one way to handle this problem, but it means that potentially interesting findings may be overlooked. In preliminary analyses, we examined 3,535 correlations (partialing out GDP), of which 177 would be expected to be significant, $p < .05$, simply by chance. However, we found 530 significant correlations, of which 272 were replicated using self-report data. Thus, it appears unlikely that our results are due entirely to chance. In the next sections we will discuss some of these associations, with particular attention to potential pitfalls in their interpretation.

These are essentially exploratory analyses. Correlations at the individual level can suggest hypotheses of similar associations at the culture level, if we assume that the distinctive contributions of culture to the variables we examine are limited. That is probably a more reasonable assumption with regard to biologically based personality traits than with regard to the criteria (such as social attitudes or drug use) that we might want to relate to traits. At present, we are not aware of any explicit theories that would guide hypotheses relating aggregate personality traits to other features of culture.

Cancer

The hypothesis that personality traits are directly or indirectly associated with cancer has been tested at the individual level in several studies. Eysenck (1980) hypothesized that high E and low N are directly associated with an increased cancer risk. However, large prospective studies have found no support for those hypotheses (e.g., Hansen, Floderus, Frederiksen, & Johansen, 2005). Still, personality traits are known to influence health risk behaviors like smoking (Paunonen 2003; Terracciano & Costa, 2004), which in turn increase cancer risk.

At the culture level, examining the association between incidence of cancer and aggregate personality traits is complicated by the influence of other macrophenomena, like GDP. Compared to the rest of the world, data from affluent countries show a much higher incidence of cancer, in part due to better diagnostic tools, in part to longer life expectancy. In less affluent countries, other causes of mortality are widespread, reducing life expectancy and the incidence of cancer. Because personality traits are also associated with GDP at the culture level, associations may be spurious.

Across the 51 cultures we examined, zero-order correlations indicated that incidence of melanoma, leukemia, breast, ovary, prostate, testicular, pancreatic, kidney, colon, rectal, lung, brain, and other cancers were consistently associated with higher E, O, and A. The correlations of a summary variable (including all except skin cancer, which is usually omitted from all-cancer indices) with E, O, and A were .43, .48, .44 for men, and .49, .49, .46 for women, respectively (all $p < .01$, $n = 51$). However, GDP was also strongly correlated with all cancer in both men ($r = .83$, $n = 51$) and women ($r = .80$, $n = 51$), which in part explains the associations with personality. Indeed, none of the above correlations remained significant when we controlled for GDP.

However, even after controlling for GDP, in both men and women the cancer summary variable was associated with lower N4: Self-Consciousness, and higher N5: Impulsiveness, O1: Fantasy, O3: Feelings, and O6: Values, findings which were replicated using self-report data. Among women, the cancer summary variable was associated also with low N6: Vulnerability, and higher E1: Warmth, E4: Activity, and A3: Altruism, and again these associations were replicated using self-report data. The pattern of facets is revealing: Low N4 and N6 and high N5, E1, E4, O1, O3, O6, and A3 are all definers of the culture-level E factor reported in Table 10.1, the factor that contrasts poorer materialist (Inglehart, 1997) with richer and longer-lived postmaterialist cultures. Apparently, controlling for GDP does not adequately account for this contrast. Such alternative hypotheses need to be carefully evaluated before any substantive interpretations of associations at the culture level are made. Overall, as in individual-level studies, it is doubtful that personality traits at an aggregate level are causally related to cancer. However, as this example should make clear, control for GDP is a minimum requirement in these analyses, and all subsequent results are net of GDP.

Life Expectancy

At the individual level, low C has been found to be associated with all-cause mortality (e.g., Weiss & Costa, 2005). At the culture level, we found measures of life expectancy, healthy life expectancy, neonatal and under-5 years survival all correlated positively with E and C (r_{GDP} ranged from .28 to .39, $n = 50$), for both men and women, but these associations were not replicated with self-report data. Consistently across observer rating and self-report data, the facets O3: Feelings, O6: Values, and low A4: Compliance were associated with life expectancy and healthy life expectancy for both men and women. In observer rating data, four of the six facets of C were associated with measures of life expectancy, and the effects for C3: Dutifulness (r_{GDP} ranged from .51 to .53, $n = 50$) were replicated with self-report data.

Substance Abuse and Obesity

Personality traits play a substantial role in substance abuse and addiction (Brooner, Schmidt, & Herbst, 2002), together with many other biological, psychological, familial, and social factors. The use of illicit drugs is a form of antisocial behavior, and thus low A should be a predictor. Substance abuse often results in many social and health-related risks, which low C individuals are more likely to incur. The fact that younger people are at higher risk for substance abuse and also lower in A and C than older adults supports these hypotheses. The emotional vulnerability and the self-medication hypotheses would predict higher scores on N for people with substance abuse. E5: Sensation Seeking and N5: Impulsivity facets might increase the risk for first use and relapse, whereas low C5: Self-Discipline and C6: Deliberation might be relevant to the continued use of drugs. Other hypotheses have also been advanced. For example, cannabis use has been associated with O (Flory, Lynam, Milich, Leukefeld, & Clayton, 2002), and with schizotypal traits (Dumas et al., 2002), which are related to high O and low E (Widiger, Trull, Clarkin, Sanderson, & Costa, 2002).

The kinds of drugs used vary widely across cultures; religious, geographical, and historical reasons seem to determine patterns of drug use. For example, Iran has one of the highest rates of consumption of opiates, but very low rates of alcohol use. With the exception of cigarette smoking, Asians seem to consume less of the drugs we examined than Europeans, Africans, and Americans.

When prevalence rates for cigarette smoking for men and women were considered separately, a higher smoking prevalence for women was found in cultures high on E and several facets, including N5: Impulsiveness (r_{GDP} = .32, $n = 43$), E6: Positive Emotions ($r_{\text{GDP}} = .44$, $n = 43$), and A3: Altruism ($r_{\text{GDP}} = .44$, $n = 43$). Those effects were replicated when using self-report data and when examining adolescent female smoking prevalence. Using observer ratings, the use of alcohol, opiates, and amphetamine was not associated with the five factors but there were significant associations of ecstasy and cocaine with E, cannabis with low C, and amphetamine with low N. However, none of these effects was replicated using self-report data. A few findings were replicated at the facet level: In cultures whose members are high on O6: Openness to Values there was a higher rate of ecstasy use ($r_{\text{GDP}} = .36$ $n = 38$); and high E3: Assertiveness was associated with amphetamine use ($r_{.GDP}$ = .33 n = 44). Overall, at the culture level we found no clear pattern across substances, and the few effects we observed did not match hypotheses generated from individual-level data. In particular, cultures low in A and C were not particularly prone to the use of drugs.

Obesity (percentage of the population with Body Mass Index > 30) was higher in cultures with higher levels of E ($r_{.GDP}$ = .42, n = 23). This finding was robust, replicated in men and women, with or without partialing GDP, and similar in self-report data. Controlling for GDP, the combined obesity measure was associated with five facets including low E4: Activity ($r_{.GDP}$ = −.54, n = 23), low O2: Aesthetics ($r_{.GDP}$ = −.54, n = 23), and high E5: Excitement Seeking ($r_{.GDP}$ = .55, n = 23), but the effects were replicated using self-report data only for E5.

Homicide, Suicide, and Accidents

Contrary to the findings of Lynn and Martin (1995), we found no association of rate of deaths due to assault with E or any other factor after controlling for GDP. Consistent with Lynn and Martin, suicide rates for females were higher in introverted cultures after controlling for GDP ($r_{.GDP}$ = −.45, n = 40), although the effect was not replicated in our self-report data. The only replicated effects across method were negative correlations of suicide rates with A3: Altruism ($r_{.GDP}$ = −.39, n = 40) and C1: Competence ($r_{.GDP}$ = −.34, n = 40), for females. Rate of deaths due to traffic accidents were related only to high A1: Trust ($r_{.GDP}$ = .41, n = 36) after controlling for GDP, and this effect was not replicated using self-report data.

Mental Health

Perhaps the most plausible hypotheses linking aggregate personality traits to national rates of illness would concern mental health. At the individual level, personality traits are related to a host of mental disorders, including mood, anxiety, and personality disorders. Camisa et al. (2005) reported that schizophrenia was associated with high levels of N and lower levels of E, O, A, and C.

However, data on cross-cultural psychiatric epidemiology are still scarce. For depressive and anxiety disorders, the largest systematic studies we could find included only about 10 countries (Demyttenaere et al., 2005; Weissman et al., 1996, 1997), which is too small a sample size for culture-level analyses. The quality of psychiatric data is also questionable. For example, in the data we examined on prevalence rates of schizophrenia (Saha, Chant, Welham, & McGrath, 2005), some of the African countries were clear outliers. There are several likely reasons for variations in the reported rates of disorders, including differences in health care systems, in the cross-cultural manifestation of the disorder, and in diagnostic criteria. Unfortunately, mental health is not typically covered by WHO international health initiatives like the Millennium Developmental Goals (but see Demyttenaere et al., 2005). And even WHO data do not escape criticism: Attaran (2005) argued that many indicators of the Millennium Developmental Goals lack valid data. For some authors "there is no solid evidence for a real difference in the prevalence of common psychiatric disorders across cultures" (Cheng, 2001, p. 1). Perhaps it is not surprising, therefore, that we found no replicable associations of personality traits with the prevalence of schizophrenia. Nevertheless, psychiatric epidemiology remains one of the most promising areas for future research on personality traits at the culture level.

Promise and Problems in Culture-Level Analyses

Culture-level correlations are very complex, and the results reported here and summarized in Table 10.2 are not easy to interpret, nor particularly impressive. At least post hoc, correlates of some variables like life expectancy and obesity seem to make sense, but many do not parallel individual-level findings. In interpreting these results there are risks of uncontrolled third variables, even when obvious candidates like GDP are controlled. Further, we do not have the luxury of replicating findings in successive samples of cultures, because the number of cultures is quite limited. For all these reasons, the findings in Table 10.2 must be viewed with considerable caution.

Failures to find associations should also be viewed cautiously. National characteristics are likely to be influenced by a host of economic, historical, and geographical forces that will often swamp the subtle influences of personality traits. Associations are most likely when the variables of interest are most directly related to personality traits at the individual level. An example is HIV stigmatization, which is associated most strongly at the individual level with conventional and dogmatic values, and which appears to be most virulent in cultures whose members collectively are low in Openness to Values (McCrae, Costa et al., 2007). Psychiatric disorders should also reflect individual-level associations on the culture level, but better and more extensive diagnostic data are needed to test this hypothesis.

However, it is also the case that our study was limited to the collection of data readily available on the Internet. Convenient as that source is, it is not a substitute for a systematic and scholarly review of the literature. Researchers may need to combine the diligence of meta-analysts with the sophistication of cross-cultural psychologists to exploit fully culture-level analyses of personality traits.

TABLE 10.2

Summary of Culture-Level Correlates

Criterion	Aggregate Personality Factor				
	N	E	O	A	C
Cancer Summary	−N4[a]	E1[ab]	O1[a]	A3[ab]	
	N5[a]	E4[ab]	O3[a]		
	−N6[ab]		O6[a]		
Life Expectancy		E	O3[a]	−A4[a]	C
		E4	O6[a]		C1
					C4
					C5
					C3[a]
Cigarette Smoking	N5	E[ab]		A3[a]	
		E6[a]			
Alcohol Use					
Opiates					
Ecstasy Use		E	O6[a]		
Cocaine Use		E			
Amphetamine Use	−N	E3[a]			
Cannabis Use					−C
Obesity	−N4	E	−O2		
	−N6	E5[a]			
		−E4			
Homicide					
Suicide		−E		−A3[ab]	−C1[ab]
Traffic Death				A1	
Schizophrenia					

Note. These are significant ($p < .05$) effects, controlling for Gross Domestic Product per cap-ita, described in the text. A total of 530 significant correlations were seen, 272 of them replicated in self-report data. See Table 1 for NEO-PI-R facet labels. Minus signs indi-cate negative associations. [a]Replicated using self-report personality data ($p < .10$). [b]Significant only for women.

Culture-Level Assessment of National Character

We conclude this section with a study in which null results from culture-level analyses were scientifically and socially important. Terracciano et al. (2005) assessed perceptions of national character in 51 cultures, using a 30-item instrument designed to parallel the 30 facets of the NEO-PI-R.

Respondents were asked to rate on a 5-point scale how likely the typical member of their own culture was to possess each trait. Aggregate ratings from a mean of 81 judges per culture were highly reliable, and the National Character Survey (NCS) scales showed a reasonable approximation to the intended FFM structure. Ratings from different sites in some cultures, and from college-age and adult judges in Italy and Ethiopia, suggested that perceptions were readily generalizable. The English thought they were reserved, Germans reported that they were industrious, and Australians asserted that they were extraverted.

However, when these NCS scores were compared to the aggregate NEO-PI-R scores from the PPOC Project, there was no evidence of agreement. Within cultures, the perceived NCS profiles did not match the assessed NEO-PI-R profiles; across cultures, none of the five factors showed a significant correlation between the two instruments. All these null findings were replicated when self-report NEO-PI-R data (McCrae, 2002) were used as the criterion for evaluating NCS perceptions. For example, Canadians believed that they were highly agreeable, whereas Americans thought Americans were quite disagreeable. In fact, however, both Canadians and Americans were near the world average on Agreeableness.

For years social scientists have debated the validity of stereotypes of all kinds; national character stereotypes in particular were sometimes thought to have at least a kernel of truth, and sometimes derided as collective fictions (Lee, Jussim, & McCauley, 1995). It was possible to resolve this issue only by having valid culture-level criteria that tell us what the people in a culture are really like, and aggregate scores from self-reports and observer ratings on the NEO-PI-R provided such criteria. Terracciano et al. (2005) showed that the widely shared perceptions of national character are unfounded stereotypes, and encouraged people to guard against these attractive, and sometimes dangerous, fictions.

MULTILEVEL ANALYSES OF PERSONALITY DATA

The history of the PPOC Project (McCrae, Terraciano et al., 2005a) offers some insights into the value of data at two levels. The analyses that preceded the PPOC Project (McCrae, 2001, 2002) used secondary analyses of NEO-PI-R self-report data gathered by other researchers for their own projects. In most cases, published means and standard deviations were used, and data from the individual level were unavailable. For the PPOC Project, individual-level data were collected. From these individual data we scored acquiescence (the sum of unreflected items from the roughly balanced NEO-PI-R) and some aspects of data quality, and used these variables, at a culture level, to help interpret culture-level findings. For example, cross-cultural differences in the strength of factor replicability were due in part to differences in the quality of the data. Strictly speaking, this is a culture-level analysis rather than a multilevel analysis, but it was made possible by the availability of individual-level data in the later project.

Because data can be analyzed at the level of the individual or of the culture, cross-cultural studies of personality would seem to yield ideal data for multilevel analyses, such as Hierarchical Linear Modeling (HLM; Raudenbush & Bryk, 2002). There are a number of different ways to approach the multilevel analysis of data. In the simplest design, individual data are grouped within cultures, and it is possible to examine whether there are cultural differences in the mean levels (and variances) of a given variable, say N. Next, one could relate the HLM-estimated culture means of an individual-level variable like N to a culture-level variable, say GDP, to examine whether mean level differences in N are predicted by GDP. This would be a more statistically sophisticated version of the culture-level analyses reported in the previous section. Third, one might consider an individual-level predictor variable, say sex, to examine whether it is related to N, whether the relationship differs across cultures, and whether culture-level variables, like GDP, explain potential differences across cultures.

Statistically, HLM and other multilevel programs involve sophisticated methods of data weighting based on Bayesian statistics, and they are likely to be increasingly used in psychology (see the chapters by Fontaine and by Selig, Card, and Little in this volume for more details on the statistical advantages of multilevel programs). Conceptually, however, the kinds of questions they address can sometimes be answered by simpler and more familiar methods, and those may suffice in the early stages of culture-level analyses.

For example, Costa, Terracciano, and McCrae (2001) were concerned with what is conceptually a multilevel problem when they examined gender differences across cultures. Within each culture, they contrasted personality scores for men and women and, at a higher level, compared cultures on these differences. Results were striking: Men and women everywhere showed the same directional pattern of differences, but the magnitude of differences varied systematically across cultures. Surprisingly, it was largest in modern, Western cultures. Costa et al. speculated that this might be due to attribution processes: Characteristics attributed to the individual in individualistic cultures might be seen instead as simply manifestations of gender role in more traditional cultures.

McCrae, Terracciano et al. (2005a) replicated those findings for gender differences and conducted similar analyses for differences between college-age and adult targets on NEO-PI-R observer ratings. Although there was some variation in the magnitude of age differences, it was not related to culture-level variables they examined in any easily interpretable way. In particular, traditional cultures did not minimize age differences, as they did gender differences.

Another conventional analysis that speaks to the relation between individual and group levels concerns the magnitude of group differences in comparison to individual differences. This is the familiar question of the percentage of variance accounted for by group factors, and it is an important issue in cross-cultural comparisons (Matsumoto, Grissom, & Dinnel, 2001). Assertions like "Norwegians are more extraverted than Hong Kong Chinese" are invariably statements about mean levels; there is a wide range of individual variation within every culture, and researchers and their readers need continual reminders of this fact to avoid thinking in stereotypes (Terracciano et al., 2005).

Table 10.3 reports an analysis of observer rating data from 51 cultures (McCrae, Terracciano et al., 2005b). For each of the five factors it shows the percentage of variance accounted for by sex, age group, culture, and their interactions. Sex and age effects are robust phenomena, and stereotypes suggest that they are relatively large in magnitude. In fact, however, they are generally smaller than the effects of culture. However, all these effects together account for only about 10% of the variance. The remaining variance is attributable to individual differences within cultures and error of measurement. Stronger effects for culture would probably be found in analyses of self-reports, because the variance between cultures is larger there (McCrae, Terracciano et al., 2005b). In fact, Poortinga and Van Hemert (2001) reported that between 14 and 16% of the variance in (self-reported) EPQ N, E, and Psychoticism scales could be attributed to culture, although

TABLE 10.3

Percentage of Variance in Observer-Rated NEO-PI-R Domain Scores Attributable to Sex, Age, and Culture

Source	Factor					Mean
	N	E	O	A	C	
Sex	2.3	0.1	0.5	1.2	0.2	0.9
Age group	0.5	3.1	4.5	0.4	7.2	3.1
Culture	3.4	3.9	5.1	4.1	3.4	4.0
Sex × Age group	0.0, *n.s.*	0.0, *n.s.*	0.0, *n.s.*	0.1	0.1	0.0
Sex × Culture	0.8	0.6	1.0	0.8	0.7	0.8
Age group × Culture	0.9	1.3	1.4	1.1	1.7	1.3

Note. $N = 12,156$. Age Group = College age vs. adult, 40+. Data from McCrae et al., 2005b. Values are partial η^2s from a three-way ANOVA. The three-way interaction is significant only for Openness, partial $\eta^2 = 0.6\%$

those values are probably inflated by age and gender differences between the cultures they examined.

The interpretation of the interaction terms in Table 10.3 is of some interest. The Sex × Culture interaction is due to the fact that gender differences are more pronounced in Western cultures. Note that this is the same finding we previously discussed as a "multilevel" result, highlighting the connection between multilevel analyses and the more familiar ANOVA. There are even larger Age Group×Culture effects, but their interpretation varies across the five domains. The largest is for Conscientiousness, and inspection of the age effects for that factor (McCrae, Terracciano et al., 2005a) shows that the difference between college-age and adult targets is smallest ($d < .30$) in developing countries (Ethiopia, Indonesia, Nigeria, Russia, and Uganda). One possible explanation for that finding is that adolescents in these countries are obliged to take on adult responsibilities earlier in life. But it is also true that data quality tends to be quite low in these countries, and real age differences may be obscured by error of measurement.

HLM analyses offer more precise statistical estimates; is it possible that the rather unimpressive results we found with simple culture-level correlations might be improved by the use of HLM methods? We examined three hypotheses that were not confirmed in the earlier analyses (homicide and E, Lynn & Martin, 1995; schizophrenia and N, Camisa et al., 2005; and opiate use and low C, Brooner, Schmidt, & Herbst, 2002) and two hypotheses that were confirmed (longevity and C, Weiss & Costa, 2005; and suicide and low E, Lynn & Martin, 1995) using HLM, to see if all five would be supported in these more sensitive analyses. In HLM, the personality traits were the outcome variables and in each analysis we included GDP as a level-2 predictor (rather than as a covariate) along with one of the other culture-level indicators (homicide rate, etc.). Aside from the fact that the association of low E with suicide rate in males showed only a trend (it was significant in females), HLM results did not differ from the simple culture-level correlations reported earlier. In this application, HLM does not seem to offer a clear advantage over traditional methods.

CONCLUSION

Psychologists have accumulated a vast catalog of personality trait correlates, many of them now summarized in terms of the FFM (e.g., Ozer & Benet-Martínez, 2006). To the extent that national levels of personality traits can be validly assessed from relatively small samples of convenience (McCrae, 2002; McCrae, Terracciano et al., 2005b) and to the extent that individual-level correlations translate directly to the culture level, we are now in a position to make inferences about a wide range of socially important outcomes for literally billions of people. Consideration of the personality profile of a culture could improve our understanding of social phenomena and the success or failure of public policy across cultures. Ideally, aggregate personality traits could guide interventions, tailoring them to the prevalent needs and traits of each population.

For example, HIV stigmatization is associated at the individual level with conservative values; societies like Zimbabwe and India score low on Openness to Values; and public policy in Zimbabwe, which preferred to ignore the problem, contributed to a devastating epidemic there (McCrae, Costa et al., 2007). There are signs of an approaching epidemic in India on an even greater scale. Knowledge of the people's likely reactions should inform a more enlightened and effective public health approach in India. For example, public health officials should recognize the paramount importance of anonymous testing and confidential treatment in a society where HIV infection is so severely stigmatized.

On the individual level, C is associated with successful smoking cessation (Terracciano & Costa, 2004). One possible inference is that anti-smoking campaigns in low-C cultures would require special incentives or sanctions (such as high cigarette taxes), because many culture members might lack the self-discipline to act prudently on health advice alone. Education itself might be effective with highly conscientious people; would it make sense to focus the world's limited public health education resources on high-C cultures? Perhaps. But our culture-level correlations did not show any association of C with smoking prevalence, so other cultural factors must be at work. At best, we might use individual-level findings as a source of hypotheses to be tested at the culture level.

Aggregate trait levels might play a role in economic planning as well. Developing countries seeking an optimal economic system might encourage individual entrepreneurs if the aggregate level of E is relatively high, but favor more collective efforts in cultures lower in E. Campaigns to increase productivity might emphasize the social contribution of work in high A cultures, but its role in personal advancement in low A cultures. Tourism promotions could highlight the treasured traditions of closed cultures and the amazing innovations of open cultures.

The practical value of personality traits at the individual level has had a very stormy history. After Mischel's (1968) critique, the very existence of traits was questioned, and until Barrick and Mount's (1991) meta-analysis, trait measures were generally derided as useless by industrial/organizational psychologists. In the past few decades we have learned much about traits and their applications in clinical, developmental, health, and industrial/organizational psychology. We are only beginning to investigate the meaning and utility of aggregate personality traits and have much to learn about the optimal criteria and methods of analysis. Only when the basic science is better understood will we be in a position to grasp the full public policy implications of personality profiles of cultures.

APPENDIX 10.A

Standardized Facet Means for 51 Cultures

	NEO-PI-R Form R Facet Means														
	N1	N2	N3	N4	N5	N6	E1	E2	E3	E4	E5	E6	O1	O2	O3
Americans	49.1	50.1	48.5	47.9	50.0	48.4	51.3	51.2	51.8	48.9	54.2	50.7	51.4	48.8	51.5
Argentines	52.0	49.2	51.8	48.2	51.6	52.1	47.0	51.6	48.6	51.4	49.5	53.2	50.7	45.9	47.4
Australians	49.8	50.3	50.1	48.7	51.1	48.6	53.5	52.3	52.4	48.8	54.9	51.6	51.5	47.8	52.5
Austrians	47.4	48.8	47.2	48.5	49.8	48.6	51.8	50.7	50.9	51.0	47.1	51.5	48.9	50.6	50.9
Batswana	48.9	51.5	52.7	50.2	49.0	51.1	45.6	49.0	50.9	46.1	50.0	48.2	47.6	48.6	46.8
Belgians	49.5	49.7	52.4	46.0	53.0	49.6	49.8	51.9	50.2	50.2	50.6	51.9	52.5	49.5	51.2
Brazilians	54.6	52.1	51.2	51.1	51.8	52.2	51.1	49.9	48.8	52.1	52.9	51.9	52.6	51.2	48.5
Burkinabé	52.0	52.9	52.6	55.0	48.9	50.9	50.0	50.3	48.2	47.3	50.7	47.8	48.5	50.7	48.1
Canadians	51.5	50.1	49.9	48.6	49.8	49.5	52.5	53.0	51.6	48.0	52.7	50.0	50.1	50.3	50.9
Chileans	51.4	48.7	49.9	47.4	49.2	50.6	49.5	50.7	51.6	50.4	49.1	54.9	52.8	50.3	51.6
Croatians	48.8	51.0	49.0	47.9	51.5	48.5	47.4	50.5	50.2	51.2	48.7	51.4	50.4	48.4	50.6
Czechs	49.8	51.4	48.8	48.7	49.3	51.1	54.3	47.1	48.2	48.1	42.9	48.9	46.1	50.9	51.9
Danes	49.3	47.3	52.9	50.1	51.9	50.1	52.1	52.0	49.5	55.3	47.2	50.6	53.2	52.0	53.4
English	50.8	50.6	50.4	48.7	51.9	48.6	53.0	50.7	51.1	49.8	53.2	53.5	54.4	50.3	55.3
Estonians	48.8	47.9	49.2	48.8	50.0	46.2	49.8	50.3	52.2	53.4	50.5	50.6	48.8	46.7	49.5
Ethiopians	47.3	50.8	51.7	51.0	49.3	52.3	46.9	49.4	47.1	48.1	50.9	48.2	48.6	50.3	46.0
Filipinos	48.3	48.0	47.7	51.4	45.7	46.9	48.7	50.5	53.8	49.2	51.2	48.4	49.0	51.1	51.2
French	53.9	51.7	52.1	51.2	51.3	51.1	48.4	46.7	47.5	51.5	47.5	47.6	52.4	49.1	49.6
French Swiss	53.2	50.9	53.0	50.9	52.4	50.5	52.5	48.2	49.1	52.4	47.1	50.3	53.5	50.4	51.6
German Swiss	46.3	45.3	44.9	48.7	47.8	45.6	52.2	48.0	49.6	51.5	43.3	52.4	53.0	55.2	57.2
Germans	47.1	47.5	46.2	48.7	48.2	47.2	52.6	50.4	50.8	51.5	46.1	50.9	51.0	55.3	54.6
H. K. Chinese	50.4	52.9	51.1	49.8	48.6	53.0	48.6	47.6	48.8	47.9	47.5	45.2	47.6	47.6	47.6
Icelanders	47.4	49.3	48.7	50.6	51.3	48.3	51.1	52.2	48.2	51.1	50.0	52.4	51.8	49.3	49.9
Indians (Telugu)	46.8	46.7	54.2	51.8	46.8	49.4	47.8	52.7	49.5	50.0	50.4	50.4	46.2	53.0	46.5
Indonesians	49.5	49.5	50.5	50.6	46.7	53.6	46.5	47.3	48.4	47.1	49.7	46.5	46.5	50.3	48.1
Iranians	48.8	49.1	51.6	48.2	47.0	52.3	46.5	51.1	48.7	47.8	53.0	48.7	47.5	54.1	48.3

Italians	52.9	52.8	52.1	50.5	53.3	53.4	46.4	46.8	48.1	50.4	46.5	46.4	52.8	52.2	48.4
Japanese	50.7	50.1	51.1	48.9	50.4	52.9	49.6	49.9	51.1	52.5	50.0	50.2	49.8	52.6	51.8
Kuwaitis	51.8	50.8	50.0	52.2	49.9	50.0	52.9	53.3	50.6	51.4	51.7	50.4	48.8	49.9	49.0
Lebanese	50.6	52.9	48.9	48.7	50.7	49.8	49.6	52.0	51.8	49.8	52.6	50.0	48.3	49.6	49.5
Malays	50.3	49.2	50.2	56.3	48.8	49.3	49.3	50.5	50.6	49.4	49.1	49.9	46.4	47.7	47.6
Maltese	53.1	52.9	52.2	51.0	51.0	51.0	51.3	49.3	49.3	51.1	50.6	48.8	48.7	48.0	51.4
Mexicans	48.7	48.3	47.1	46.4	47.7	48.0	45.5	48.8	51.3	49.7	49.3	51.5	50.2	49.8	46.5
Moroccans	50.6	52.3	53.3	53.8	49.9	53.4	42.6	47.5	49.4	48.5	50.8	44.7	48.5	49.0	45.5
N. Irish	51.4	50.3	50.9	49.7	50.9	47.7	55.1	52.7	50.8	49.5	52.9	52.1	50.5	44.5	53.8
New Zealanders	48.9	50.2	50.0	48.4	49.6	48.4	52.4	51.9	50.0	48.5	54.9	50.6	50.7	47.7	50.7
Nigerians	46.7	50.5	52.7	51.3	48.6	51.4	42.8	47.8	48.7	46.5	51.4	45.4	47.8	49.9	44.6
P. R. C. Chinese	46.1	48.2	49.6	49.8	47.4	50.0	47.5	50.0	50.1	49.8	47.9	48.0	47.6	50.3	46.5
Peruvians	49.5	47.6	48.7	50.3	51.1	50.4	48.2	49.0	50.8	49.4	51.0	50.5	50.5	48.5	47.3
Poles	50.0	49.3	51.4	52.2	52.4	50.5	49.8	49.3	49.5	50.4	47.8	48.1	49.4	48.1	49.2
Portuguese	53.5	49.5	50.1	49.3	51.8	50.2	51.5	50.2	49.4	49.6	52.6	49.4	52.6	50.5	51.8
Puerto Ricans	50.2	50.0	49.3	47.9	48.5	49.6	49.6	49.9	50.5	53.6	54.0	52.6	50.2	50.5	48.6
Russians	50.0	49.8	49.7	54.1	50.5	54.0	48.0	45.3	47.6	47.2	49.0	45.5	48.7	51.2	48.4
S. Koreans	48.9	48.3	49.4	51.2	48.1	50.4	50.4	52.2	52.9	49.5	49.4	51.9	49.5	50.3	52.9
Serbians	48.8	50.8	47.5	48.2	52.2	47.7	48.9	49.9	47.9	49.9	49.7	48.4	51.0	51.5	52.8
Slovaks	49.5	51.2	48.6	48.0	51.4	50.5	51.1	48.8	48.0	49.7	48.0	50.1	48.9	47.9	47.8
Slovenians	51.1	50.0	49.3	49.9	50.2	50.0	49.4	49.6	49.1	52.1	49.0	49.7	48.7	49.0	49.7
Spaniards	51.6	46.3	49.5	49.9	50.8	48.8	50.5	50.6	51.4	50.0	46.3	51.7	49.8	49.4	49.0
Thais	51.0	50.6	50.3	48.6	48.7	49.6	48.8	48.4	49.2	48.4	49.8	51.6	48.4	48.8	46.2
Turks	47.8	51.0	49.6	53.2	50.6	50.7	51.4	50.9	51.8	51.1	51.1	52.0	49.6	49.6	51.1
Ugandans	47.9	50.7	52.0	52.5	49.0	51.0	45.7	49.6	49.6	47.5	50.7	47.4	48.4	50.5	46.4

(continued)

APPENDIX 10.A

Standardized Facet Means for 51 Cultures (*Continued*)

	NEO-PI-R Form R Facet Means														
	O4	O5	O6	A1	A2	A3	A4	A5	A6	C1	C2	C3	C4	C5	C6
Americans	49.2	51.3	52.5	50.7	49.7	51.3	49.6	50.7	48.0	51.0	49.4	48.5	49.5	50.8	49.0
Argentines	47.5	46.8	48.8	49.4	51.2	51.3	48.9	54.3	51.5	50.6	47.6	51.1	52.6	52.0	48.0
Australians	49.7	52.4	53.4	52.0	51.9	52.1	49.3	51.4	47.7	51.0	47.6	48.4	47.9	49.4	47.5
Austrians	49.1	51.7	50.5	51.5	49.0	51.6	50.6	48.7	51.6	54.5	52.8	52.9	50.0	53.2	50.5
Batswana	51.6	48.4	45.0	47.2	47.7	43.8	52.8	49.3	47.5	44.7	49.6	44.1	46.2	49.3	50.3
Belgians	49.8	49.5	52.2	50.9	50.6	49.7	47.3	52.2	50.7	47.4	47.7	48.6	49.6	49.0	48.4
Brazilians	48.0	48.4	48.7	49.2	49.1	51.3	50.7	51.7	50.6	51.6	50.7	51.8	51.5	50.1	49.7
Burkinabé	51.5	50.1	45.3	47.1	48.3	49.2	51.8	50.3	56.3	46.6	49.9	49.1	49.7	48.8	51.2
Canadians	47.4	50.4	50.7	49.7	49.7	52.3	49.9	49.9	49.3	50.7	50.3	49.9	49.8	50.5	50.9
Chileans	49.1	51.8	50.2	53.2	49.6	51.7	51.0	47.8	52.6	54.1	49.9	52.8	53.6	52.6	50.4
Croatians	48.6	49.5	50.9	50.2	49.1	50.7	47.8	50.5	48.5	50.6	50.5	49.5	52.4	49.7	48.3
Czechs	49.7	49.6	52.1	48.7	55.1	54.2	50.9	54.0	52.9	49.0	48.3	53.9	50.7	50.3	50.5
Danes	54.1	52.3	56.7	54.8	52.7	52.0	50.6	50.5	54.9	53.1	47.4	50.4	47.9	48.6	47.9
English	53.2	51.2	55.9	51.6	49.8	52.6	49.1	51.1	49.2	51.3	49.0	48.8	48.6	49.4	47.8
Estonians	46.4	47.4	50.9	50.7	48.7	48.8	47.4	48.6	49.0	49.7	51.4	49.7	50.0	50.6	48.9
Ethiopians	51.0	49.8	45.8	48.9	44.0	45.7	50.7	48.6	45.0	46.0	50.8	44.3	47.7	47.7	51.8
Filipinos	54.7	51.7	43.4	45.5	46.6	50.2	49.0	47.0	48.1	53.0	51.4	51.1	54.0	52.3	51.8
French	50.2	50.7	54.1	48.1	52.6	50.9	50.7	52.5	51.9	48.0	48.3	48.9	47.0	48.4	47.1
French Swiss	50.7	50.0	52.6	49.1	53.8	53.1	51.7	53.4	53.6	48.5	49.2	50.6	48.5	50.2	47.4
German Swiss	55.1	55.4	56.8	53.2	52.1	54.9	53.8	50.1	52.4	55.9	52.2	54.8	51.3	53.7	51.4
Germans	52.4	52.3	52.7	52.7	49.5	51.5	51.6	50.0	52.5	54.3	51.8	53.6	50.4	52.3	50.5
H. K. Chinese	48.0	48.0	46.9	47.4	46.0	44.9	47.8	45.7	48.7	46.1	51.2	49.6	48.5	49.1	50.3
Icelanders	50.4	50.7	54.8	53.5	51.4	52.3	53.8	51.2	49.2	50.2	49.5	51.5	51.6	49.7	50.5
Indians (Telugu)	46.8	51.8	43.8	52.2	49.9	47.4	54.1	49.1	54.2	47.8	53.9	51.3	53.7	50.2	52.8
Indonesians	51.5	49.2	46.1	49.4	48.6	46.7	49.4	49.8	47.3	45.5	51.3	48.4	50.2	47.8	52.4
Iranians	49.7	47.4	49.0	50.3	47.4	45.0	51.2	45.4	50.2	47.4	48.7	47.3	49.4	45.9	48.5

Italians	52.6	50.1	51.3	47.0	49.0	48.1	45.7	48.7	49.7	47.0	47.2	48.2	47.9	48.8	48.1
Japanese	52.4	49.5	46.1	50.4	51.5	44.4	52.3	46.6	46.6	48.0	48.6	48.9	50.6	48.9	47.9
Kuwaitis	46.9	51.5	43.7	51.9	55.0	53.9	49.0	47.8	49.8	51.0	50.5	51.9	52.9	50.7	49.9
Lebanese	50.6	49.6	47.8	44.5	48.6	49.5	46.1	46.8	47.4	48.3	50.7	49.1	49.4	50.5	50.8
Malays	48.8	50.3	45.1	49.8	53.3	46.8	52.3	51.5	53.7	49.8	53.1	52.1	53.1	48.6	54.6
Maltese	49.0	49.3	50.7	46.4	51.1	51.5	48.2	51.7	48.5	51.3	50.1	50.9	48.9	51.3	49.8
Mexicans	49.4	50.8	49.6	49.6	46.4	47.6	49.8	46.8	48.8	51.3	49.6	50.3	52.0	51.7	52.0
Moroccans	51.4	49.3	45.7	46.6	44.8	42.3	50.4	49.2	45.3	43.9	47.6	43.8	44.9	45.9	48.2
N. Irish	49.2	48.0	52.1	51.4	53.1	54.9	50.3	54.7	51.1	50.6	47.8	49.1	46.6	49.0	47.9
New Zealanders	50.0	51.0	54.3	51.7	51.5	51.4	49.7	52.5	47.5	51.9	48.0	48.5	48.6	50.3	48.0
Nigerians	52.4	49.6	46.0	46.9	45.6	42.7	50.8	47.8	47.1	45.0	47.7	44.2	47.0	46.3	50.2
P. R. C. Chinese	50.2	49.6	51.3	49.3	48.6	45.5	50.2	46.5	49.5	48.3	48.9	48.0	47.4	48.6	52.0
Peruvians	50.2	50.1	47.9	48.2	48.9	50.0	49.8	46.4	49.2	49.4	48.3	48.6	50.5	49.3	49.1
Poles	50.3	49.8	48.0	49.7	49.3	47.6	48.5	49.0	46.8	48.3	51.5	48.4	49.9	48.5	47.9
Portuguese	50.9	50.3	51.2	51.3	49.3	50.6	51.1	52.3	51.8	51.5	51.5	51.1	51.4	50.2	49.9
Puerto Ricans	49.8	50.5	48.9	47.5	50.4	52.0	49.6	49.0	49.7	53.1	49.2	52.1	53.4	52.8	51.8
Russians	48.9	48.7	49.4	51.6	48.5	48.4	48.9	50.5	49.6	47.1	51.0	49.3	48.3	47.3	51.6
S. Koreans	52.0	49.7	49.1	52.8	50.4	47.3	51.0	46.6	50.3	48.4	49.1	49.3	45.7	50.7	50.4
Serbians	48.5	50.6	51.9	50.1	49.3	49.9	47.5	46.3	49.8	52.8	50.1	51.9	52.2	51.6	50.3
Slovaks	51.5	47.0	51.4	49.9	51.6	49.7	49.0	52.7	49.0	49.7	50.2	49.0	47.8	48.4	51.0
Slovenians	47.8	49.5	51.0	49.9	49.2	50.3	48.8	50.6	47.1	51.4	51.5	51.3	52.0	51.2	52.1
Spaniards	47.9	47.1	53.1	51.2	48.6	50.2	50.4	54.4	50.6	52.7	51.2	51.7	51.3	52.1	51.3
Thais	51.6	47.8	48.6	49.9	48.1	49.8	49.0	47.8	52.5	49.5	48.8	49.4	49.2	48.8	51.2
Turks	49.0	45.9	52.4	51.0	54.5	54.5	46.7	49.9	51.6	50.9	51.6	52.0	51.1	49.9	50.2
Ugandans	53.0	50.4	46.0	46.0	47.6	45.8	53.0	48.5	48.5	47.4	50.2	44.8	48.5	48.3	51.5

APPENDIX 10.B

Standardized Facet Standard Deviations for 51 Cultures

	NEO-PI-R Form R Facet Standard Deviations														
	N1	N2	N3	N4	N5	N6	E1	E2	E3	E4	E5	E6	O1	O2	O3
Americans	9.6	10.5	10.4	10.0	10.4	9.7	10.2	10.0	10.0	8.6	10.5	10.3	9.6	9.8	9.8
Argentines	9.2	10.0	9.6	9.4	9.8	10.5	11.5	10.6	10.4	11.4	9.4	11.4	10.2	9.5	9.1
Australians	9.8	10.7	10.8	10.0	9.9	10.4	9.5	10.1	10.7	9.4	10.0	10.5	9.5	9.9	9.9
Austrians	12.4	10.5	11.7	11.6	10.9	11.6	10.5	10.8	12.2	10.3	9.6	10.4	12.0	10.4	11.3
Batswana	7.4	7.3	8.0	8.4	8.1	8.4	10.5	10.3	8.6	8.1	8.7	8.8	7.4	7.6	8.3
Belgians	10.1	9.8	10.1	10.0	9.7	10.2	8.9	9.2	10.0	9.7	9.1	9.5	11.3	11.0	10.3
Brazilians	8.7	10.0	10.8	10.8	11.1	10.5	10.1	11.3	8.6	10.4	10.2	10.9	10.6	10.3	8.9
Burkinabé	7.3	8.3	8.1	9.1	7.7	7.9	9.3	8.5	8.9	8.3	7.7	8.0	7.5	6.9	7.4
Canadians	9.5	9.6	8.9	8.9	9.1	9.5	10.3	10.1	10.9	8.5	10.4	9.5	10.3	9.3	9.2
Chileans	10.7	11.1	10.3	10.5	11.5	10.6	11.2	10.2	9.9	10.5	9.1	11.6	11.4	11.2	11.6
Croatians	10.0	9.1	9.4	10.2	8.9	10.1	9.9	10.0	11.5	9.8	9.9	10.0	10.6	9.6	9.8
Czechs	10.9	10.8	10.5	11.4	12.5	11.1	9.8	11.6	11.7	10.5	10.7	10.1	12.0	11.9	12.3
Danes	12.0	10.3	12.0	11.3	10.7	11.7	10.2	10.2	10.8	10.2	10.2	11.1	10.3	10.8	12.1
English	10.9	10.7	10.5	10.5	10.8	10.2	10.6	10.1	10.4	9.3	10.5	9.7	11.5	10.6	9.9
Estonians	10.2	11.7	10.9	11.0	10.6	10.3	12.0	11.7	13.0	15.0	10.6	12.0	12.3	12.7	10.7
Ethiopians	6.9	7.5	7.4	7.8	7.4	8.2	9.0	8.0	7.7	8.0	7.7	7.6	6.8	7.4	8.4
Filipinos	8.0	10.1	9.3	8.4	9.6	8.6	9.5	9.6	8.8	10.5	9.2	9.6	9.0	7.4	8.8
French	11.2	10.9	11.3	10.3	10.5	11.3	10.5	10.6	9.8	10.5	9.2	9.8	10.5	10.1	9.4
French Swiss	12.8	11.7	11.3	10.4	10.4	11.2	10.1	10.8	11.1	10.7	9.7	11.0	10.8	11.3	10.7
German Swiss	11.2	10.1	11.4	11.2	8.9	9.8	9.1	11.0	11.7	10.6	9.5	10.4	10.8	10.5	11.4
Germans	10.1	8.7	9.7	9.8	9.0	8.7	7.8	9.1	10.8	10.5	9.3	9.0	9.8	8.9	9.4
H. K. Chinese	10.0	10.3	9.8	9.8	10.1	9.8	8.5	7.8	9.7	8.4	9.0	8.7	7.9	9.3	8.4
Icelanders	9.9	9.2	9.5	9.3	9.7	9.0	10.3	10.3	10.2	10.7	9.4	10.5	8.7	9.9	9.1
Indians (Telugu)	8.9	7.7	7.7	8.3	8.8	9.0	8.3	9.5	7.7	8.6	8.3	7.4	7.2	9.2	7.9
Indonesians	11.7	10.4	9.0	9.3	8.3	10.0	9.4	9.2	8.1	8.5	9.3	10.0	7.7	8.6	8.3
Iranians	11.0	10.7	11.4	11.9	12.9	11.6	10.3	9.7	10.2	10.3	10.8	11.4	10.0	10.3	10.0

Italians	10.3	9.8	10.3	10.5	10.6	9.5	9.7	9.3	9.1	9.6	9.3	9.4	10.8	9.6	10.6
Japanese	11.5	11.2	10.0	9.1	11.5	8.7	10.5	10.2	10.7	10.7	9.6	9.5	8.7	8.5	9.1
Kuwaitis	9.1	9.7	8.9	8.7	7.1	9.9	9.2	8.8	9.8	7.6	8.8	8.0	8.5	9.3	8.2
Lebanese	9.3	9.0	8.3	8.5	8.3	9.4	9.5	9.3	9.5	8.7	9.1	8.4	9.2	9.9	8.6
Malays	7.6	9.3	7.3	7.1	8.7	8.5	8.9	7.7	7.4	7.8	7.3	8.3	7.0	7.7	7.6
Maltese	9.8	10.7	10.9	11.7	10.5	10.6	9.8	10.8	11.2	9.4	10.4	10.7	10.9	11.5	11.4
Mexicans	9.1	8.9	10.0	10.0	9.7	9.9	10.2	9.9	9.1	9.9	8.7	10.4	8.3	8.7	9.5
Moroccans	7.4	5.9	6.7	7.7	6.9	7.5	7.4	7.1	6.7	7.6	8.3	8.3	7.7	8.0	8.2
N. Irish	10.0	11.5	11.6	11.2	10.7	9.9	8.6	9.3	11.5	9.9	10.5	10.2	10.1	10.4	9.8
New Zealanders	10.8	11.5	11.5	10.8	9.6	9.7	9.6	10.5	10.8	9.1	10.6	11.5	11.5	11.3	10.0
Nigerians	7.7	7.5	7.2	7.3	7.5	8.6	8.8	8.8	7.3	8.2	9.0	9.2	7.9	7.1	8.4
P. R. C. Chinese	9.1	8.5	8.0	9.4	9.8	9.0	8.8	8.9	9.2	8.9	8.2	9.5	8.5	8.6	9.5
Peruvians	8.2	9.4	9.1	8.4	8.4	10.1	9.0	8.5	8.5	9.3	9.2	9.8	7.8	7.5	9.0
Poles	10.3	9.7	9.9	10.0	9.9	10.4	10.8	9.6	8.9	10.9	10.6	9.4	9.7	10.8	11.2
Portuguese	9.2	9.4	10.0	10.2	10.9	9.7	9.4	9.6	8.7	9.4	9.0	7.7	9.5	9.4	8.7
Puerto Ricans	9.2	10.3	10.3	9.7	11.7	9.7	10.2	9.9	9.9	9.8	11.0	9.8	8.3	9.4	9.1
Russians	9.5	8.0	8.1	8.6	8.1	8.5	8.2	9.4	9.8	10.7	8.5	7.9	8.9	8.9	8.6
S. Koreans	7.2	10.7	8.7	9.2	9.4	8.7	9.1	10.3	9.1	9.3	10.0	9.8	9.9	8.9	9.9
Serbians	10.8	8.7	10.1	9.5	10.9	9.6	10.4	9.3	9.1	11.0	10.6	10.2	11.1	11.6	11.8
Slovaks	9.4	9.1	9.3	8.9	9.7	9.8	7.8	8.3	8.6	8.5	9.2	7.2	8.3	9.1	9.4
Slovenians	10.3	9.1	10.1	10.6	11.0	10.6	9.0	9.4	9.6	10.4	10.2	10.2	11.1	10.6	10.6
Spaniards	11.1	10.8	11.4	10.0	10.7	11.5	11.0	11.2	11.1	12.1	9.6	10.8	11.8	11.7	10.7
Thais	10.1	11.0	9.8	10.0	11.0	10.6	10.8	10.5	10.2	11.2	10.4	10.7	9.9	9.9	10.7
Turks	9.9	11.4	9.5	9.7	10.8	10.1	9.5	10.3	9.7	11.4	11.2	11.2	11.4	10.2	9.0
Ugandans	7.5	7.6	7.4	7.5	7.9	8.4	8.5	8.5	8.5	8.3	7.3	8.3	7.8	8.2	9.0

(continued)

APPENDIX 10.B

Standardized Facet Standard Deviations for 51 Cultures (Continued)

	NEO-PI-R Form R Facet Standard Deviations														
	O4	O5	O6	A1	A2	A3	A4	A5	A6	C1	C2	C3	C4	C5	C6
Americans	9.5	9.6	10.6	10.4	9.7	10.5	10.5	9.9	9.6	10.4	9.6	9.9	9.2	10.1	9.5
Argentines	10.4	10.8	8.5	10.7	9.4	11.3	10.5	10.9	10.6	10.5	9.4	10.0	11.2	10.6	10.8
Australians	10.6	10.6	10.0	9.8	9.6	10.1	10.8	11.1	8.6	10.4	10.1	10.1	9.6	11.2	9.7
Austrians	13.1	11.0	10.1	12.8	8.9	9.8	10.4	8.9	11.6	8.9	11.2	9.2	10.3	11.0	10.9
Batswana	8.7	8.2	7.6	7.7	9.9	8.9	9.6	9.8	10.0	10.0	9.0	9.8	9.8	10.8	9.5
Belgians	9.0	10.3	7.9	9.7	10.8	8.2	9.5	10.6	9.2	7.4	9.5	9.3	9.7	9.5	10.5
Brazilians	10.0	9.9	10.2	10.9	9.1	10.3	10.6	10.3	9.7	9.7	12.4	10.2	10.5	9.7	12.0
Burkinabé	7.5	8.2	7.2	8.5	9.3	8.5	8.9	10.0	10.3	9.3	7.9	9.8	9.0	7.9	9.6
Canadians	9.1	9.2	10.3	10.3	8.7	10.0	10.6	10.7	9.4	9.9	9.0	9.3	9.8	10.6	9.9
Chileans	10.3	12.9	12.9	11.4	9.4	9.9	11.3	10.2	11.7	10.0	9.9	9.3	9.6	10.5	11.1
Croatians	9.6	11.1	9.4	9.9	9.7	10.3	10.3	11.5	9.9	10.5	9.5	10.0	10.6	11.3	10.1
Czechs	11.9	10.8	9.9	10.3	11.5	9.7	11.7	11.8	10.1	10.2	11.8	10.6	11.5	11.5	11.3
Danes	11.2	12.2	9.4	10.9	10.6	10.3	10.6	10.9	11.1	10.1	9.5	10.7	10.3	12.0	10.5
English	10.6	10.8	9.8	11.1	10.5	10.2	11.2	10.4	9.5	10.0	10.4	9.5	8.7	10.6	9.6
Estonians	11.6	12.3	10.5	10.8	11.3	10.7	10.7	11.9	10.8	10.5	10.7	10.1	12.5	10.9	10.5
Ethiopians	7.6	7.3	8.5	8.0	7.1	8.2	7.9	8.0	8.3	10.3	7.5	7.9	8.2	8.6	8.4
Filipinos	10.1	8.6	9.7	9.1	9.7	10.1	10.3	7.8	10.5	10.1	10.2	9.5	10.3	10.0	9.3
French	10.9	11.5	9.2	11.0	10.8	9.3	9.6	11.1	10.7	9.2	10.7	9.6	9.6	9.7	9.5
French Swiss	10.9	10.7	9.7	11.6	10.9	9.4	10.3	11.6	12.1	9.6	11.8	9.6	9.9	10.0	10.0
German Swiss	12.4	10.6	10.4	10.2	8.4	8.4	9.3	8.7	10.3	8.2	9.1	8.7	9.1	9.7	9.0
Germans	10.6	8.6	8.9	8.7	8.2	7.9	9.1	8.7	9.1	8.0	9.3	8.0	9.5	8.9	8.6
H. K. Chinese	9.7	10.4	7.8	9.9	9.7	9.7	9.7	8.3	8.9	9.3	9.8	8.7	9.3	8.4	9.7
Icelanders	10.3	9.8	9.2	8.3	9.7	9.4	10.0	9.0	8.9	9.5	9.0	9.6	10.4	10.4	10.4
Indians (Telugu)	8.0	7.0	7.7	7.7	8.1	8.0	9.4	6.8	11.6	8.5	8.3	9.9	8.6	8.2	7.9
Indonesians	9.6	8.8	8.9	9.4	9.8	9.9	8.4	8.7	8.9	9.1	8.9	10.7	9.4	9.4	10.0
Iranians	10.5	10.3	9.5	12.7	12.2	10.4	10.7	11.8	11.2	12.3	10.7	12.9	12.2	11.1	12.6

Italians	10.9	10.6	10.4	9.6	10.4	8.8	8.4	9.9	10.7	9.9	10.3	10.1	9.1	10.2	10.5
Japanese	9.1	10.2	8.4	9.8	10.2	10.7	11.4	9.7	9.0	9.3	10.7	8.7	10.5	8.7	10.0
Kuwaitis	7.6	8.4	7.5	9.0	10.2	9.3	8.3	6.7	8.3	9.3	8.2	9.7	9.0	8.7	8.6
Lebanese	8.2	9.9	9.3	9.7	9.9	9.5	9.7	11.1	8.5	9.9	8.6	9.5	8.7	9.7	9.4
Malays	7.0	6.6	7.2	7.0	8.6	7.6	8.4	7.6	8.0	8.6	8.8	9.0	8.1	7.3	8.3
Maltese	8.7	11.4	11.3	11.1	11.2	10.5	11.6	12.0	10.0	9.5	10.3	10.0	9.6	10.6	10.5
Mexicans	9.4	10.0	9.6	9.4	8.3	9.5	9.2	8.1	9.7	10.8	9.3	9.5	9.7	9.8	9.9
Moroccans	7.4	7.2	9.0	6.5	6.7	7.7	7.3	6.6	9.4	8.9	8.0	8.8	7.3	8.0	6.8
N. Irish	9.6	10.6	9.6	10.9	11.4	9.5	11.5	10.7	9.5	10.5	9.5	8.8	10.9	11.3	10.0
New Zealanders	10.3	10.7	9.8	10.2	10.1	10.2	11.2	10.7	9.0	10.2	9.8	10.7	9.9	10.4	9.4
Nigerians	8.6	5.8	8.8	7.0	7.1	6.9	7.5	7.6	9.3	9.5	7.2	10.4	8.0	8.5	8.1
P. R. C. Chinese	9.3	8.3	9.9	9.1	8.7	8.4	7.9	8.0	10.6	9.0	8.6	9.1	8.7	8.4	9.3
Peruvians	7.6	8.7	9.0	8.2	9.2	9.2	8.7	6.9	8.5	10.2	7.5	8.6	9.3	9.3	8.9
Poles	11.1	11.1	8.6	9.9	10.4	10.0	9.6	10.0	8.2	10.7	10.6	11.7	9.1	10.5	10.1
Portuguese	10.4	9.5	9.2	9.2	9.5	10.4	10.4	10.1	9.5	10.2	11.4	9.8	9.7	10.0	11.1
Puerto Ricans	8.6	10.3	9.4	10.5	8.9	9.9	9.8	8.2	10.1	9.0	7.9	10.5	9.7	9.1	10.1
Russians	7.9	8.6	7.2	8.4	8.1	7.7	7.7	8.8	8.4	8.7	10.7	8.5	9.8	10.1	8.8
S. Koreans	10.6	9.9	10.3	9.1	9.6	9.7	8.8	8.2	10.9	10.0	10.8	10.0	10.0	9.7	8.9
Serbians	10.5	12.0	10.1	11.7	11.5	11.2	10.6	11.6	10.8	10.2	10.1	10.7	11.0	11.0	11.2
Slovaks	9.5	9.2	9.3	9.0	10.9	8.9	9.7	9.7	8.6	8.6	11.1	10.1	9.1	9.4	9.9
Slovenians	9.9	11.3	9.7	9.7	9.7	10.1	9.2	9.7	9.7	9.8	8.9	10.6	10.6	11.0	10.6
Spaniards	11.6	11.8	11.8	11.9	9.6	10.9	10.5	11.4	10.3	10.2	10.4	9.3	10.1	11.4	11.9
Thais	9.9	8.9	8.7	8.9	10.3	11.1	10.6	9.0	11.0	10.3	10.0	10.4	11.5	9.5	10.1
Turks	10.7	10.8	11.3	9.3	10.0	9.5	10.4	10.7	9.0	9.3	12.3	9.8	10.9	10.1	9.7
Ugandans	7.3	7.1	8.0	7.3	10.1	9.1	8.2	8.4	8.1	9.9	8.6	9.9	8.9	8.8	8.6

APPENDIX 10.C

Standardized Facet Means and Standard Deviations for Self-Report Data in Three Cultures

NEO-PI-R Facet Scale	Burkinabé[a]		French Swiss[a]		Poles[b]	
	M	SD	M	SD	M	SD
N1: Anxiety	58.5	7.6	55.7	11.4	52.8	10.3
N2: Angry hostility	56.5	8.4	51.4	10.4	50.5	9.4
N3: Depression	59.1	7.8	54.6	10.2	55.1	8.6
N4: Self-consciousness	60.0	8.3	53.3	10.2	54.5	9.8
N5: Impulsiveness	48.5	8.1	53.4	10.6	47.7	9.6
N6: Vulnerability	58.7	9.8	54.0	12.6	55.6	11.5
E1: Warmth	45.2	9.6	49.3	10.4	45.4	10.5
E2: Gregariousness	50.5	10.1	48.9	11.4	49.5	10.7
E3: Assertiveness	45.8	7.6	46.5	10.2	45.8	8.8
E4: Activity	44.0	9.7	49.8	11.0	52.5	10.9
E5: Excitement seeking	48.6	8.8	45.8	10.9	44.2	11.3
E6: Positive emotions	43.8	10.9	51.6	11.5	46.5	10.2
O1: Fantasy	47.5	8.8	56.4	10.6	47.7	9.0
O2: Aesthetics	54.0	7.9	53.9	9.7	50.2	8.8
O3: Feelings	43.3	9.3	52.7	10.1	45.8	10.4
O4: Actions	52.5	8.9	53.4	10.9	50.0	10.9
O5: Ideas	51.6	7.7	51.2	10.4	47.6	9.3
O6: Values	41.2	8.1	51.5	10.1	44.8	9.7
A1: Trust	38.8	9.6	45.9	12.8	46.2	10.0
A2: Straightforwardness	45.7	10.0	49.9	12.5	47.7	10.7
A3: Altruism	44.9	10.1	48.4	10.6	43.0	11.1
A4: Compliance	51.2	10.4	51.0	11.2	48.1	10.9
A5: Modesty	50.8	9.4	52.9	11.3	51.3	10.8
A6: Tender-mindedness	59.5	10.7	56.8	11.9	46.7	9.4
C1: Competence	39.4	9.5	42.0	10.1	43.1	10.0
C2: Order	48.7	8.5	47.0	12.0	51.7	10.3
C3: Dutifulness	46.0	10.2	48.2	11.5	48.4	10.3
C4: Achievement striving	53.1	9.1	48.7	9.8	50.7	8.8
C5: Self-discipline	43.3	8.9	44.4	11.6	46.6	9.3
C6: Deliberation	52.5	10.4	47.3	11.4	47.4	11.1

Note. Factor means for Burkinabé and French Swiss samples are given in Rossier, Dahourou, and McCrae (2005). Factor means for Poles are 54.0, 45.4, 47.4, 48.0, and 49.6 for N, E, O, A, and C, respectively. [a]Personal communication, J. Rossier, August 19, 2004. [b]Personal communication, J. Siuta, June 9, 2005.

Author Note

The research was supported in part by the Intramural Research Program of the NIH, National Institute on Aging. Robert R. McCrae receives royalties from the Revised NEO Personality Inventory. We thank the members of the Personality Profiles of Cultures Project, who provided data and are listed as coauthors of three publications that report the basic analyses (McCrae et al., 2005a, 2005b; Terraccciano et al., 2005).

Notes

1. As is often the case, *ceteris paribus* conceals many important qualifications. For example, it implies that the groups are based on random selection; more relevant here, it also implies that the variables show scalar equivalence across the whole population. That would normally be assumed if subgroups from a single culture were analyzed. In cross-cultural comparisons equivalence is in question, and if there are serious violations of scalar equivalence, Allik's prediction should not hold. Conversely, confirmations of his prediction when data are sampled across cultures are consistent with the hypothesis of scalar equivalence. Note, however, that artifacts that affect equally all variables that define a factor—say, adding two points to each Agreeableness facet in some cultures—would violate scalar equivalence but not alter the factor structure (see McCrae et al., 2005b, Footnote 8).
2. Acquiescence does not lead to changes in mean scores when half of the items in a scale are worded negatively, and this is the case with the NEO-PI-R.
3. E, O, and A are not related to income at the individual level (e.g., Judge, Higgins, Thoresen, & Barrick, 1999). In this sense, the meaning of the aggregate personality factors differs from that of the individual-level factors. We do not regard GDP as intrinsically related to aggregate personality, however; their confluence is probably an historical accident. Partialing GDP in the culture-level analyses makes them more comparable to individual-level analyses and more psychologically meaningful.
4. Cancer incidence rates were obtained from the International Agency for Research on Cancer (IARC), which is part of the WHO. The data for the 51 cultures were obtained from the GLOBCAN 2002 database (http://www-dep.iarc.fr/). Annual prevalence of drug abuse for opiates (overlapping cultures, $n = 45$), cocaine ($n = 38$), cannabis ($n = 45$), amphetamine ($n = 44$), and ecstasy ($n = 38$) were obtained from the 2005 World Drug Report of the UN Office on Drugs and Crime (http://www.unodc.org/unodc/en/world_drug_report.html). Latest (1994–2004) smoking prevalence data for 47 overlapping cultures, from WHO sources, were retrieved from the statistics website of the British Heart Association (http://www.heartstats.org/datapage.asp?id=889).

   Data on adolescent tobacco use ($n = 28$) and adult alcohol consumption ($n = 49$) were obtained from the Millennium Development Goal Indicators database of the UN with the latest available data as of April 2005 (http://millenniumindicators.un.org/unsd/mi/mi_goals.asp). The same database provided indicators of life expectancy (n = 50), healthy life expectancy (n = 50), neonatal (n = 50) and under-5 years mortality (n = 50), and obesity separately for men (n = 30) and women (n = 33). Combined gender obesity data (n = 23) were retrieved from the Organization for Economic Co-operation and Development (OECD; http://www.oecd.org/dataoecd/7/38/35530193.xls).

A combined obesity measure using the average of men's and women's rates from WHO integrated with OCED data provided a combined overlapping sample of 40 cultures. The latest (as of June 2004) suicide rates for men and women in 40 overlapping cultures were retrieved from WHO website (http://www.who.int/mental_health/prevention/suicide/en/Figures_web0604_table.pdf). Schizophrenia prevalence data (n = 26) were taken from the literature review of Saha et al. (2005), Table S4 (http://medicine.plosjournals.org/archive/1549-676/2/5/supinfo/10.1371_journal.pmed.0020141.st004.doc).

When separate estimates for men and women, or minimum and maximum, or multiple studies from the same country were available, the average was computed. When multiple estimates for point, period, or lifetime were available, the longest interval was considered. Rates of deaths due to assault and transport accidents (latest 1995–2002, n = 36) were obtained from the UN 2002 *Demographic Yearbook System* (http://unstats.un.org/unsd/demographic/products/dyb/dyb2.htm).

REFERENCES

Allik, J., & McCrae, R. R. (2004). Toward a geography of personality traits: Patterns of profiles across 36 cultures. *Journal of Cross-Cultural Psychology, 35,* 13–28.

Attaran, A. (2005). An immeasurable crisis? A criticism of the Millennium Development Goals and why they cannot be measured. *PLoS Medicine, 2,* e318.

Barrick, M. R., & Mount, M. K. (1991). The Big Five personality dimensions and job performance: A meta-analysis. *Personnel Psychology, 44,* 1–26.

Brooner, R. K., Schmidt, C. W., & Herbst, J. H. (2002). Personality trait characteristics of opioid abusers with and without comorbid personality disorders. In P. T. Costa, Jr., & T. A. Widiger (Eds.), *Personality disorders and the Five-Factor Model of personality* (2nd ed., pp. 249–268). Washington, D.C.: American Psychological Association.

Camisa, K. M., Brockbrader, M. A., Lysaker, P., Rae, L. L., Brenner, C. A., & O'Donnell, B. F. (2005). Personality traits in schizophrenia and related personality disorders. *Psychiatry Research, 133,* 23–33.

Cheng, A. T. (2001). Case definition and culture: Are people all the same? *British Journal of Psychiatry, 179,* 1–3.

Cheung, F. M., & Leung, K. (1998). Indigenous personality measures: Chinese examples. *Journal of Cross-Cultural Psychology, 29,* 233–248.

Costa, P. T., Jr., & McCrae, R. R. (1980). Influence of Extraversion and Neuroticism on subjective well-being: Happy and unhappy people. *Journal of Personality and Social Psychology, 38,* 668–678.

Costa, P. T., Jr., & McCrae, R. R. (1992). *Revised NEO Personality Inventory (NEO-PI-R) and NEO Five-Factor Inventory (NEO-FFI) professional manual.* Odessa, FL: Psychological Assessment Resources.

Costa, P. T., Jr., Terracciano, A., & McCrae, R. R. (2001). Gender differences in personality traits across cultures: Robust and surprising findings. *Journal of Personality and Social Psychology, 81,* 322–331.

Demyttenaere, K., Bruffaerts, R., Posada-Villa, J., Gasquet, I., Kovess, V., Lepine, J. P. et al. (2004). Prevalence, severity, and unmet need for treatment of mental disorders in the World Health Organization World Mental Health Surveys. *JAMA: Journal of the American Medical Association, 291,* 2581–2590.

De Raad, B., & Peabody, D. (2005). Cross-culturally recurrent personality factors: Analyses of three factors. *European Journal of Personality, 19,* 451–474.

De Raad, B., & Perugini, M. (Eds.). (2002). *Big Five assessment.* Göttingen, Germany: Hogrefe & Huber Publishers.

Diener, E., Diener, M., & Diener, C. (1995). Factors predicting the subjective well-being of nations. *Journal of Personality and Social Psychology, 69,* 851–864.

Dumas, P., Saoud, M., Bouafia, S., Gutknecht, C., Ecochard, R., Dalery, J. et al. (2002). Cannabis use correlates with schizotypal personality traits in healthy students. *Psychiatry Research, 109,* 27–35.

Eysenck, H. J. (1947). *Dimensions of personality.* London: Routledge & Kegan Paul.

Eysenck, H. J. (1980). *The causes and effects of smoking.* Beverly Hills, CA: Sage.

Flory, K., Lynam, D., Milich, R., Leukefeld, C., & Clayton, R. (2002). The relations among personality, symptoms of alcohol and marijuana abuse, and symptoms of comorbid psychopathology: Results from a community sample. *Experimental and Clinical Psychopharmacology, 10,* 425–434.

Hansen, P. E., Floderus, B., Frederiksen, K., & Johansen, C. (2005). Personality traits, health behavior, and risk for cancer: A prospective study of a Swedish twin cohort. *Cancer, 103,* 1082–1091.

Haven, S., & Ten Berge, J. M. F. (1977). *Tucker's coefficient of congruence as a measure of factorial invariance: An empirical study* (Heymans Bulletin No. 290 EX): University of Groningen.

Hofstede, G. (2001). *Culture's consequences: Comparing values, behaviors, institutions, and organizations across nations* (2nd ed.). Thousand Oaks, CA: Sage.

Hofstede, G., & McCrae, R. R. (2004). Personality and culture revisited: Linking traits and dimensions of culture. *Cross-Cultural Research, 38,* 52–88.

Huang, C. D., Church, A. T., & Katigbak, M. S. (1997). Identifying cultural differences in items and traits: Differential item functioning in the NEO Personality Inventory. *Journal of Cross-Cultural Psychology, 28,* 192–218.

Inglehart, R. (1997). *Modernization and postmodernization: Cultural, economic, and political change in 43 societies.* Princeton, NJ: Princeton University Press.

Judge, T. A., Higgins, C. A., Thoresen, C. J., & Barrick, M. R. (1999). The Big Five personality traits, general mental ability, and career success across the life span. *Personnel Psychology, 52,* 621–652.

Kroeber, A. L. (1917). The superorganic. *American Anthropologist, 19,* 163–213.

Lee, Y.-T., Jussim, L. J., & McCauley, C. R. (1995). *Stereotype accuracy: Toward appreciating group differences.* Washington, D.C.: American Psychological Association.

Lynn, R., & Martin, T. (1995). National differences for thirty-seven nations in Extraversion, Neuroticism, Psychoticism and economic, demographic and other correlates. *Personality and Individual Differences, 19*, 403–406.

Markon, K. E., Krueger, R. F., & Watson, D. (2005). Delineating the structure of normal and abnormal personality: An integrative hierarchical approach. *Journal of Personality and Social Psychology, 88*, 139–157.

Matsumoto, D., Grissom, R. J., & Dinnel, D. L. (2001). Do between-culture differences really mean that people are different? A look at some measures of cultural effect size. *Journal of Cross-Cultural Psychology, 32*, 478–490.

McCrae, R. R. (2001). Trait psychology and culture: Exploring intercultural comparisons. *Journal of Personality, 69*, 819–846.

McCrae, R. R. (2002). NEO-PI-R data from 36 cultures: Further intercultural comparisons. In R. R. McCrae & J. Allik. (Eds.), *The five-factor model of personality across cultures* (pp. 105–125). New York: Kluwer Academic/Plenum.

McCrae, R. R., & Costa, P. T., Jr. (1992). Discriminant validity of NEO-PI-R facets. *Educational and Psychological Measurement, 52*, 229–237.

McCrae, R. R., & Costa, P. T., Jr. (1999). A five-factor theory of personality. In L. A. Pervin & O. P. John (Eds.), *Handbook of personality: Theory and research* (2nd ed., pp. 139–153). New York: Guilford.

McCrae, R. R., & Costa, P. T., Jr. (2003). *Personality in adulthood: A five-factor theory perspective* (2nd ed.). New York: Guilford.

McCrae, R. R., Costa, P. T., Jr., Martin, T. A., Oryol, V. E., Senin, I. G., & O'Cleirigh, C. (2007). Personality correlates of HIV stigmatization in Russia and the United States. *Journal of Research in Personality, 41*, 190–196.

McCrae, R. R., Terracciano, A., & 78 Members of the Personality Profiles of Cultures Project. (2005a). Universal features of personality traits from the observer's perspective: Data from 50 cultures. *Journal of Personality and Social Psychology, 88*, 547–561.

McCrae, R. R., Terracciano, A., & 79 Members of the Personality Profiles of Cultures Project. (2005b). Personality profiles of cultures: Aggregate personality traits. *Journal of Personality and Social Psychology, 89*, 407–425.

Mischel, W. (1968). *Personality and assessment*. New York: Wiley.

Muthén, B. O. (1991). Multilevel factor analysis of class and student achievement components. *Journal of Educational Measurement, 28*, 338–354.

Muthén, B. O. (1994). Multilevel covariance structure analysis. *Sociological Methods & Research, 22*, 376–398.

Ozer, D. J., & Benet-Martínez, V. (2006). Personality and the prediction of consequential outcomes. *Annual Review of Psychology, 57*, 8.1–8.21.

Paunonen, S. V. (2003). Big Five factors of personality and replicated predictions of behavior. *Journal of Personality and Social Psychology, 84*, 411–424.

Paunonen, S. V., Keinonen, M., Trzebinski, J., Forsterling, F., Grishenko-Roze, N., Kouznetsova, L. et al. (1996). The structure of personality in six cultures. *Journal of Cross-Cultural Psychology, 27*, 339–353.

Piedmont, R. L., Bain, E., McCrae, R. R., & Costa, P. T., Jr. (2002). The applicability of the five-factor model in a Sub-Saharan culture: The NEO-PI-R in Shona. In R. R. McCrae & J. Allik (Eds.), *The five-factor model of personality across cultures* (pp. 155–173). New York: Kluwer Academic/Plenum.

Poortinga, Y. H., & Van Hemert, D. A. (2001). Personality and culture: Demarcating between the common and the unique. *Journal of Personality, 69*, 1033–1060.

Ramírez-Esparza, N., Gosling, S. D., Benet-Martínez, V., Potter, J., & Pennebaker, J. W. (2006). Do bilinguals have two personalities? A special case of cultural frame switching. *Journal of Research in Personality, 40*, 99–120.

Raudenbush, S. W., & Bryk, A. S. (2002). *Hierarchical linear models: Applications and data analysis methods* (2nd ed.). Thousand Oaks, CA: Sage.

Rossier, J. (2005). A review of the cross-cultural equivalence of frequently used personality inventories. *International Journal for Educational and Vocational Guidance, 5*, 175–188.

Saha, S., Chant, D., Welham, J., & McGrath, J. (2005). A systematic review of the prevalence of schizophrenia. *PLoS Medicine, 2*, e141.

Salgado, J. F. (1997). The five-factor model of personality and job performance in the European Community. *Journal of Applied Psychology, 82*, 30–43.

Spiro, M. E. (1999). Anthropology and human nature. *Ethos, 27*, 7–14.

Steel, P., & Ones, D. S. (2002). Personality and happiness: A national-level analysis. *Journal of Personality and Social Psychology, 83*, 767–781.

Terracciano, A., Abdel-Khalak, A. M., Ádám, N., Adamovová, L., Ahn, C.-K., Ahn, H.-N. et al. (2005). National character does not reflect mean personality trait levels in 49 cultures. *Science, 310*, 96–100.

Terracciano, A., & Costa, P. T., Jr. (2004). Smoking and the five-factor model of personality. *Addiction, 99*, 472–481.

Tupes, E. C., & Christal, R. E. (1992). Recurrent personality factors based on trait ratings. *Journal of Personality, 60*, 225–251. (Original work published 1961)

Van de Vijver, F. J. R., & Leung, K. (1997). Methods and data analysis of comparative research. In J. W. Berry, Y. H. Poortinga, & J. Pandey (Eds.), *Handbook of cross-cultural psychology: Vol 1: Theory and method* (pp. 257–300). Boston: Allyn & Bacon.

Van de Vijver, F., & Poortinga, Y. H. (2002). Structural equivalence in multilevel research. *Journal of Cross-Cultural Psychology, 33*, 141–156.

Weiss, A., & Costa, P. T., Jr. (2005). Personality predictors of cardiovascular disease and all-cause mortality. *Psychosomatic Medicine, 67*, 724–733.

Weissman, M. M., Bland, R. C., Canino, G. J., Faravelli, C., Greenwald, S., Hwu, H. G. et al. (1996). Cross-national epidemiology of major depression and bipolar disorder. *Journal of the American Medical Association, 276*, 293–299.

Weissman, M. M., Bland, R. C., Canino, G. J., Faravelli, C., Greenwald, S., Hwu, H. G. et al. (1997). The cross-national epidemiology of panic disorder. *Archives of General Psychiatry, 54*, 305–309.

Widiger, T. A., Trull, T. J., Clarkin, J. F., Sanderson, C., & Costa, P. T., Jr. (2002). A description of the DSM-IV personality disorders with the Five-Factor Model of personality. In P. T. Costa, Jr. & T. A. Widiger (Eds.), *Personality disorders and the five-factor model of personality* (pp. 89–99). Washington, D.C.: American Psychological Association.

Yik, M. S. M., Russell, J. A., Ahn, C.-K., Fernández Dols, J. M., & Suzuki, N. (2002). Relating the five-factor model of personality to a circumplex model of affect: A five language study. In R. R. McCrae & J. Allik (Eds.), *The five-factor model of personality across cultures* (pp. 79–104). New York: Kluwer Academic/Plenum.

11

Acquiescence, Extreme Response Bias and Culture: A Multilevel Analysis

Peter B. Smith and Ronald Fischer

In Schwartz's (1992) analysis of the core elements of culture, achieving coordination with others is postulated as one of three basic challenges that any culture must address. This chapter focuses on one particular aspect of communication, through which cultural groups foster needed harmony and acquiescence among their members, and on identifying what may encourage some cultures to do so more than others. Of course, reaching agreement is not the only goal of a society. In pursuit of the other challenges that are entailed in life, it is often also necessary to assert one's individuality and difference from others. A second goal for this chapter is to explore the cultural contexts in which this assertiveness becomes a priority. Brewer (1991) has formulated an individual-level theory of "optimal distinctiveness," focused upon the way in which persons may find a balance between their conflicting motives to stand out and to be included with others. Individual ways of handling this dilemma vary, but cultures have evolved in ways that press individuals toward distinctive definitions of what is an acceptable balance. In some settings, the press is toward overt harmony and compliance with the expectations and opinions of others. In other cultural settings, the press is more toward self-presentation as someone who is confident, distinctive, and therefore to be valued highly.

This cultural press is accomplished through the totality of cultural socialization processes. In particular, it is accomplished by both formal and informal training through childhood and through continuing adult experiences in how to communicate effectively with others. It is the premise of this chapter that culture-members' trained styles of habitual communication are reflected in the way that they respond to the survey questionnaires that we ask them to complete, particularly those that use a Likert-scale response format. Consistently acquiescent responses to a series of survey items corresponds to a habitual emphasis upon inclusion with others, generalized to include the researcher, who has entered the life space of the respondent. On the other hand, consistent use of the extreme response categories to a series of survey items corresponds to a habitual emphasis upon representing oneself as decisive, separate, and distinctive, or at least as exemplifying qualities that do not rest upon a need for endorsement by others.

In accomplishing the goals of this chapter, it will be necessary to distinguish clearly between response style toward others as an expression of individual-level personality traits and as a property of the culturally specified systems of communication within which individuals operate. We explore each perspective in turn.

INDIVIDUAL-LEVEL RESPONSE STYLES

Persons differ in how they choose to address one another. These differences are apparent in everyday behavior, and have long been of interest to students both of personality (Adorno, Frenkel-Brunswik, Levinson, & Sanford, 1950; Couch & Keniston, 1960) and of social psychology, especially the area of conformity (Asch, 1951).

Acquiescence

By acquiescence we mean a person's consistent tendency to record agreement rather than disagreement with communications that are addressed to him or her, independent of the content of the communication. Particular interest has been elicited in the differences in the degree to which persons exhibit acquiescent responses to survey questionnaires because acquiescent responses threaten the validity of all measures other than that of acquiescence itself. In fact, surveys constructed with the direct purpose of measuring acquiescent responses have been few and far between. Our concern here is with the occurrence of acquiescence and other forms of response bias within data derived from scales that have been designed to measure a wide variety of other psychological attributes.

Acquiescent responding is likely to be a function both of respondent personality and of situational factors such as item format and the context within which surveys are administered. Different survey instruments may not always evoke acquiescence by the same type of respondents (Ferrando, Condon, & Chico, 2004), but where the same instrument is used in numerous locations, the effect of dispositional factors will be greater. In particular, survey instruments with items that are all positively worded will confound acquiescent responding attributable to personality factors with acquiescent responding that is due to the social desirability of the statements within the survey (Cheung & Rensvold, 2000). This is particularly problematic for cross-culturalists, because many survey instruments that are in current use contain only positively worded items.

The recent consensus that most of the major dimensions of personality can be summarized within the Big Five dimensions has made it more possible to determine the types of person most likely to exhibit acquiescence. Since the NEO-PI-R and NEO-FFI instruments comprise equal numbers of positively and negatively worded items they can be correlated with response styles derived from other measures that contain only positively worded items. Consistently positive responses to positively worded items could indicate either acquiescence or a desire to respond in a socially desirable manner. However, social desirability and acquiescence cannot be equated, because there may be circumstances in which it is desirable to disagree with positively worded items. Socially desirable responding has been frequently investigated. Indeed, a meta-analysis of 233 studies by Ones, Viswesvaran, and Reiss (1996) concluded that socially desirable responding is associated with high conscientiousness and low neuroticism. Ones et al. argue that since high conscientiousness and low neuroticism are positive attributes, socially desirable responding does not threaten the validity of psychometric tests for selection purposes. However, the great majority of studies included in this meta-analysis were conducted in the United States, where a positive self-presentation is said to be highly valued. We do not know whether desirable responding would be characteristic of similar personalities in other cultural contexts, such as those that value modesty. Neither do we know the personality correlates of acquiescent responding, either in the United States or elsewhere.

Sorrentino (2005) has developed an individual-level personality measure of uncertainty-orientation. Those who score high on certainty-orientation do not seek out uncertain or risky settings and when faced with uncertainty, they are more likely to acquiesce to guidance from peers or leaders. Sorrentino found many more certainty-oriented respondents among Japanese students than among Canadian students. He proposes that responses to certainty or uncertainty will be affected not just by the individual's orientation, but also by the orientation that is prevalent in the culture within which the individual is located. Thus a certainty-oriented Japanese person located in the highly uncertainty-avoidant Japanese culture is expected to react differently from a certainty-oriented Canadian person located in the low uncertainty-avoidant Canadian culture. Sorrentino studied reports of mood rather than acquiescence, but he did obtain the predicted effects. For instance, certainty-oriented Japanese persons reported more active than passive emotions, whereas certainty-oriented Canadian persons reported more passive than active emotions.

Even within the United States, researchers using the Asch conformity paradigm have illustrated the manner in which the social context can induce acquiescent responding. Although personality attributes do have some influence in this setting (Crutchfield, 1955), it is the basic experimental manipulation from a unanimous but incorrect group of peers that is the major cause of conforming responses. Thus, to obtain a full understanding of the meaning of an individual's acquiescence, we must give equal attention to the individual and to the contextual demands that he or she may experience.

Extreme Responding

Extreme responding is the consistent tendency of a person to respond decisively to communications that are addressed to him or her. In other words, it involves more frequent statements of both agreement and of disagreement, depending on the item content, and less frequent use of the more equivocal judgments represented by the items toward the center of a series of Likert rating scales. There is no reason to predict any association between acquiescence and extremity, since one is operationalized as frequent use of just *one* end of a series of rating scales, whereas the other is operationalized as frequent use of *both* ends.

Extreme responding was identified as a problem long ago (Cronbach, 1946), but in contrast to acquiescent bias, it has until recently been studied rather less by cross-culturalists (Cheung & Rensvold, 2000; Clarke, 2000). Indeed, some might argue that extreme responding should not be thought of as a bias in relation to individuals, since it does provide the researcher with a somewhat better prospect than does acquiescent responding of identifying distinctive attributes of individual respondents and of the range of variations within a sample of respondents. In the context of the present discussion, we should entertain the possibility that extreme response bias is seen as less problematic than acquiescent bias because it is more culturally compatible with the more individualist cultures within which psychometric testing has been most strongly developed. However, extreme bias is just as problematic as acquiescence as soon as one starts to compare mean scores of different samples. In studying extreme responding at the individual level cross-culturally, we can best understand its incidence by examining its correlates separately within each nation, rather than by comparing means across nations. Chen, Shin-Ying, and Stevenson (1995) adopted this approach, sampling high school students in Canada, the United States, Japan, and Taiwan. They found that extreme responding was correlated with a measure of individualism in each of these four nations.

So, extreme response bias may be an expression of individual personality traits but, like acquiescence, its expression is also responsive to context. Hui and Triandis (1989) showed that among bilingual Hispanic respondents, both the language of response and the number of points on Likert response scales affected the proportion of extreme responses. Greater extremity was found when responding in Spanish than in English, suggesting that Hispanic cultures may exert a stronger press toward extremity.

The conventional wisdom among cross-cultural researchers over the past two decades has been that response bias is a source of error and that our studies of culture can best progress if we find ways to discount it. Among psychometricians, the construction of scales with equal numbers of positively worded and negatively worded items has long been a favored procedure for eliminating acquiescent bias. However, cross-cultural researchers have been loath to adopt this solution, rightly or wrongly believing that willingness to disagree with negatively worded items varies across cultures, and that negatively worded items are more difficult to translate into different languages. Consequently, the alternative strategy of within-subject standardization has been widely adopted (Van de Vijver & Leung, 1997). Pioneered by Hofstede (1980), within-subject standardization has the advantage of controlling for both acquiescence and extremity. It has the disadvantage that it eliminates the independence from one another of the scores used to accomplish the standardization (Fischer, 2004). Even more importantly from the present perspective, it may eliminate from our data part of the variance that we are trying to study, if such response styles are related to systematic cultural differences rather than being a simple measurement artifact. The studies reported in the present chapter seek to shed light on these dilemmas by examining within a large sample of survey data the circumstances under which acquiescent and extreme bias are found to occur. In using our results to achieve a conclusion on when the use of within-subject standardization is advisable and when it is not, we need to consider more fully what exactly we mean by a culture of acquiescence or of extremity.

CULTURE AND RESPONSE STYLE

Until very recently, the dominant theme of cross-cultural research has become the exploration of the contrast between nations that are characterized as collectivistic and high on power distance versus those Western nations that are characterized as individualistic and low on power distance. As Hofstede's (1980) study first indicated, nations high on collectivism were usually also high on power distance, and little subsequent progress has been made in differentiating the two dimensions, possibly because of an overly restricted sampling of nations (Smith, Bond, & Kagitcibasi, 2006). At least in terms of Hofstede scores, East Asian nations are by no means the highest in the world on collectivism and power distance. However, the comparisons that have typically been made between North American and East Asian samples have identified several important differences in communication styles. East Asians are shown to have more interdependent self-construals (Kashima et al., 2005), greater concern for others' face (Oetzel et al., 2001), greater embarrassability (Singelis, Bond, Sharkey, & Lai, 1999), greater concern for relationship harmony (Kwan, Bond, & Singelis, 1997), a more indirect communication style (Holtgraves, 1997), more restrictive rules for emotional expression (Argyle, Henderson, Bond, Iizuka, & Contarello, 1986), and less competitive negotiation styles (Morris et al., 1998). Furthermore, several of these studies have shown that at the individual level, interdependent self-construal is a significant predictor of these effects. We do not have full information at present as to how many of these findings may be specific to East Asia or can be said to characterize all nations scoring relatively high on collectivism and power distance. Let us assume for the moment that they do. While not all individuals within any of these cultural groups will be in accord with these aggregated effects, each person must choose how to behave within a context in which *most* persons do accord with these effects. Thus, we may expect that members of nations scoring high on collectivism and power distance will experience a greater cultural press toward acquiescence, while members of nations scoring low on collectivism and power distance will experience a greater press toward extreme responding. This will find expression in terms of modesty and harmony in the former case and in terms of assertion and confidence in the latter case.

An initial test of these ideas is provided by Bond and Smith's (1996) meta-analysis of studies employing versions of the Asch conformity paradigm. They identified 133 Asch replications, of which 36 had been conducted in 17 different nations outside the United States. After discounting the effects of variations in experimental design that were found within the U.S. studies, they found significant variations across nations in the proportion of conforming responses. While these differences might conceivably have been explicable in terms of differential recruitment of personality types in different countries, a more concise and plausible explanation is that there are nation-level differences in the frequency and desirability of acquiescent behaviors, and that these differences were reflected in the results obtained from the Asch replications. Bond and Smith found that higher conformity levels by nation were significantly predicted by nation-level indicators of collectivism (Hofstede, 1980; Trompenaars, 1993) and conservatism (Schwartz, 1994).

This meta-analysis does provide some initial suggestions as to the parts of the world in which acquiescent responding may be more frequent. However, it covered few nations and did not address the basic question as to how best to conceptualize culture-level acquiescence. Is an acquiescent culture simply a large group of persons in which the majority favors acquiescence to others? Recent attempts to define culture in ways that better represent the interrelatedness of the elements in a social system suggest a more adequate conceptualization. The essence of a culture is that it is characterized by a set of shared meanings that are applied by its members to the interpretation of what goes on around them. The behavior pattern that social scientists interpret as acquiescence does have a shared meaning within the social science community, but the behaviors to which it refers are open to a broader variety of interpretations in the wider world. Asch's (1951) classic study is typically thought of as a study of conformity, but within more collectivist cultural contexts it would be equally possible to interpret it as a study of tact or sensitivity. Acquiescent behavior can thus serve a variety of social functions dependent upon the priorities and interpretive schemas that prevail within a given cultural context.

An important aspect of Hofstede's (1980) pioneering study was his realization that if we wish to study nations as cultures, we must establish the coherence of the available data at the level of nations, not at the level of individuals. We can average the scores of individuals within one or more nations on a measure of individual acquiescence, but if we do so, we shall have a "citizen mean" for each nation, not a nation-level mean (Smith et al., 2006). To obtain a nation-level mean, the available indicators of a concept must be separately aggregated to the nation level, so that their structure at that level can be determined. For instance, estimates of acquiescence may be available from responses to each of several different scales. To better understand the distinction between a citizen mean and a nation-level mean, visualize a matrix in which several estimates of acquiescence for each respondent are arrayed within rows in a matrix. The citizen mean is the mean of the row means. The nation-level scores are the column means. The way in which separate column means cluster together at the nation level tells us the extent to which there is a consistent meaning to a concept at that level of analysis. Thus, we can only speak of nation-level acquiescence or extremity if we can find coherence between aggregated (i.e., nation-level) indicators of individual-level acquiescence and extremity.

Smith (2004) compared the indices of acquiescence that had been computed by six research teams, each of which had conducted surveys in 34 or more nations. In five instances, these indices provided a single citizen mean for each nation (Bond, Leung et al., 2004; Hofstede, 1980; House et al., 2004; Schwartz, 1994; Smith, Peterson et al., 2002). In the remaining instance, Van Hemert, Van de Vijver, Poortinga, and Georgas (2002) were able to establish the nation-level structure of the items defining the Lie scale in the Eysenck Personality Questionnaire. The Lie scale is strictly speaking a measure of social desirability rather than acquiescence, but those who have used it cross-culturally have not made any tests of the extent to which the items comprising the scale are in fact socially desirable. The scale may measure social desirability, but it certainly taps acquiescence, since all items are positively worded. These different surveys had separately focused upon values, beliefs, and self-reported behaviors, as well as the Lie scale, and they had sampled divergent populations at different times. Nonetheless, nation-level correlations between the six indices of acquiescence were all positive, with many of them sizable and strongly significant. It was not possible to confirm the nation-level structure of acquiescence by undertaking a nation-level factor analysis of these indices because the number of nations common to all six surveys was too few. Even so, this result provides empirical support for the contention that some nations do have a stronger culture of acquiescence than others. Unfortunately, we do not yet have available data that would permit an analysis of this type that focuses upon extreme response bias.

Having established convergence between the available measures of acquiescence, Smith (2004) then attempted to identify the characteristics of those nations which exhibited greater acquiescence. This was done primarily by regressing acquiescence on the most recently measured nation-level dimensions, namely those provided by the GLOBE group of researchers (House et al., 2004). House et al. asked their respondents to characterize their nation "as it is" and "as it should be" on a series of items that were used to define nine different dimensions of national culture.

Two of the GLOBE dimensions refer to collectivism, because these researchers found that the items that they had intended to define collectivism factored separately. These dimensions were named as "in-group collectivism" and "institutional collectivism." Both of these dimensions are potentially of interest to the analysis of response styles, but it is necessary to look beyond the labels assigned by the GLOBE researchers to these dimensions to gain a clearer understanding of what they may be measuring. The four items defining the in-group collectivism scale refer to pride in group members' accomplishments and loyalty to one's group. This scale appears close to Hofstede's conceptualization, and nation-level scores for "as is" in-group collectivism are correlated with Hofstede collectivism at $r = +0.77$ across the 47 nations in common between the two samples. In contrast, the four items defining the "as is" institutional collectivism scale refer to the degree to which leaders and institutions are perceived to foster loyalty and commitment, but there is no indication in the items as to their specific focus. Although it was not the original intention of the GLOBE researchers to identify a new dimension of cultural variation, these items proved unrelated to the in-group collectivism items and do not appear close to Hofstede's conceptualization of collectivism. The items appear more targeted upon cultural contexts in which some degree of centralized control is present, and may perhaps resemble the cultural dimension of tightness-looseness that was first identified by Pelto (1968) and has been studied more recently by Gelfand, Nishi, and Raver (2006). Among Hofstede's four dimensions, "as is" institutional collectivism correlates significantly only with Uncertainty Avoidance at $r = -0.53$.

The two aspects of communication style that were identified as acquiescent and extreme response styles will be most evident within different contexts. We can expect acquiescence to be stronger in nations that score high on in-group collectivism. It is within in-group contexts that the need for harmony will provide the strongest press. In contrast, we can expect extreme response bias to be greatest in contexts where risk-taking and individual salience are positively valued. These circumstances are less likely to be found within in-group contexts. However, they are more likely in the less structured circumstances that might be afforded by low institutional collectivism and low uncertainty avoidance. Smith (2004) found that the score for "as-is" in-group collectivism was indeed a strongly significant predictor for acquiescence in each of the five independent databases that he sampled. He did not examine extreme response bias.

Johnson, Kulesa, Cho, and Shavitt (2005) studied the relationship of the Hofstede dimensions to both acquiescence and extreme responding among a sample of 18,000 survey respondents drawn from 19 nations. After controlling for individual-level demographic variance using hierarchical linear modeling, they found that extreme response bias was significantly associated with high power distance and high masculinity at the nation level. In a smaller sample drawn from just 10 nations, they found acquiescence to be significantly associated with low GNP, high collectivism, high femininity, low uncertainty avoidance and low power distance.

The result for collectivism is consistent with that obtained by Smith (2004), but the result for power distance is significantly reversed. The pattern of findings obtained by Johnson et al. is hard to comprehend, since power distance and collectivism scores are correlated −0.61 among the 10 nations that they sampled. The reported association of high power distance with high extreme responding is also contrary to the expected relationship that is proposed in this chapter. It seems likely that the results of Johnson et al. were affected by multicollinearity of their indices of collectivism, power distance, and GNP. Indeed, they also report a low but positive correlation between the raw means for acquiescence and power distance in their 10-nation sample. Their results may also have been affected by the restricted number of nations sampled, and by the particular group of nations that they sampled. Further investigations are required in order to clarify these divergent results.

The results obtained by Smith indicate significant predictive power of three of Hofstede's original nation-level dimensions, while Johnson et al. also obtained a significant effect for masculinity-femininity. Smith also obtained effects with both of the GLOBE project collectivism dimensions. For an exploratory study it is appropriate to include all available nation-level dimensions from these two surveys as well as those identified by Schwartz (1994).

STUDY 1: EXTREME RESPONDING BY MANAGERS

As a first step in this direction, the databank of Smith et al. (2002) was used to construct an index of extreme response bias. This is the only database among the six sampled by Smith (2004) that is amenable to creating such an index. The index was based upon the same 64 ratings on 5-point scales that had been used earlier to create an index of acquiescence. Acquiescence was defined as mean positive endorsement across all 64 items. In the present analysis, this score was reduced by 1 and then multiplied by 30 to yield a range (0–120) directly comparable to the extremity measure. For extremity, respondents were assigned two points for each rating at points 1 or 5 on each scale and one point for each rating at scale points 2 and 4 and no points for ratings at scale point 3. This weighting was preferred to an index based solely on extreme scores, as it makes fullest use of the information that can be derived from the responses. Data were available from 8,733 respondents from 56 nations. Bias estimates for individuals were aggregated to the nation level and correlated with available nation-level indices of values.[1] The results are shown in Table 11.1, along with a reanalysis of the data presented by Smith (2004) for acquiescence, now including some additional nations, and providing also a fuller exploration of Schwartz's value domains.

Across this much larger sample of nations, the associations between power distance and masculinity and extreme response bias obtained by Johnson et al. are not replicated. Extreme responding is shown to be asso-

TABLE 11.1

Correlations Between Extreme Responding, Acquiescence, and Nation-Level Indices

Culture dimensions	Extreme Response	Acquiescence
H: Individualism	.10	−.37**
H: Power distance	−.10	.29*
H: Uncertainty avoidance	.13	.00
H: Masculinity	.10	−.18
G: Performance orientation	−.16	.05
G: Future orientation	.04	−.06
G: Assertiveness	.14	−.11
G: Institutional collectivism	−.47**	.09
G: In-Group collectivism	−.16	.45**
G: Gender equality	−.05	−.08
G: Humane orientation	−.15	.24
G: Power distance	.06	.30
S: Harmony	−.11	−.32*
S: Embeddedness	−.19	.45*
S: Hierarchy	−.03	.38*
S: Mastery	.18	.00
S: Affective autonomy	.32*	−.21
S: Intellectual autonomy	−.13	−.44**
S: Egalitarianism	.08	−.46**

Note. H = Hofstede (2001), $N = 56$; G = GLOBE study (House et al., 2004), $N = 42$; S = Schwartz (2004), $N = 43$.

ciated with the GLOBE measure of low "as is" institutional collectivism and with Schwartz's measure of affective autonomy, but no links with the Hofstede dimensions are found. In relation to acquiescence, the enlarged sample shows correlations with collectivism and power distance that are now somewhat weaker, but remain significant. As would be expected, acquiescence is predicted by the GLOBE dimension of "as is" in-group collectivism, and is also linked positively with Schwartz's measures of embeddedness and hierarchy, and negatively with intellectual autonomy and egalitarianism. The weaker but still significant negative correlation with harmony is less easy to explain.

In considering further why these results do not accord with those of Johnson et al., an additional possibility that is central to the theme of this book is worthy of investigation. Johnson et al. used hierarchical linear modeling to control for individual-level demographical correlates of response biases, whereas the analyses reported in Table 11.1 used uncorrected citizen means. Johnson et al. found few uniform effects of the three demographic variables that they analyzed, but there was significant random variance in their effects across nations. The demographic variables upon which they focused were age, gender and job tenure. Individuals' positioning on these attributes might be expected to relate to biased responding, if they were associated with the dimensions of values for which there is a hypothesized linkage with bias. It is plausible that there would be such linkages. Further investigations are necessary, in which variance due to demographic factors has been controlled. This opportunity for clarification requires a sample for which individual-level demographic data are available.

STUDY 2: PREDICTING ACQUIESCENCE

Formulation of Hypotheses

Hierarchical linear modeling permits a closer examination of the ways in which demographic attributes, individual propensities and cultural context may combine to induce varying degrees of response bias. By examining variations across nations in the extent of individual-level predictors of bias, we can determine the extent to which cultural press has moderating effects on the relationships that are found. No doubt there are numerous individual-level factors that can affect types and extent of response bias. We can do no more here than focus on orientations derived from individualism and collectivism, since this distinction was found to be relevant by both Smith (2004) and Johnson et al. (2005). In order to express these issues in the clearest possible way, we do best to follow the lead of those who have argued that we need different terms to refer to attributes of individuals and of nations, even where the terms are conceptually related (Smith et al., 2006; Triandis, 1995). We refer to individuals who favor individualism as independent. We refer to individuals who favor collectivism as interdependent. To put our question more specifically, are interdependent persons even more acquiescent when they are located in a collectivist cultural context? It is plausible that they would be, because they would be aware of locally salient cultural norms as to how best to communicate with others. Conversely, independent persons in a collectivist context would be more likely to express dissent, and hence be less acquiescent. Similarly, it is possible that acquiescence would be stronger in more relationship-oriented cultural contexts labeled by Hofstede as feminine, and less so in more competitive, masculine cultures.

In a parallel way, independent persons may show even more extreme bias within certain types of cultural context. If extremity is a product of wishing to appear distinctive and decisive, we could expect such effects to be maximized in cultural contexts where there are few established pathways for persons to become involved in new groups. These are the circumstances that appear to be tapped by the GLOBE measure of (low) institutional collectivism. Furthermore, extremity could be favored by an environment that encourages risk taking and novelty. There is current confusion as to how best to measure uncertainty avoidance, but validly measured low uncertainty avoidance as well as high masculinity could provide contexts of this type. Low institutional collectivism, low uncertainty avoidance, and high masculinity could also discourage interdependent persons from wishing to appear distinctive. Our discussion of these types of interaction between individual propensities and their cultural context suggests two hypotheses:

> Hypothesis 1: *Respondents' endorsement of interdependence will be positively related to acquiescence, and this effect will be stronger in nations with low individualism and high femininity.*

> Hypothesis 2: *Respondents' endorsement of independence will be positively related to extremity, and this effect will be stronger in cultures characterized by low nation-level institutional collectivism, low uncertainty avoidance and high masculinity.*

Method

To test these hypotheses, two series of HLM analyses were conducted. Study 2 tested Hypothesis 1, while Study 3 tested Hypothesis 2. Both studies required an individual-level measure of independence/interdependence. Such a measure was created from within the databank reported by Smith et al. (2002), selecting the 38 nations from whom this data had been collected. The measure comprised the mean of responses to three survey items: *I do better working alone than in my work team; If the team is slowing me down, it is better to leave it and work alone,* and *In most cases, to cooperate with someone whose ability is lower than mine is not as desirable as doing the thing on my own.* Responses were given on 5-point Likert scales. Since these items were all phrased in terms of independence, any acquiescent bias in responding to them would yield effects contrary to the hypotheses. Hence, no standardization was necessary. To yield an interdependence index, each item was reverse-coded. Nation-level means for these three items were factor analyzed, in order to create a nation-level index of collectivism. The three items yielded a single factor with eigenvalue 2.37, accounting for 79% of variance. This factor score correlated at $r = +0.99$ with the aggregated individual-level measure of interdependence, so there is no indication in this instance of separate structures at different levels of analysis. In other words, it is a strong etic, as Leung and Bond (1989) termed this sort of construct. Among the nations in common, this collectivism index correlated at $r = -0.34, p < .05$, and at $r = +0.50, p < .001$, with Hofstede's individualism and power distance indices respectively; at $r = 0.48, p < .01$, with GLOBE "as is" in-group collectivism; and at $r = 0.58, p = .001$, and at $r = -0.65, p < .001$, with Schwartz's embeddedness and intellectual autonomy indices, respectively.

Details of the sample used are given in Table 11.2. Preliminary analyses indicated that the principal sources of demographic variability between samples were in terms of age, gender, state ownership of one's employing organization, and working in sales. Indices of these attributes were therefore first controlled in an individual-level analysis. The nation-level aspects of the hypotheses were then tested several times, drawing separately on the established nation-level predictors provided by Hofstede (2001), Schwartz (1994) and the GLOBE project (House et al., 2004), as well as the nation-level collectivism index provided by the respondents to the present survey. Controlling for variance attributable to individual-level factors before entering nation-level predictors can provide much more precise estimates of the ways in which the separate variables at these two levels of analysis do or do not interact with one another. We used HLM (Raudenbush & Bryk, 2002; Raudenbush, Bryk, Cheong, & Congdon, 2000) for testing our hypotheses. In the results presented below, coefficient gamma represents the magnitude of effects attributable to a given predictor at a nation level (Raudenbush & Bryk, 2002).

Using Hofstede Predictors

In testing hypothesis 1 with Hofstede dimensions as predictors, it is important to avoid the multicollinearity effects that may have confused earlier analyses. Consequently although power distance has been indicated as a predictor of acquiescence, it was not entered into the analyses.

TABLE 11.2

Samples Used in the HLM Analysis

Nation	N	Mean age	% Male	% State	% Sales	Acquies-cence	Extremity
Australia	185	36.8	74	57	30	2.88	59.7
Belarus	333	42.4	58	84	3	2.89	61.2
Brazil	177	34.8	55	46	9	3.10	54.8
Bulgaria	162	41.7	62	54	17	3.14	57.4
China	119	33.7	55	53	32	3.04	42.1
Colombia	96	39.1	70	39	22	2.96	61.3
Czech Republic	71	41.7	84	6	20	2.86	54.7
Finland	118	43.6	91	20	44	2.97	57.0
France	257	41.2	73	30	23	3.03	58.9
Germany	80	43.5	93	7	29	2.90	55.9
Greece	102	43.4	74	34	38	3.14	65.2
Hong Kong	83	31.5	59	33	48	3.07	55.5
Hungary	100	41.7	72	51	27	3.10	57.7
India	101	37.9	96	76	25	3.41	61.0
Indonesia	109	40.8	89	26	14	3.15	49.8
Iran	93	36.2	98	76	24	3.30	43.5
Italy	130	46.5	98	44	10	2.78	51.4
Jamaica	88	33.1	38	51	37	3.06	57.9
Japan	95	45.9	98	55	15	3.10	49.0
Mexico	297	33.4	76	5	54	3.08	55.9
Netherlands	112	40.1	88	21	42	3.05	51.9
Nigeria	186	38.4	70	45	38	3.43	59.4
Philippines	36	33.1	54	52	16	3.37	51.5
Poland	103	45.9	62	63	16	3.15	40.6
Portugal	213	42.7	72	42	8	2.84	61.3
Romania	82	44.3	67	70	21	2.83	62.0
Singapore	99	39.5	51	70	17	3.20	59.4
Slovakia	38	38.1	76	49	24	2.95	52.5
South Africa	250	35.6	78	22	49	3.02	63.9
South Korea	296	36.8	100	0	27	3.25	43.5
Spain	43	36.9	59	48	17	3.08	59.4
Sweden	106	47.6	66	23	35	3.05	46.7
Turkey	64	34.2	71	0	23	2.96	55.1
Uganda	230	35.5	76	44	40	3.07	59.4
Ukraine	108	39.2	43	48	20	2.88	62.4
United Kingdom	141	39.1	77	24	29	2.75	60.7
United States	341	34.7	61	23	24	3.14	57.5
Zimbabwe	56	36.9	87	25	21	2.76	66.3
Total	5,054	38.4	71	39	28	3.08	55.4

In nations within which high power distance provides a press toward acquiescence, we presumed that an equally strong press is provided by low individualism.

We used Hofstede's (2001) scores for nations, employing the West Africa score for Nigeria, the East Africa score for both Uganda and Zimbabwe, and the score for Russia for both Belarus and Ukraine. This permitted inclusion of all 38 nations in the present sample. We used grand-mean centering for age and interdependence, but left the dummy variables for male respondent, state employees, and sales uncentered. In all of the analyses presented in this chapter, we report estimations of fixed effects based on robust standard errors. The individual-level analysis indicated that age, gender, and interdependence had a significant effect on acquiescent responding: older participants were less likely to acquiesce (γ = $-.097$, $p < .001$); male respondents were somewhat less likely to respond acquiescently (γ = -1.185, $p = .05$); and more strongly endorsed interdependence was associated with greater acquiescence ($\gamma = 1.428$, $p < .01$). The effects of state versus private employment and sales were not significant. There was significant variation in the variance of both the intercept (the mean level of acquiescence: $\chi^2(35) = 119.83$, $p < .001$) as well as the effect of interdependence: $\chi^2(35) = 93.82$, $p < .001$ and sales: $\chi^2(35) = 57.04$, $p < .01$. Having controlled both for the effects of these demographic variables and for interdependence, 13.92% of the remaining variance in acquiescence was due to nation. The significant variance component for the intercept indicates that nations' characteristics may be able to explain levels of acquiescence. This allows us to explore the variability of the mean for acquiescence and the effect of interdependence on acquiescence across nations. Variation in the effects of interdependence also suggests that interdependence may provide at least part of the explanation. We allowed these variance components to vary across nations, but set the variance components for age, males, and state employees as fixed.

In the second step of the analysis, we tried to predict the nation-level variation in mean acquiescence as well as any differences in the relation of individualism with mean acquiescence. First, using grand-mean centered indicators for Hofstede's individualism, uncertainty avoidance and masculinity-femininity indices, a significant effect for individualism on acquiescence was found: ($\gamma = -.066$, $p < .05$). Lower individualism was associated with higher mean acquiescence overall. This effect explained 35.42% of the variance between nations. The effect for uncertainty avoidance was not significant ($\gamma = -.015$, $p > .10$), nor was the effect of masculinity-femininity ($\gamma = .003$, $p > .10$). Investigating variation in the relation of interdependence to acquiescence, when entering the cross-level effect of Hofstede's individualism index only, no significant effect was found: $\gamma = -.025$, $p = .12$. Although not significant, the effect was in the predicted direction in that the effect of interdependence at the individual level becomes stronger in increasingly more collectivist nations. When entering the other two dimensions, neither of the variables alone or in combination was able to predict a significant amount of variance.

Using the Three-Item Collectivism Index

We noted above that the three-item collectivism index prepared from the Smith et al. (2002) databank and computed at the nation level correlated at only +0.34 with Hofstede collectivism. It may therefore provide a conceptually different basis for testing hypotheses about nation-level effects of collectivism than does the traditional Hofstede index. Moreover, it has the virtue that it is based upon the responses of the specific individuals who contributed to the Smith et al. databank. The demographic profiles of samples from different nations were less well matched than were the profiles in Hofstede's national samples, but those who did provide the present data should reflect locally relevant aspects of collectivism. The individual-level analysis is identical to the one reported above for Hofstede, since the same nations were used for this analysis. Using the nation-level collectivism score to predict variation across nations, greater national collectivism was again associated with more acquiescent responding, $\gamma = 1.882$, $p < .05$. However, the cross-level interaction between collectivism and interdependence was not significant, although the effect was again in the predicted direction, $\gamma = .679$, *ns*. Thus, in this analysis, acquiescence is affected by both interdependence and collectivism, but there is no interaction between them.

Using GLOBE Predictors

Using the 30 nations in the present sample for which GLOBE scores were available, 14.82% of the variance in individual-level acquiescence was due to nation, after adjusting for interdependence and demographic variables. As before, grand-mean centered age was a significant predictor, but gender was only marginally significant ($p < .07$). The effects of interdependence and sales on acquiescence at the individual level varied across nations, as did the intercept (the mean level of acquiescence across nations). As before, we set all variance components except those for the intercept, interdependence, and sales as fixed in the analyses next reported. In testing hypotheses with the GLOBE predictors, it is again important to avoid multicollinearity, since nation-level scores on several of the GLOBE dimensions are quite strongly correlated with one another. We used only the two GLOBE "as is" collectivism indicators. In-group collectivism was a significant predictor of mean acquiescence, $\gamma = 2.917$, $p < .01$. In addition, the effect of institutional collectivism was marginally significant, $\gamma = 2.791$, $p = .06$. Both effects were in the predicted direction, associating high nation-level collectivism with greater acquiescence, even after controlling for the effects of interdependence and demographics. Taken together, 13.76% of nation-level variation was explained by these two indicators.

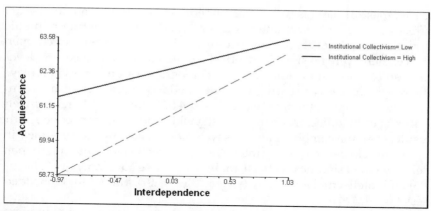

FIGURE 11.1 Interaction between institutional collectivism and interdependence as predictors of acquiescence.

Investigating the interaction between nation-level indicators and individual-level interdependence, the cross-level effect for institutional collectivism was significant ($\gamma_{institutional} = -1.925$, $p < .05$), while that for in-group collectivism was not ($\gamma_{in-group} = .643$, $p > .10$). The plot of the interaction in Figure 11.1 shows that overall the level of acquiescence is higher in nations where institutional collectivism is strong, but that the effect of interdependence is actually stronger in nations that are low in institutional collectivism. At first sight, this effect may appear opposite to our hypotheses, but we need to bear in mind that despite the name assigned to it by the GLOBE researchers, institutional collectivism taps variance that is largely independent of Hofstede collectivism. GLOBE in-group collectivism is much more similar to Hofstede collectivism, as noted above, and the cross-level interaction between in-group collectivism and interdependence is in the same direction as was found in the Hofstede analysis reported above. If the analysis is repeated entering in-group collectivism but not institutional collectivism, the interaction effect for in-group collectivism becomes marginally significant, ($p = .10$). This suggests that the effect of in-group collectivism is to some extent masked by low institutional collectivism.

Using Schwartz Predictors

Across the 31 nations of which we had nation-level means for the Schwartz values, 13.40% of the variance of acquiescence at the individual-level was due to nation, when controlling for demographic variables and interdependence. The result is similar to that reported above for the Hofstede analysis, only the effect of sales on acquiescence responding was invariant across these 31 nations. When embeddedness, intellectual autonomy, and affective autonomy were entered using grand-mean centering to predict both the mean level of acquiescence and their interaction with interdependence, there were no significant effects of these values on the mean levels of acquiescence, after adjusting for demographics and individual-level interdependence. The coefficients for embeddedness, affective autonomy, and intellectual autonomy were 4.648, 4.524 and −2.681, respectively. Entering each indicator separately also yielded no significant effect, so the results from the combined analysis were not affected by multicollinearity problems. However, tests for interactions between values and interdependence, yielded significant effects for both affective autonomy ($\gamma = 3.021$, $p < .05$) and intellectual autonomy ($\gamma = −4.335$, $p < .01$), but not for embeddedness ($\gamma = −1.709$, $p > .10$).

The first important point to note is that these interactions are in opposite directions and therefore resemble the apparently contradictory patterns obtained with Hofstede and GLOBE scores. As Figure 11.2 shows, greater intellectual autonomy at the nation-level is associated with a flat relationship between interdependence and acquiescence. In contrast, in nations characterized by low emphasis on intellectual autonomy, interdependence is strongly related to acquiescence. This effect therefore resembles the trend found in the Hofstede analysis above. In contrast, Figure 11.3 shows that in nations with a strong emphasis on affective autonomy, independence is positively related to acquiescence, whereas this relationship is much weaker where affective autonomy is low, after adjusting for demographics. Therefore, this finding resembles the pattern observed for "as is" institutional collectivism as measured by the GLOBE project. It is worth noting that when the Schwartz predictors are entered separately, the pattern of results is identical, but then only the effect for affective autonomy remains significant ($p < .05$). Therefore, the effects of intellec-

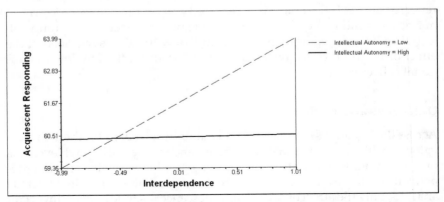

FIGURE 11.2   Interaction between intellectual autonomy and interdependence as predictors of acquiescence.

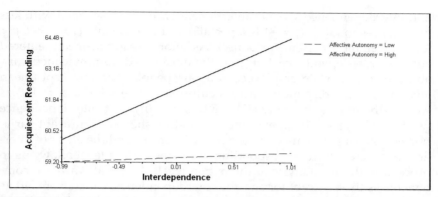

FIGURE 11.3 Interaction between affective autonomy and interdependence as predictors of acquiescence.

tual autonomy are visible only when we control for the closely related concept of affective autonomy.

Discussion of Study 2

The findings for Hofstede collectivism, GLOBE "as is" in-group collectivism and the new three-item collectivism index all concur in indicating that greater nation-level collectivism is associated with a tendency to agree with items independent of their item content. Second, we find two contrasting findings for the interactions with individual-level interdependence. First, individual-level interdependence, just like nation-level collectivism, is always positively related to acquiescence. However, this effect differs depending on ways of measuring the cultural context. In nations low on Schwartz's intellectual autonomy, a stronger effect of interdependence on acquiescence is found. In contrast, in nations high on Schwartz's affective autonomy we also find stronger relationships between interdependence and acquiescence. These results suggest that we have identified two separate sets of circumstances in which acquiescence is maximized. This conclusion can be examined more closely when we have presented a parallel set of analyses concerning extreme response bias.

STUDY 3: PREDICTING EXTREME RESPONDING

Using Hofstede Predictors

Using all 38 nations, 11.08% of variation in extreme responding at the individual-level was due to nation, after controlling for demographics and interdependence. Greater interdependence was associated with less extreme responding (γ = −1.149, p < .05) and salespeople (γ = 1.999, p < .01) showed more extreme responses. As before, we grand-mean centered age and interdependence, but used the uncentered dummy-coded variables for males, state employees and salespeople. The intercept (mean level of extreme responding across cultures) ($\chi^2(35)$ = 80.75, p < .001) as well as the effects of age ($\chi^2(35)$ = 59.22, p < .01), and interdependence ($\chi^2(35)$ = 64.16, p < .01), on extreme responding showed significant variation across nations. This variation in the intercept and the effect of interdependence on extreme responding at the individual level allows us to proceed with our analysis at the nation level. We set all variance components as fixed, except for age and interdependence, which were left as random. At the nation level, none of the variables significantly predicted extreme responding (individualism: γ = .043, p > .10; uncertainty avoidance: γ = .035, p > .10; masculinity-femininity: γ = .007, p > .10). Neither did we observe any cross-level interactions between any of the nation-level indicators and interdependence as predictors of extreme responding ($\gamma_{\text{individualism}}$ = −.005; p >.10; $\gamma_{\text{uncertainty avoidance}}$ = −.013; p > .10; $\gamma_{\text{masculinity-femininity}}$ = −.029; p > .10).

Using the Three-Item Collectivism Index

The individual-level results were identical for this analysis. Entering nation-level collectivism to predict mean levels of extreme responding, no significant effect was found, γ = .011, p > .10. However, the interaction with interdependence was strongly significant, γ = 1.826, p < .001. As shown in Figure 11.4, in more collectivistic nations, interdependence showed a min-

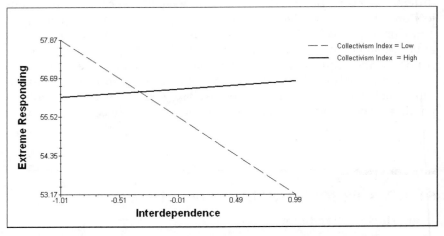

FIGURE 11.4   Interaction between nation-level collectivism and interdependence as predictors of extreme responding.

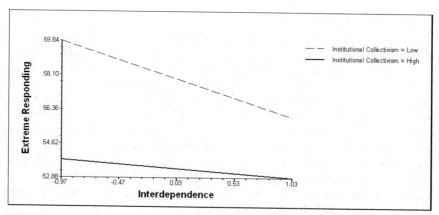

FIGURE 11.5 Interaction between institutional collectivism and interdependence as predictors of extreme responding.

imal relationship with extreme responding. In contrast, in more individualistic nations, individuals who were interdependent were less extreme in their responses, whereas the more independent individuals showed more extreme response tendencies.

Using GLOBE Predictors

Across the 30 nations for which GLOBE scores were available, about 12.87% of the variance was due to nation, after adjusting for level 1 variables. The effect for working in sales was significant, but there was only a marginally significant effect for interdependence ($p < .07$). As before, the intercept, age, and interdependence showed significant variation across nations, allowing us to proceed with our analysis. We left these variance components as random and set all other components as fixed. Entering both the "as is" measures centered around the grand mean, institutional collectivism was a strongly significant predictor ($\gamma = -7.836$, $p < .001$), as was in-group collectivism: $\gamma = -3.621$, $p < .01$. Greater institutional collectivism were thus both associated with less extreme responding. The two predictors explained 40.94% of the variation due to nation. When interactions with interdependence were entered, the effect for institutional collectivism was significant: ($\gamma = 2.510$, $p < .05$), but the effect for in-group collectivism was not, $\gamma = .749$, $p > .10$. As Figure 11.5 shows, in nations high on institutional collectivism, there was little effect of interdependence on extreme responding. However, resembling the results reported above for nation-level collectivism, in nations low on institutional collectivism, there was a negative effect of interdependence on extreme responding.

Using Schwartz Predictors

Across the 31 countries for which we had Schwartz values data, 10.04% of the variance in extreme responding was due to nation, after adjusting for demographics and interdependence. Greater interdependence was associated with less extreme responding and working in sales was associated with more extreme responding. As before, the intercept, age and interdependence showed significant variation across nations, allowing us to proceed with our analysis. Testing effects of grand-mean centered nation-level indicators on extreme responding at the individual level, significant effects were found for affective autonomy ($\gamma = 5.464$, $p < .05$), and intellectual autonomy ($\gamma = -7.182$, $p < .01$), but not for embeddedness, $\gamma = -3.549$, $p > .10$. Greater affective autonomy was associated with greater response extremity, whereas intellectual autonomy was associated with lesser extremity. These variables together explained 37.50% of the nation-level variance in extreme responding. When entering each predictor individually, the effect for affective autonomy was only marginally significant ($p = .08$), but in the same direction, whereas the effect for intellectual autonomy remained significant.

Tests for the cross-level interactions between Schwartz values and interdependence showed significant interaction effects for embeddedness ($\gamma = 10.674$, $p < .05$) and for affective autonomy ($\gamma = 5.210$, $p < .05$), but the effect for intellectual autonomy was only marginally significant, $\gamma = 2.718$, $p = .08$. Resembling the effects observed previously, as illustrated in Figure 11.6, in settings where embeddedness values are endorsed, interdependence showed a positive relationship with extreme responding. In contrast, in settings low in embeddedness, the relationship was negative, with independent persons showing more extreme responses, and interdependent persons showing less extreme responses. The results for affective autonomy are shown in Figure 11.7. In settings high for affective autonomy, the relationship between interdependence and extreme responding was close to zero. However, in nations low on affective autonomy, interdependent persons are low on response extremity, whereas independent persons select more extreme responses. It should be noted that although the effects for embeddedness and affective autonomy were in the same direction, when entering each value individually and adjusting for demographics, neither cross-level interaction effect was significant.

Discussion of Study 3

Extreme response bias is associated with low individual-level interdependence, and with high nation-level institutional collectivism and affective autonomy, but low nation-level intellectual autonomy. In addition, there

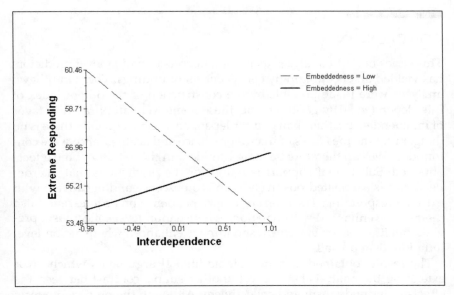

FIGURE 11.6 Interaction between embeddedness and interdependence as predictors of extreme responding.

are interaction effects whereby independent persons within individualistic nations are particularly prone to use more extreme response options within nations that are individualistic and nations that are low on institutional collectivism.

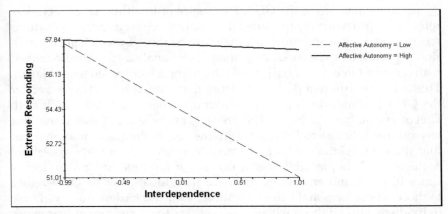

FIGURE 11.7 Interaction between affective autonomy and interdependence as predictors of extreme responding.

CONCLUSION

This series of HLM analyses using parallel sets of nation-level predictors has yielded an encouragingly consistent set of findings. These multilevel analyses were made possible by the construction of the 3-item index of interdependence. By good fortune, these items were all phrased in favor of independence rather than of interdependence. Consequently there is no danger that the measures of interdependence and acquiescence were confounded. We can therefore be more confident in the validity of the effects obtained. Substantial support is found for the predictions that interdependence is associated positively with acquiescence and negatively with extreme responding. The effect of interdependence on acquiescence also seems to be enhanced within nations where nation-level collectivism prevails, but its effect on extreme responding is enhanced where nation-level individualism prevails.

The results obtained also provide additional arguments which favor extending the analysis beyond yet another simple contrast between the effects of individualism and collectivism. Although the predicted effects of uncertainty avoidance and femininity were not found, the GLOBE predictors did indicate that there are some additional ways in which nation-level cultural press may encourage particular response styles. Low institutional collectivism was much the strongest predictor of extreme responding, and it also interacted significantly with interdependence in predicting heightened acquiescence. Similar effects were obtained with Schwartz's affective autonomy. How can we best understand the circumstances that demonstrate these effects?

The items that define the GLOBE measure of institutional collectivism refer to the provision of structures that facilitate collective action. Nations scoring low on this measure will therefore be those in which such provision is perceived to be modest. In the present analysis the lowest ranked nations were Greece and Italy, while the highest were Sweden and Japan. This is a very different dimension from that tapped by Hofstede, and by the GLOBE dimension of "as is" in-group collectivism (on which both Greece and Italy score high). The present results showed that in nations low on institutional collectivism extreme responding was maximal but that those individuals who had interdependent values were also more acquiescent. It is plausible that a context of low institutional collectivism will favor and encourage assertive individuals, but be challenging to those whose personal values are more toward interdependence. These individuals will be those who are reliant on others and prefer teamwork rather than working alone, but who are in a context where collective action is not strongly practiced. The resulting uncertainties around one's work roles would be highly challenging and uncertainty inducing. Sorrentino

(2005) argued that individuals in ambiguous situations will seek guidance from both peers and leaders when answering questions. The present survey included items that referred to reliance on a wide variety of sources of guidance in the work setting. Responses that indicated reliance on all available sources of guidance would yield an enhanced acquiescence score, which is consistent with the result obtained.

The results for affective autonomy suggest a related scenario. Schwartz's measure of affective autonomy is defined by hedonistic values such as enjoying life and having an exciting life. High affective autonomy predicted greater extremity, but where affective autonomy was low independence was associated with increased extremity. Persons endorsing independent values may find living in a nation low on affective autonomy a challenging experience, so that we can again speculate that they may respond by enhancing their attempts to present themselves as distinctive.

The interaction between intellectual autonomy and interdependence might be explained in a somewhat similar fashion. Intellectual autonomy refers to a highly stimulating environment where people search for new ideas and new experiences. Individuals who prefer working with others rather than alone are likely to show greater agreement (higher acquiescence), since they will have a particularly strong need to establish links with others in this challenging type of context.

Putting these speculations together, we can formulate a view as to the ways in which individuals' personal dispositions and the cultural contexts within which these individuals are located may interact. First, collectivism provides a press toward acquiescence, while individualism provides a press toward extreme responding. Second, there are consistent congruence effects, in that interdependent persons become even more acquiescent in collectivistic settings, whereas independent persons respond even more extremely in individualistic settings. Third, the analysis points toward the view that individualism and collectivism are not monolithic attributes of cultures such as nations. Different aspects of individualism and collectivism can be associated with different types of effects. While individualism and collectivism as defined by the values measures of Hofstede and others show congruence effects, the more behaviorally anchored measure of "as is" institutional collectivism shows a significant contrast effect.

These conclusions must be considered tentative, because the characterizations of nations that were used in most of our analyses were derived from samples that differed substantially from those containing the individuals whose response bias was examined. Effects could be stronger or weaker when there is a closer match between samples. Nonetheless, the effects obtained proved broadly replicable across the samples that provided the predictors.

The results have implications both for cross-cultural methodology and for our conceptualization of culture. In terms of methodology, the continuing use of cross-cultural survey instruments that contain only positive wordings cannot be defended. The developing field of cross-cultural psychology requires measures of the cultural orientation of individuals that are not confounded with a predisposition to communicate in particular ways. Translation of measures that have both positively and negatively keyed items, such as the Big Five personality inventory has yielded versions with adequate factor structure within many language versions (McCrae, Terracciano et al., 2005). Such scales are more likely to be valid if the reversed items are not simple negations of the positive items. Even among scales that do contain adequately worded positive and negative items, the effects of acquiescent responding will not be totally discounted, since acquiescent respondents tend to agree with the negatively keyed items more than do non-acquiescent respondents. This can lead to the emergence of separate factors for responses to positively and negatively keyed items among samples of highly acquiescent respondents (Wong, Rindfleisch, & Burroughs, 2003). Where responses are available to a broad range of uncorrelated items, some forms of ipsatization can overcome this difficulty (Fischer, 2004). Where this is not possible, it may be preferable to construct items in ways that elicit choices rather than statements of agreement or disagreement (Wong et al., 2003).

Our suggestion that acquiescence and extreme response should be taken out of individual-level measures of cultural orientation should not be read as endorsing the view that these indices are artifactual and of no interest. On the contrary, they provide sample instances of the styles of communication that prevail in different cultural settings (Smith, 2004), whose occurrence may be used in testing hypotheses in the way that has been done in this chapter. The important point is not to confound such indices with measures of other attributes of cross-cultural interest.

Our results also bear upon the themes that are explored throughout this book. Acquiescence and extreme responding are individual acts that are carried out within particular cultural contexts. We have used characterizations of nations based upon aggregation of individuals' values and perceptions of behaviors to formulate a view that cultures "press" individuals to communicate in particular ways. However, we cannot argue that it is useful to speak simply of acquiescent cultures or of extreme response cultures. We have identified a series of cross-level interactions which indicate that to understand acquiescence or extremity we need to take account both of individuals' predispositions and of their cultural context. We have even found interactions with opposing signs when using different predictors that derive from cultural values or from perceptions of prevailing behaviors. Thus a given national culture could evoke either acquiescence or extremity depending on the facet of that national culture which had greatest relevance for a particular type of individual.

Author Note

We thank Michael Bond, Tim Johnson, Viv Vignoles, and the editors for helpful comments on earlier drafts.

Note

1. The use of "citizen mean" scores for acquiescence and for extreme response bias does not accord with the argument presented earlier that nation-level scores should be based upon separate items that have been aggregated to the nation level. As a test of the extent to which use of nation-level scores might yield different results, the following procedure was employed. Respondents had completed eight ratings in respect of each of eight different work events. If acquiescence has differing meanings in different contexts, some variation would be expected in the amount of acquiescence elicited by differing events. Separate acquiescence scores were computed for the ratings referring to each of the events and these scores were then aggregated to the nation-level. Factor analysis yielded a one-factor solution, eigenvalue 6.82, explaining 85.2% of variance. This factor score correlated with the acquiescence citizen mean at $r = +0.97$. A similar procedure for extreme response bias yielded a single factor, eigenvalue 6.62, explaining 82.8% of variance. This correlated with the extreme bias citizen mean at $r = +1.00$.

REFERENCES

Adorno, T. W., Frenkel-Brunswik, E., Levinson, D. J., & Sanford, R. N. (1950). *The authoritarian personality*. New York: Harper.

Argyle, M., Henderson, M., Bond, M. H., Iizuka, Y., & Contarello, A. (1986). Cross-cultural variations in relationship rules. *International Journal of Psychology, 21*, 287–315.

Asch, S. E. (1951). Effects of group pressure upon the modification and distortion of judgments. In H. Guetzkow (Ed.), *Groups, leadership and men.* (pp. 177–190). Pittsburgh: Carnegie Press.

Bond, M. H., Leung, K., & 67 co-authors (2004). Culture-level dimensions of social axioms and their correlates across 41 cultures. *Journal of Cross-Cultural Psychology, 35*, 548–570.

Bond, R. A., & Smith, P. B. (1996). Culture and conformity: A meta-analysis of studies using Asch's (1952, 1956) line judgment task. *Psychological Bulletin, 119*, 111–137.

Brewer, M. B. (1991). The social self: On being the same and different at the same time. *Personality and Social Psychology Bulletin, 17*, 475–482.

Chen, C., Shin-Ying, L., & Stevenson, H. W. (1995). Response style and cross-cultural comparisons of rating scales among East Asian and North American students. *Psychological Science, 6*, 170–175.

Cheung, G. W., & Rensvold, R. B. (2000). Assessing extreme and acquiescent response sets in cross-cultural research using structural equations modeling. *Journal of Cross-Cultural Psychology, 31*, 187–212.

Clarke, I. (2000). Extreme response style in cross-cultural research: An empirical investigation. *Journal of Social Behavior and Personality, 15*, 137–152.

Couch, A. S., & Keniston, K. (1960). Yeasayers and naysayers: Agreeing response set as a personality variable. *Journal of Abnormal and Social Psychology, 60*, 151–174.

Cronbach, L. J. (1946). Response sets and test design. *Educational and Psychological Measurement, 6*, 475–494.

Crutchfield, R. A. (1955). Conformity and character. *American Psychologist, 10*, 191–198.

Ferrando, P. J., Condon, C., & Chico, E. (2004). The convergent validity of acquiescence: An empirical study relating balanced scales and separate acquiescence scales. *Personality and Individual Differences, 37*, 1331–1340.

Fischer, R. (2004). Standardization to account for cross-cultural response bias: A classification of score adjustment procedures and review of research in JCCP. *Journal of Cross-Cultural Psychology, 35*, 263–282.

Gelfand, M., Nishi, L., & Raver, J. (2006). On the nature and importance of cultural tightness-looseness. *Journal of Applied Psychology, 91*, 1225–1244.

Hofstede, G. (1980). *Culture's consequences: International differences in work-related values*. Beverly Hills, CA: Sage.

Hofstede, G. (2001). *Culture's consequences: Comparing values, behaviors, institutions and organizations across nations* (2nd ed.). Thousand Oaks, CA: Sage.

Holtgraves, T. (1997). Styles of language use: Individual and cultural variability in conversational indirectness. *Journal of Personality and Social Psychology, 73*, 624–637.

House, R. J., Hanges, P. J., Javidan, M., Dorfman, P. W., Gupta, V., & GLOBE associates (2004). *Leadership, culture and organizations: The GLOBE study of 62 nations.* Thousand Oaks, CA: Sage.

Hui, C. H., & Triandis, H. C. (1989). Effects of culture and format on extreme response style. *Journal of Cross-Cultural Psychology, 20*, 296–309.

Johnson, T. P., Kulesa, P., Cho, Y. I., & Shavitt, S. (2005). The relation between culture and response styles. *Journal of Cross-Cultural Psychology, 36*, 264–277.

Kashima, Y., Kashima, E., Chiu, C.Y., Farsides, T., Gelfand, M., Hong, Y. Y. et al. (2005). Culture, essentialism and agency: Are individuals universally believed to be more real entities than groups? *European Journal of Social Psychology, 35*, 147–170.

Kwan, V. S. Y., Bond, M. H., & Singelis, T. M. (1997). Pancultural explanations for life satisfaction: Adding relationship harmony to self-esteem. *Journal of Personality and Social Psychology, 73*, 1038–1051.

Leung, K., & Bond, M. H. (1989). On the empirical identification of dimensions for cross-cultural comparisons. *Journal of Cross-Cultural Psychology, 20*, 133–152.

McCrae, R. R., Terracciano, A. et al. (2005). Universal features of personality traits from the observer's perspective: Data from 50 cultures. *Journal of Personality and Social Psychology, 88*, 547–561.

Morris, M. W., Williams, K. Y., Leung, K., Larrick, R., Mendoza, M. T., Bhatnagar, D. et al. (1998). Conflict management style: Accounting for cross-national differences. *Journal of International Business Studies, 29*, 729–747.

Oetzel, J. G., Ting-Toomey, S., Masumoto, T., Yochi, Y., Pan, X. H., Takai, J. et al. (2001). Face and facework in conflict: A cross-cultural comparison of China, Germany, Japan and the United States. *Communication Monographs, 68,* 235–258.

Ones, D. S., Viswesvaran, C., & Reiss, A. D. (1996). Role of social desirability in personality testing for personnel selection: The red herring. *Journal of Applied Psychology, 81,* 660–679.

Pelto, P. (1968). The difference between "tight" and "loose" societies. *Transaction, 5,* 37–40.

Raudenbush, S. W., & Bryk, A. S. (2002). *Hierarchical linear models* (2nd ed.). London: Sage.

Raudenbush, S., Bryk, A., Cheong, Y. F., & Congdon, R. (2000). *Hierarchical linear and nonlinear modelling.* Lincolnwood, IL: Scientific Software International.

Schwartz, S. H. (1992). Universals in the structure and content of values: Theoretical advances and empirical tests in 20 countries. In M. P. Zanna (Ed.), *Advances in Experimental Social Psychology* (Vol.25, pp. 1–65). Orlando, FL: Academic.

Schwartz, S. H. (1994). Beyond individualism/collectivism: New cultural dimensions of values. In U. Kim, H. C. Triandis, C. Kagitcibasi, S. C. Choi, & G. Yoon (Eds.), *Individualism and collectivism: Theory, method and applications* (pp. 85–119). Thousand Oaks, CA: Sage.

Schwartz, S. H. (2004). Mapping and interpreting cultural differences around the world. In H. Vinken, J. Soeters, & P. Ester (Eds.), *Comparing cultures: Dimensions of culture in a comparative perspective* (pp. 43–73). Leiden, the Netherlands: Brill.

Singelis, T. M., Bond, M. H., Sharkey, W. F., & Lai, C. S. Y. (1999). Unpackaging culture's influence on self-esteem and embarrassability: The role of self-construals. *Journal of Cross-Cultural Psychology, 30,* 315–341.

Smith, P. B. (2004). Acquiescent response bias as an aspect of cultural communication style. *Journal of Cross-Cultural Psychology, 35,* 50–61.

Smith, P. B., Bond, M. H., & Kagitcibasi, C. (2006). *Understanding social psychology across cultures: Living and working in changing world.* London: Sage.

Smith, P. B., Peterson, M. F., Schwartz, S. H., Ahmad, A.H., Akande, D., Andersen, J.A. et al. (2002). Cultural values, sources of guidance and their relevance to managerial behavior: A 47 nation study. *Journal of Cross-Cultural Psychology, 33,* 188–208.

Sorrentino, R. M. (2005). Uncertainty orientation and social behavior: Individual differences within and across cultures. In R. M. Sorrentino, D. Cohen, J. M. Olson & M. P. Zanna (Eds.) *Culture and social behavior: The Ontario symposium* (Vol. 10, pp. 181–206). Mahwah, NJ: Lawrence Erlbaum.

Triandis, H. C. (1995). *Individualism and collectivism.* Boulder, CO: Westview.

Trompenaars, F. (1993). *Riding the waves of culture.* London: Economist Books.

Van de Vijver, F. J. R., & Leung, K. (1997). *Methods and data analysis for cross-cultural research.* Thousand Oaks, CA: Sage.

Van Hemert, D. A., van de Vijver, F. J. R., Poortinga, Y. H., & Georgas, J. (2002). Structural and functional equivalence of the Eysenck Personality Questionnaire within and between nations. *Personality and Individual Differences, 33,* 1229–1249.

314 *Multilevel Analysis of Individuals and Cultures*

Wong, N., Rindfleisch, A., & Burroughs, J. E. (2003). Do reverse-worded items confound measures in cross-cultural research? The case of the material values scale. *Journal of Consumer Research, 30,* 72–91.

12

Multilevel Issues in International Large-Scale Assessment Studies on Student Performance

Petra Stanat and Oliver Lüdtke

The primary goal of international large-scale assessment studies is to provide countries with comparative data on the outcomes of their school systems. They describe performance levels of students in selected grades or age groups in order to supply benchmarking information to policy makers, researchers, practitioners, and the general public. A central feature of these studies is their multilevel structure (e.g., Raudenbush & Bryk, 2002). This feature is highly relevant for designing and implementing the assessments as well as for analyses of the data. Multilevel issues are omnipresent in international large-scale assessment studies and the number of levels that could be taken into account is particularly large, ranging from the individual student to the larger society.

Figure 12.1 shows an extended version of a framework for indicators of teaching and learning that was initially developed by a Task Force of the Organisation for Economic Cooperation and Development (OECD) (Baumert, Blum & Neubrand, 2004). Based on Bronfenbrenner's (1979) ecological model of human development, the model assumes that a number of environmental layers interact in determining the outcomes of teaching and learning processes. The societal level forms the most encompassing layer. It includes a number of factors that may be of importance for teaching and learning outcomes, such as the value societies place on learning and education, the status of schools as an institution, or the reputation of teachers (Baumert, et al., 2004). Despite their potential relevance for explaining the results from international comparisons of student performance, the role of these factors is rarely explored. This is probably partly due to the lack of a theoretical framework linking societal factors to processes of teaching and learning as well as to the difficulty of measuring these factors (Baumert et al., 2004; Stanat & Lüdtke, 2007).

The system level of the model also involves a host of variables that can be assumed to affect teaching and learning. They include structural features of school systems (e.g., the onset of compulsory schooling, tracking, and accountability systems) and characteristics of the teacher workforce (e.g., age, experience, and qualification). Due to the policy focus of international large-scale assessment studies, especially those carried out by the OECD, attempts of explaining between-country differences of student performance often concentrate on system-level factors.

At the community level, features of the catchment area (e.g., the community's socioeconomic situation and the proportion of immigrant families not speaking the language of instruction at home) or local resources allocated to schools are relevant. These have a direct impact on schools that form the next layer in the model and that have been studied extensively in research on school effectiveness and school development (e.g., Teddlie & Reynolds, 2000). Nested in the school layer is the classroom level, which includes such factors as the learning climate and the implemented curriculum. The most proximal determinants of teaching and learning processes, finally, which form the center of the model, encompass background characteristics and actions of students and teachers, such as students' prior knowledge in a specific school subject and their motivation to learn, as well as teachers' pedagogical content knowledge and their motivation to teach (Baumert et al., 2004).

Although international large-scale assessment studies do not provide comprehensive information on all layers of the framework, they offer a unique analytical potential that allows for the simultaneous consideration

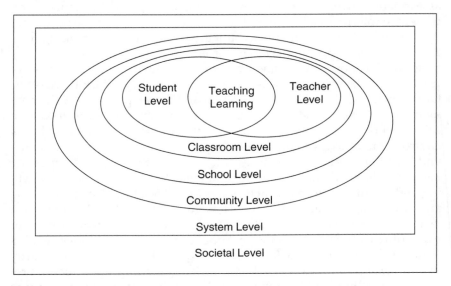

FIGURE 12.1 Multilevel framework for indicators of teaching and learning

of factors at different levels and their interactions. At the same time, the multilevel structure of the studies entails a number of methodological challenges and potential pitfalls that need to be taken into account at different stages of a research project.

The present chapter describes some of the most important conceptual and methodological issues associated with the multilevel structure of international large-scale assessment studies on student performance. The next section provides a description of central aspects of their design and implementation. Subsequently, we discuss specific multilevel issues in the analysis of data from international large-scale assessments and in the interpretation of their results. The final section describes a few studies that have used the data to explore basic research questions. These include analyses of determinants of student performances at different levels as well as analyses of the validity of psychological theories in different countries. As the OECD's Programme for International Student Assessment (PISA) builds on previous international studies of student performance and can be considered to represent the current state of the art, most illustrations and examples in this chapter are from this study.

DESIGN AND IMPLEMENTATION OF INTERNATIONAL LARGE-SCALE ASSESSMENT STUDIES ON STUDENT PERFORMANCE

In the 1950s, international organizations such as the UNESCO and the OECD began to collect and document comparative data on selected features (e.g., national curricula) of school systems in a number of countries. As an indicator of the systems' effectiveness, the proportion of students reaching different levels of education in terms of certificates was used. Soon, however, researchers came to the realization that nominally comparable educational certificates may be associated with highly varying levels of student performance (Postlethwaite, 1999). A group of educational researchers met in 1958 to discuss the possibilities of assessing learning outcomes in an international context. This ultimately resulted in the First International Mathematics Study (FIMS) in which a total of 12 countries participated (Husén, 1967).

The First International Mathematics Study as well as the majority of subsequent international assessments were planned and conducted under the auspices of the International Association for the Evaluation of Educational Achievement (IEA)—an international foundation involving research institutions and government representatives of the member countries. More recently, the OECD has begun to assess student performance as well. The

OECD has been providing comparative data on the resources and structures of educational systems and on participation rates at different levels of education since 1991. These data are published on a regular basis in *Education at Glance* (e.g., OECD, 2006). With the programme for international student assessment (*PISA*), the OECD aims at supplementing this information with indicators of learning outcomes within the countries' school systems.

As we pointed out before, a main goal of international large-scale assessments is to provide cross-national benchmarking information on overall student performance. The units of analysis are the school systems of the countries involved in a given study; these are compared in terms of selected learning outcomes. From the perspective of this goal, international large-scale assessments are *level-oriented studies* that aim at drawing conclusions about the absolute level of the target variables in the different countries (e.g., Van de Vijver & Tanzer, 1997). These types of intercultural comparisons are particularly vulnerable to systematic *bias* and require that the variables are measured with a high degree of *equivalence* (Van de Vijver & Tanzer, 1997). More specifically, it does not suffice that the performance tests used in the assessment measure the same construct in all countries (*structural equivalence*) and that the measurement units are comparable (*measurement unit equivalence*), but it is also necessary that the origin of the scale is the same in all groups that are compared (*scalar/full-scale equivalence*). Only under this condition is it permissible to interpret differences between students' test scores in different countries (Van de Vijver & Tanzer, 1997).

To ensure that full-scale equivalence is reached it is necessary to consider a number of multilevel issues in designing and implementing the assessments. This is particularly relevant to the definition of assessment domains, to the development of measurement instruments as well as to population definitions and sampling.

Definition of Assessment Domains

The interpretability and usefulness of results from international comparisons of student performance depend on the definition of the assessment domains and their operationalization in test items. In order to reach meaningful results, it is necessary to consider between-country differences in the relevance of the domains.

Among the tests that have been employed in the past, two types can be distinguished: curriculum-oriented tests and literacy tests (e.g., Mullis et al., 1998). An attempt is made when developing curriculum-oriented tests, to identify a common core of learning goals within the curricula of participating countries and to assess this common core with test items. In this case, the main criterion for construct validity is the extent to which the test items match the internationally shared curriculum. This approach was used in most of the IEA projects. For example, in the Third International Mathematics and Science Study (TIMSS) for the population of students in lower secondary schools, judgments by curriculum experts confirmed that the mathematics test was valid in terms of the countries' national curricula. With some restrictions, this was also the case for the science test (Beaton, Martin et al., 1996).

Literacy tests aim at assessing knowledge and skills that are judged to be important for mastering authentic problems (OECD, 1999, 2003). The concept of literacy is based on a functional view of competencies in language, mathematics, and science that is most prevalent in Anglo-American countries. It is assumed that students need to develop basic competencies in these domains in order to function successfully in modern society. Thus, literacy tests are based on normative premises about the relevance of knowledge and skills for students' lives (for a critique of literacy tests, see, for example, Prais, 2003).

Although other studies have used literacy tests as well, the approach is most consistently implemented in PISA. The definitions of the assessed competencies are laid out in a framework that was developed jointly by international and national expert groups (OECD, 1999, 2003). As was the case for most conceptual decisions in PISA, this process was closely monitored by educational policy representatives from the participating countries. The discussions resulted in a general agreement that the competencies defined in the PISA framework and assessed with the PISA tests constitute central prerequisites for life success that students in modern societies should have acquired by the end of compulsory schooling. This assumption presupposes a high level of cross-cultural validity of the literacy concept used in PISA. However, the extent to which the assessed competencies do, in fact, contribute to students' future success within each of the participating countries is unclear. In order to test the predictive validity of the PISA test, it would be necessary to carry out longitudinal studies that follow up on students after they have made the transition from school to work.

Test and Questionnaire Development

Based on the definition of the assessment domain, test items have to be developed that are equivalent across countries. Again, this requires the consideration of factors that may potentially bias students' responses and, as a result, the outcomes of the assessment. These factors include characteristics of language and culture-specific experiences. Although biases associated with differences between such characteristics are mainly taken into account at the country level, they may also be located at the level of subgroups within countries, such as different immigrant groups or groups with different socioeconomic backgrounds.

The task of developing cross-culturally equivalent items is particularly challenging for literacy tests. These tests aim at ensuring authenticity by embedding items in real-life contexts. Such contextualized items are highly vulnerable to cultural bias. To avoid that the item development process will result in culturally narrow tests, the PISA items are generated in close cooperation between international and national expert groups (e.g., Wu, 2002). A large proportion of the items is based on stimulus materials and items that were submitted by participating countries. Based on feedback from national experts in the participating countries, a first selection is chosen from this item pool. In addition to the subject-related quality of the items, criteria for this selection include ratings of students' likely familiarity with the context used to embed the items and the extent to which it seems possible to translate the items into the respective test language. This first selection is then submitted to the translation process (see below) and pretested in an extensive field trial involving all participating countries. The international PISA consortium performs extensive analyses with the field trial data to ensure that the tests meet the criterion of full-scale equivalence (OECD, 2001, 2004). Based on these analyses, which we describe in more detail below, the final pool of items is selected for the main study.

In addition to performance tests, large-scale assessment studies also employ questionnaires to collect background information at several levels. The questionnaire framework used in PISA 2003, for example, distinguishes four levels (the education system as a whole, educational service providers/schools, instructional settings/classrooms, and individuals involved in the learning activities) and three types of indicators (output and outcome of education and learning, policy levers and contexts, and antecedents and constraints of policy) (OECD, 2005, p. 35). These two dimensions form a matrix with 12 cells for most of which PISA collects information with student and school questionnaires (e.g., classroom size, school resources, perceived school climate, motivation related to learning) as well as from other OECD data sources, such as those used for the *Education at a Glance* series. The PISA questionnaires also include measures of psychological variables. In the PISA 2000 assessment cycle, for example, 26 countries implemented scales on prerequisites of self-regulated learning (e.g., motivational orientations, learning strategies) as an international option (Artelt, Baumert, Julius-McElvany, & Peschar, 2003). In PISA 2003, the scores for questionnaire indices representing latent traits were, for the most part, derived through scaling based on item response theory (OECD, 2005).

In the past, international large-scale assessment studies have invested much less effort and care into the development of background questionnaires than in the development of performance tests. Although this is still the case today, the most recent studies have made an attempt to explore the cross-national comparability of the questionnaire items as well (OECD, 2005). In PISA 2003, the international consortium performed confirmatory factor analyses (CFA) and multigroup modeling with the field trial data to ensure that the factorial structures of the questionnaire constructs are invariant across countries. However, these analyses can only confirm structural equivalence of scales. Full-scale equivalence cannot be assumed for the questionnaire constructs measured in the studies and between-country comparisons in terms of their level should therefore be interpreted with caution.

Translation of Tests

Various approaches to translation are available that aim at ensuring equivalence among the national versions of measurement instruments in studies involving cross-cultural comparisons (Harkness, 2003; Van de Vijver & Hambleton, 1996). In the past, the most common approach was to translate the material into the national languages and then back into the language of the original material (Brislin, 1986). Deviations between the original and the back translation are interpreted as indications for possible inaccuracies. This procedure is quite effective when it comes to identifying clear translation mistakes or interpretation problems. However, it also has a few limitations that are associated with the lack of an isomorphic relationship between different languages. More specifically, even if the back translation of a test were to succeed in reproducing the original verbatim, this would not necessarily mean that the national version of the test is equivalent. Frequently, the back translation approach results in translations that remain too close to the syntax and vocabulary of the original and that therefore seem unnatural (Grisay, 2002).

An alternative approach is to translate the original instrument more than once and subsequently to reconcile the different versions. According to Harkness (2003), this process should start with the phases of *translation, review, adjudication* followed by *pretesting* and *documentation* ("TRAPD" approach). Harkness recommends working with a team of translators and reviewers who not only have a very good command of both languages but are also familiar with the specific study and the principles of test and questionnaire construction as well as with a larger group of experts (including the translators and reviewers) that is responsible for making the final translation decisions. With some deviations, the TRAPD approach is also implemented in PISA (Grisay, 2002, 2003). In addition to translators and reviewers, the team involved in the translation process includes national education experts on the PISA assessment domains (reading, mathematics, and science) and school teachers.

Differential Item Functioning

In international large-scale assessment studies, it is standard procedure to pretest a larger number of items in participating countries to generate an empirical basis for their selection. The item selection process involves a number of criteria. It has to be ensured that the items cover the entire construct as well as an adequate range of difficulty. In addition, it is necessary to make sure that the items function in similar ways across countries. To confirm that this is the case, the pretest data are used to test for differential item functioning (DIF) which is inferred from the relationship between students' scores on the individual items and their overall test scores. If the scores on an item vary between persons from different countries even though they have reached the same overall test score, DIF is said to exist (for an overview of different approaches to identifying DIF, see Camilli & Shepard, 1994; Holland & Wainer, 1993). Often, DIF is due to translation errors, such as differences in the difficulty of the vocabulary used, which can easily be fixed. At other times, the source of DIF is more substantial and cannot be eradicated. In these cases, the item will have to be discarded.

In the item selection process within PISA, DIF is not only tested at the level of countries but also at the level of subgroups within countries (Adams & Carstensen, 2002; OECD, 2005; Wu, 2002). The main focus of these analyses is on differential results for students from families with higher and lower socioeconomic status (SES). Because some countries differ considerably in terms of the social structure of their populations, DIF at the level of socioeconomic subgroups may also impair the transnational equivalence of the tests. Thus, an item which, compared to the overall test, is harder for low SES students than for high SES students would tend to disadvantage countries with proportionately fewer wealthy families. This might occur, for example, if understanding an item would require specific experiences (e.g., traveling by plane) that are less common among persons with lower SES.

As discussed in more detail below, the meaning of results in international large-scale assessment studies on student performance may differ across levels. This is also the case for differential item function. In international assessment studies, DIF is typically used as an indicator for item bias, and it is thus interpreted as reflecting validity problems that need to be removed by modifying or eliminating the item. Viewed from the perspective of curricula or instruction, however, DIF may also provide substantive information on specific strengths and weaknesses in student performance that helps to differentiate the findings. Using data from PISA, Klieme and Baumert (2001) demonstrated how DIF can be used to identify and describe cultures of mathematics education in the countries that participated in the assessment. This presents an example for the more general problem that the application of one-dimensional models to test development and international comparisons may result in the loss of valuable information on between-country differences (Goldstein, 2004).

DIF analyses allow for the identification of cross-cultural differences in the relative difficulty at the level of individual items but not at the level of the overall tests (Sireci, 1997). It would be quite conceivable that the difficulty of a reading literacy test, for example, may be systematically affected by certain characteristics of the respective test languages, such as the complexity of their grammar. This would invalidate the assumption of full-scale equivalence (Van de Vijver & Tanzer, 1997) that needs to be met in order to compare the absolute levels of student performance across countries.

To gain some indication for the extent to which test languages influence students' reading performance, Grisay (2002) performed a series of analyses with the French and English versions of the reading test used in PISA 2000. As would be expected, the findings showed that some of the texts used in the test were considerably longer in French than in English. In order to estimate the effect of this difference, the author grouped the texts in terms of the extent to which the two versions differed (French version less than 5%, 6–10%, 11–20%, or more than 20% longer). An analysis of variance with the probability of a correct answer as the dependent variable revealed a significant interaction between language and the difference in length between the two versions. There was an overall tendency for the probability of a correct answer to be lower for the French version across all four groups of texts, yet this difference increased with larger deviations in the length of the text.

Findings such as these suggest that results from international comparisons of student performance are influenced by characteristics of the different languages involved. In fact, some authors doubt that it is possible to reach cross-cultural equivalence for tests of reading literacy based on translations of standardized material (e.g., Bonnet, 2002; Bonnet et al., 2003). To explore the extent to which translated items result in systematic performance disadvantages, Artelt and Baumert (2004) performed DIF analyses with the reading literacy test from the PISA 2000 assessment. The findings of these analyses showed that students reached higher scores on items that originated from their own countries (see also Allalouf, 2003; Budgell, Namburty & Douglas, 1995; Gierl & Khaliq, 2001). However, the authors concluded that the effect of this pattern on the results of the overall comparisons between countries was relatively small. They recommend the use of test materials from a variety of different countries in order to prevent the bias that may potentially be associated with the origin of an item.

Sampling

Multilevel issues in international large-scale assessment studies are also prevalent in sampling. The goal of sampling in these studies is to achieve representativeness at the level of selected student populations. The populations are typically defined in terms of grade level or in terms of age. The TIMSS study for students in upper secondary school, for example, used a grade-based population definition including all students in the final year of full-time secondary education across general and vocational tracks

(Mullis et al., 1998). In contrast, PISA defines its student population based on age, including all students between the ages of 15 years, 3 months and 16 years, 2 months at the time of testing (Krawchuk & Rust, 2002; OECD, 2005). Because 15-year-olds in most countries are approaching the end of compulsory schooling, this population definition was chosen to capture the yield of education systems shortly before students could potentially enter the labor market.

In sampling from the defined student populations in international assessment studies, the multilevel structure of school systems has to be taken into account. Because students are nested in schools, sampling requires at least a two-stage plan. In determining the sample size, it is also necessary to adjust for effects of clustering (Kish, 1965). Due to such factors as geographical variations, selection processes based on tracking, and shared instruction, students within schools tend to be more similar to one another than students between schools. Therefore, the efficiency of a cluster sample is lower than that of a simple random sample. At the same time, the lower degree of efficiency of cluster samples is, to some extent, compensated by stratifications that are used in international large-scale assessment studies in order to represent important structural features of countries' school systems (Lohr, 1999). These features can be located at different levels, such as the level of school types (e.g., public and private schools and schools of different confessions) or at the level of subnational entities (regions, states, provinces, etc.). Which levels and structural features have to be taken into account varies across countries. Therefore, international assessment studies involve individual sampling plans for each country that are developed in cooperation between the international and the national project managements (e.g., Krawchuk & Rust, 2002; OECD, 2005).

Whether or not the sampling procedure results in representative samples across countries can have effects on the validity of the international comparisons. More specifically, between-country differences in population coverage and sample participation rates can bias the results substantially. Therefore, the most recent large-scale assessment studies have set relatively high standards for inclusion at different levels. At the level of student populations, an attempt is made to achieve full coverage of all students who are able to participate in the assessment. In PISA, for example, it was possible to exclude certain schools (e.g., if carrying out the assessment in the school would have been exceedingly difficult for geographical or administrative reasons) and students (e.g., if they were unable to participate in the assessment due to severe intellectual or functional disabilities). However, the overall exclusion rates were not to exceed 2.5% of the total target population of 15-year-olds.

In terms of sample participation rates, minimum requirements are typically defined at the level of schools (or classrooms) and students. In PISA, for example, the response rate had to reach at least 85% at the level of schools. If the initial rate ranged between 65 and 85%, countries were permitted to select substitute schools. At the level of students, at least 80% of the sample had to participate. These requirements led to an exclusion of the Netherlands from most analyses in PISA 2000 and of the United Kingdom from most analyses in PISA 2003.

MULTILEVEL ISSUES IN ANALYSES OF DATA FROM INTERNATIONAL LARGE-SCALE ASSESSMENTS OF STUDENT PERFORMANCE

In analyses of datasets involving multilevel structures, two general approaches can be distinguished (Muthén, 1994; Raudenbush & Bryk, 2002). The first approach views the multilevel structure as a "nuisance factor" and treats it accordingly. Due to the multistage sampling employed in international large-scale assessment studies, observations are not independent, as students within schools tend to be more similar to one another than to students from different schools. Applying common statistical analyses to these correlated observations will typically overestimate the effective sample size, thus resulting in an underestimation of the standard error and in overly liberal significance testing (Kish, 1965). Therefore, it is necessary to adjust the standard error in analyses of data from cluster samples to account for the design effect. Several adjustment procedures are available, most of which have been developed by researchers working with survey data (Lohr, 1999; Muthén & Satorra, 1995).

Instead of viewing the hierarchical data structure as a nuisance factor, the second approach is specifically interested in the different levels and treats them as objects of analysis. This approach has been around in educational research for about three decades (Burstein, 1980; Cronbach, 1976). In analyses of students within classrooms, for example, the observed interindividual differences are composed of variance stemming from two sources: variability at the level of individuals and variability at the level of classrooms (assuming a two-level structure of the data). This can be illustrated by decomposing the individual score of a student into two components. If, for example, a student evaluates the quality of instruction in his or her mathematics class, the individual evaluation score Y_T can be decomposed into the mean evaluation score of all students in the class Y_B and the deviation Y_W of the student's evaluation from the class mean. The two components added together represent the observed individual score of the student: $Y_T = Y_W + Y_B$. Based on this relationship, Cronbach (1976) argued that analyses involving students within classrooms should not be based on the confounded value Y_T but on its two independent parts Y_W und Y_B (see also the critical discussion of aptitude-treatment research by Cronbach & Webb, 1975).

The following subsections focus on the second general approach to analyzing hierarchical data, as this is the more interesting one from a psychological perspective. First, we describe basic types of questions that can be explored with multilevel analyses of data from international large-scale assessment studies. Second, we discuss a number of methodological problems and challenges that confront researchers in performing such analyses.

Research Questions of Multilevel Analyses

A major appeal of multilevel analyses lies in the possibility of exploring relationships among variables located at different levels simultaneously, with the dependent variable always being located at the lowest level. In outlining different types of questions that can be examined with multilevel analyses of large-scale assessment data, we focus on two-level models, such as students (individual level) nested in countries (group level).

In exploring the role of a context (e.g., classroom, school, or country) for an individual-level variable, different types of group-level variables can be distinguished (see also Van de Vijver, Poortinga, & Van Hemert, this volume). The first type can be measured directly, such as the amount of educational spending in a country or the size of a country's population. These directly measurable variables that cannot be broken down to the individual level are often referred to as "global" or "integral" variables (Blakely & Woodward, 2000). They have to be distinguished from group-level variables that are generated by aggregating variables from a lower (typically the individual) level. For example, students' school climate ratings may be aggregated at the school level in order to use the resulting mean as an indicator for the school's collective climate (see Fischer, this volume). Variables that are obtained through the aggregation of scores at the individual level are known as "contextual" or "analytical" variables.

In two-level modeling, three types of contextual effects can be distinguished (see Figure 12.2, adapted from Blakely & Woodward, 2000; see also Snijders & Bosker, 1999). The first type is the *direct cross-level effect* (see Figure 12.2, model 1). In this case, the variable Z has a direct effect on the variable Y while simultaneously controlling for the individual-level variable X. Within international large-scale assessment studies such as PISA, one could, for example, ask whether the amount of educational spending in the participating countries (Z) has an effect on students' reading performance (Y) when parental support (X) is controlled. It is assumed that the relationship between reading performance and parental support is constant across countries and that only the *level* of reading performance covaries with the amount of educational spending. This type of model

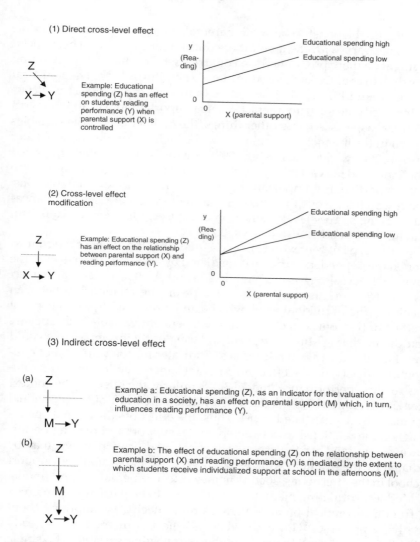

FIGURE 12.2 Types of contextual effects in two-level modeling

is referred to as *random-intercept model* (Raudenbush & Bryk, 2002). If the context factor were generated by way of aggregating individual scores X, it would represent the classical contextual analysis model (e.g., Blalock, 1984; Firebaugh, 1978).

A second type of contextual effect is the *cross-level effect modification* (see Figure 12.2, model 2). It asks whether a context factor influences the relationship between variables. This effect describes the extent to which the context factor Z moderates the association between the individual-level variables X and Y. In international large-scale assessment studies, for example, the relationship between parental support and reading performance may vary with the amount of educational spending. The association might be more pronounced in countries where educational spending is low than in countries where educational spending is high. The statistical literature on multilevel analyses refers to this effect as *cross-level interaction*. In specifying such an interaction, it is important to pay attention to a few critical aspects. Among other things, the main effects of the variables involved in the interaction should always be included in the model (Bauer & Curran, 2005; Snijders & Bosker, 1999), and the issue of centering applied to the independent variable (group mean centering vs. grand mean centering) is particularly important in models with cross-level interactions. Some researchers argue that group-mean centering increases the chances of identifying a cross-level interaction effect (see, for example, Hofmann & Gavin, 1998; Raudenbush & Bryk, 2002).

The third type of contextual effect assumes that the effect of the context factor on the dependent variable is mediated by additional variables at the individual level (see Figure 12.2, models 3a and 3b). It represents an *indirect cross-level effect* on an outcome variable or on the relationship between variables at the individual level, which can be revealed by showing that the effect of the context factor Z on the dependent variable Y disappears when the mediator M is controlled. In terms of the example, this could mean that educational spending, as an indicator for the valuation of education in a society, has an effect on parental support which, in turn, influences reading performance (model 3a). Similarly, the effect of the context factor Z on a relationship between two variables X and Y at the individual level may also be mediated by M. Thus, the effect of educational spending (Z) on the relationship between parental support and reading performance, as outlined for the cross-level effect modification above, may be mediated by the extent to which students receive individualized support at school in the afternoons, such as homework or remedial support (model 3b). Models postulating mediation effects tend to be particularly interesting from a theoretical point of view as they specify assumptions about underlying processes. However, whereas a host of methods are already available for testing mediation hypotheses involving variables at a single level, this is not the case for mediation analyses within multilevel models. The development of appropriate methods is currently an area of intensive research (e.g., Bauer, Preacher, & Gill, 2006; Krull & MacKinnon, 2001).

Thus far, the models presented in this section have focused on multilevel analyses as generalizations of regression analyses. A different type of investigation involves factor analytical models exploring differences in factor structures between countries and across levels. One approach explores the equivalence of factor structures in different countries. This type of analysis is typically used to compare the measurement properties of an instrument, such as the PISA literacy tests, between countries or cultures. Another approach examines the extent to which the factor structure varies across different levels of analysis. Thus, the factor structure of the literacy tests at the individual student level and at the country level could be compared. To our knowledge, this analysis has not yet been performed, even though previous research has shown that a different factor structure may emerge already on the class or school level as compared to the individual level (e.g., Härnqvist, Gustafsson, Muthén, & Nelson, 1994; Muthén, 1991). For the most part, the correlations tend to be stronger at the aggregate level than at the individual level (see, for example, Ostroff, 1993). Reasons for this include the increased reliability of measures at higher levels of analysis and differences in the processes underlying correlations at different levels (Snijders & Bosker, 1999). Therefore, one would expect the factor structure to be less differentiated at the country level than at the individual level. Due to methodological advances in the integration of structural equation and multilevel modelling, simultaneous analyses of factor structures and relationships among variables at different levels within a single model should become more prevalent in the future (Mehta & Neale, 2005; Skrondal & Rabe-Hesketh, 2004).

Methodological Challenges

This subsection discusses some of the potential pitfalls that can be associated with the interpretation of results from multilevel analyses of large-scale assessment data. The first potential pitfall is the *shift of meaning* of variables that may occur at different levels of analysis. A variable that was initially measured at the individual student level does not necessarily retain its meaning after it was aggregated at a higher level (see also Van de Vijver, Poortinga, and Van Hemert, this volume). As a result, it is not permissible to generalize relationships between variables that were identified at one level (e.g., the student level) to another level (e.g., the country level). One of the most remarkable and, from a psychological perspective, most interesting illustrations of this problem was presented by Shen and Pedulla (2000). Using data from the TIMSS cohort of lower secondary students, the authors examined the relationship between students' self-evaluated mathematics ability, which was assessed with the item "I usually do well in mathematics," and students' actual mathematics performance both within as well as between the 40 participating countries. As would be expected, the findings revealed a positive relationship between mathematics self-concept and mathematics performance at the individual level within all countries. The within-country correlations ranged from $r = .12$, $p < .01$, to $r = .47$, $p < .01$. The corresponding analysis at the country level, however, showed a negative correlation of $r = -.57$, $p < .01$. The authors attribute this reversal in the relationship to cultural differences in self-evaluations of ability. According to this interpretation, students from East Asian countries such as Korea, Hong Kong, or Singapore tend to evaluate their achievement more critically than their peers from different cultural backgrounds. Thus, by aggregating the self-concept measure at the country level, the indicator changed its meaning. At the country level, it no longer represented self-evaluations of ability but rather the tendency of cultural groups to be self-critical or modest. This illustrates that psychological and other constructs that distinguish individuals within populations may not necessarily be meaningful when it comes to distinguishing populations. It implies that instruments which were initially developed and validated for the measurement of constructs at the individual level need to be validated again if they are to be used at a higher level.

Closely related to the shift-of-meaning problem is the concept of the *ecological fallacy* that was coined by Robinson (1950). This concept points out that it is often inadequate to generalize a relationship which was found on an aggregate level to the individual level (cf., King, 1997).[1] Robinson illustrates the issue with correlations between illiteracy and skin color in the United States. At the level of the nine census districts in the U.S., the correlation between the proportion of illiterate individuals and the proportion of Black residents was $r = .95$. As Robinson (1950) points out, however, it would be wrong to interpret this association as proof of an almost perfect linear relationship. In fact, based on the absolute numbers at the individual level summarized in a 2×2 table, the relationship was reduced to $r = .20$.

Because large-scale assessment studies provide access to both individual and group-level data for many variables, ecological fallacies can be avoided for many research questions (e.g., the relationship between interest in reading and reading performance) by analyzing the different levels simultaneously with multilevel modeling. In other cases, however, researchers working with data from large-scale assessment studies have to choose which level of aggregation for a given variable is theoretically the most plausible. Bliese (2000), Chan (1998), as well as Kozlowski and Klein (2000) provide theoretical and methodological rationales for choosing among different aggregation levels for a construct (see also Fischer, this volume).

A further challenge is the extent to which all relevant levels can be taken into account. In studies such as TIMSS or PISA, this tends to be only partly possible. As was pointed out before, these studies are mainly interested in providing precise estimates of student performance and in comparing these estimates across countries. In sampling students and analyzing the data, the multilevel structure of the educational system is only partly taken into account. PISA, for example, sampled schools and subsequently students within schools (15-year-olds). The dataset does not include any information to tell the researcher which students are in the same class or which students have the same teacher in a given school subject. Therefore, it is impossible to study effects of instructional factors or class characteristics. More importantly, the findings of analyses at the level of schools may be biased as well. Van den Noortgate, Opdenakker and Onghena (2005) showed mathematically as well as with simulation studies that ignoring levels in random intercept models (i.e., models that explore variations in the level of a variable only, not in relationships between variables) may affect estimates of variance components and standard errors (see also Moerbeek, 2004; Opdenakker & Van Damme, 2000). These findings suggest that proportions of between-school variance are overestimated in a study like PISA, because it does not take the class level into account. The variance associated with the class level will be attributed to neighboring levels. Thus, the possibilities for drawing conclusions about the relative role of different levels (students, teachers, classes, schools) in international large-scale assessment studies on student performance are limited if levels are omitted.

A main goal of psychological research is to explain interindividual variations in human experiences and behaviors. International large-scale assessments studies, however, are primarily interested in providing descriptions of between-country differences in student performance. Theoretical models of student performance that take into account country-level characteristics and cultural factors are rare, and the number of empirical studies that have explored possible explanations of between-country differences is still small (see below). The issue of testing explanatory models is closely tied to the question whether it is at all possible to draw causal conclusions on the basis of data from international assessment studies. Multilevel analyses are no silver bullet—they are as limited by similar methodological problems as ordinary regression models (Gelman, 2006). These problems include the omission of important variables in the model as well as the assumption that the independent variables are exogenous with regard to the dependent variable. In addition, potential explanatory factors at the country level are often highly interrelated such that it is difficult (or even impossible) to disentangle them empirically. A considerable improvement would be to implement longitudinal designs (see, for example, the criticism of international large-scale assessments by Goldstein, 2004), yet this has only been done within individual countries (e.g., Canada and Germany), not internationally.

To conclude this section, we would like to point out a more general limitation. Multilevel analyses presuppose that the variables included in the model are comparable across countries. However, specific features of individual countries will almost inevitably be neglected (Esping-Andersen & Przeworski, 2001). For example, countries use different approaches to ability grouping, such as general or subject-specific tracking or streaming, each with varying numbers of ability levels. Moreover, the extent to which different curricula are implemented within each of the tracks varies as well. It is often impossible to develop indicators that allow researchers to take such complex between-country differences into account in multilevel analyses. Therefore, it is important to supplement the quantitative perspective of statistical multilevel analyses with a qualitative perspective in order to generate more in-depth information on single cases (see, for example, the ethnographical studies of selected school systems by Stevenson & Nerison-Low, 1997) and to combine the strengths of both approaches (King, Keohane, & Verba, 1994). For example, countries that deviate substantially from their predicted value in a multilevel analysis (Bowers & Drake, 2005) could, in a subsequent step, be submitted to an intensive ideographical analysis which also takes into account the country's historical complexity.

Taken together, the naturally occurring multilevel structure of data from international large-scale assessment studies on student performance offers unique opportunities for exploring a host of research questions. At the same time, it confronts researchers with a series of challenges requiring decisions that often lack a clear rationale. Despite these complications, studies such as PISA provide some of the best cross-cultural datasets that can be used to explore comparative research questions. In the next section, we describe a few studies that have performed such analyses.

SELECTED MULTILEVEL ANALYSES OF DATA FROM INTERNATIONAL LARGE-SCALE ASSESSMENTS OF STUDENT PERFORMANCE

The comparative analyses that have been carried out to date can be subdivided into two groups: The first group explored determinants of student performance at various levels, while the second group tested the validity of psychological theories across countries and cultures.

Determinants of Student Performance

Determinants of student performance in international large-scale assessment studies can be located at various levels (see Figure 12.1). They may involve characteristics of individuals, classrooms or schools, and school systems as well as factors located at the societal or state levels. In addition to mean student performance, some analyses have tried to explain performance gaps between different student groups, such as female and male students, students from families with lower and higher socioeconomic status, or native students and immigrant students.

Analyses exploring determinants of student performance at the levels of countries and school systems have to deal with small sample sizes and a host of confounded variables whose effects cannot be separated. Nevertheless, if conducted carefully, these analyses can provide some indications for potential causes of between-country differences in absolute levels of student performance or in the size of performance gaps. Good examples for this type of investigation were presented by the economist Woessmann and his colleagues (e.g., Fuchs & Woessmann, 2007; Hanushek & Woessmann, 2005; Woessmann, 2001, 2003; Woessmann & West, 2006) who performed several reanalyses of the TIMSS and PISA data. Based on an econometric model of educational outcomes that focuses on institutional characteristics and their incentive structures, Fuchs and Woessmann (2007) derived an international production function model of student performance and applied it to the PISA data (for a very similar analysis of the TIMSS data see Woessmann, 2003). This model includes variables at the level of students (grade, age, and gender) and their families (e.g., immigration background, parental education and work status, and books at home), at the level of schools (e.g., availability of instructional material, student-teacher ratio, and school autonomy with regard to such aspects as textbook selection or budget allocation), at the level of the community (size of a school's community location), at the level of the school system (e.g., existence of external exit exams, standardized testing, and average educational expenditure per student), and at the level of the country (Gross Domestic Product [GDP] per capita). In addition, the authors explored a number of cross-level interactions between a feature of the school system deemed to be central (external exit exam) on the one hand and characteristics of individual schools (several aspects of school autonomy and private vs. public operation and funding) on the other hand. Among the institutional factors, external exams (cf., Bishop, 1997), several aspects of school autonomy (with regard to textbook choice, hiring of teachers, and within-school budget allocations), and private school management (but not private funding) were associated with higher student performance. Also, educational spending was positively related to achievement, although the relationship was relatively weak and disappeared when four countries with very low levels of spending were excluded from the analyses (see also Hanushek, 2003; Woessmann, 2003). In terms of the cross-level interactions explored in the study, the findings showed that the positive effects of school autonomy were more pronounced in systems with external school leaving exams than in systems without such exams. Overall, the model tested by Fuchs and Woessmann (2007) explained 85% of the between-country variance in student performance, with approximately 25% attributable to institutional factors.

Several studies have used data from large-scale assessment studies to explore the relationship between student performance and student background characteristics in international comparison. These concerned differences in performance related to gender (e.g., Van Langen, Bosker, & Dekkers, 2006), socioeconomic background (e.g., Marks, 2006; Marks, Cresswell, & Ainley, 2006), and immigrant background (e.g., Stanat & Christensen, 2006). Again, in trying to determine factors that may moderate these performance gaps, most of the analyses focused on institutional or structural factors at the levels of school systems or states, such as tracking of students into school types or immigration and integration policies.

Validity of Psychological Theories across Countries

The number of studies that have explored potential causes of between-country differences in student performance is relatively small, and most of these studies have concentrated on the role of institutional factors. The number of analyses that have been carried out from a more psychological perspective is even smaller. Cross-cultural psychology in particular has been surprisingly reluctant to get involved in international large-scale assessment projects and to work with their data.

One study that used data from international assessments to explore a psychological construct at the country level was performed by Lynn and Mikk (2007). Based on previous work by Lynn and Vanhanen (2002), who had gathered intelligence data for 113 countries from studies reporting nonverbal IQ test results, the authors set out to establish the validity of the notion of "national IQs" which they operationalized as the average intelligence scores within a country. To validate the construct, they correlated the mean IQ scores with mean mathematics and science performance of fourth grade and eighth grade students in the TIMSS 2003 assessments (Martin, Mullis, Gonzales & Chrostowski, 2004; Mullis, Martin, Gonzalez & Chrostowski, 2004). The analyses were based on the data from 25 countries for grade 4 and 46 countries for grade 8 and revealed very strong correlations ranging from .85 and .93 without correction for attenuation and from .92 to 1.0 with correction for attenuation. In addition, the relationships between mean achievement and mean IQ were consistently higher than the relationships between mean achievement and a number of school characteristics (e.g., teacher qualifications, school climate perceived by principals, and percentage of students whose parents have completed university). The authors interpret this pattern as providing strong support for the validity of the national IQs construct which is also related to countries' GDP. They suggest that the correlations among IQ, GDP, and test scores in mathematics and science "arise from a complex network of relationships" where the "most fundamental are national IQs and per capita GDP (as a measure of per capita income)" (Lynn & Mikk, 2007). According to this line of reasoning, the association between these two factors is reciprocal, and they jointly influence student achievement in mathematics and science.

The studies by Lynn and colleagues (Lynn & Mikk, 2007; Lynn and Vanhanen, 2002) have been criticized on various grounds, such as the use of IQ data from studies with nonrepresentative, often very small and highly heterogeneous samples (e.g., Hunt & Sternberg, 2006). Also, although they cite research showing that education affects both domain-specific performance in school subjects as well as general cognitive abilities (e.g., Blair,

Gamson, Thorne, & Baker, 2005; Ceci, 1991), they largely ignore this relationship in their assumptions about causal relationships.

Another way in which psychologists have utilized data from international large-scale assessments is to explore the generalizability of psychological theories across countries and cultures. These types of analyses can provide valuable information on the extent to which a given psychological model is universally valid or might need to be specified to account for cross-cultural variations (Sue, 1999). Marsh and Hau (2004) tested the predictions of the internal/external frame of reference (I/E) model of self-concept in the 26 countries that participated in PISA 2000 and had implemented the questionnaire on prerequisites of self-regulated learning as an international option. The I/E model posits that academic self-concepts are determined by comparisons based on two different frames of reference (e.g., Marsh & Yeung, 2001): Within the external frame of reference, students compare their own performance in a school subject with the performance of their peers. Within the internal frame of reference, in contrast, students compare their own performance across different school subjects. In line with these assumptions, it has repeatedly been shown that verbal and mathematical achievement levels are not only positively related to the corresponding self-concepts but also negatively related to the noncorresponding self-concepts (for a review, see Skaalvik & Skaalvik, 2002). Thus, good relative mathematics performance predicts higher mathematics self-concept but lower verbal self-concept, and good relative verbal performance predicts higher verbal self-concept but lower mathematics self-concept.

Marsh and Hau (2004) conducted structural equation modeling (SEM) with the PISA data to test the invariance of the I/E model across countries. Using a multigroup comparison approach, they successively introduced additional parameter restrictions and evaluated the change in model fit. The findings revealed that even the most restrictive model assuming invariance of all parameters across countries resulted in a good fit of the data. The authors interpret these findings as strong evidence for the cross-national validity of the I/E model. However, they also acknowledge that the diversity of the countries included in the analyses is limited, including only one country from Central America (Mexico), South America (Brazil), and Asia (Korea) respectively.

In another analysis, Marsh and Hau (2003) examined the cross-national validity of the big-fish-little-pond-effect (BFLPE) on academic self-concept that results from the social comparison processes specified in the I/E model. The BFLPE posits that, due to social comparison processes, the self-concept of an individual student will be affected by the performance level of his or her reference group (Marsh & Parker, 1984). More specifically, given the same level of mathematics performance, a student should develop a less positive self-concept within a high-performing group than within a low-performing group. Thus, the BFLPE predicts that a student's self-concept in a school subject will be positively related to his or her own individual achievement level but negatively related to the average achievement level of the class or school he or she is attending. Again, using the PISA 2000 data Marsh and Hau explored the generalizability of these predictions. This required the simultaneous consideration of three levels: the levels of students, schools, and countries. They performed a multilevel analysis to estimate the extent to which the effect of average school performance (level 2) on student performance (level 1) varies in international comparison (level 3).

Although the results provided general support for the BFLPE, they also indicated that the effect varies cross-nationally. This was confirmed by separate estimations of the model for each of the 26 countries included in the study. The findings showed that, although the effect of mean achievement at the school level on students' academic self-concept varied in size, it reached significance in all countries, except in Hungary and Korea. The authors conclude that "the BFLPE may approach what Segall et al. [1998, p. 1102] referred to as a 'nearly universal psychology, one that has pan-human validity'—one of the goals of cross-cultural research" (Marsh & Hau, 2003, p. 373; for critiques of the study see Dai, 2004; Plucker et al., 2004).

Artelt (2005) used the PISA 2000 data to explore the constructs of extrinsic and intrinsic aspects of motivation. She examined the extent to which instrumental motivation related to reading and interest in reading show similar factor structures and associations with reading achievement across countries. A multigroup confirmatory factor analysis revealed that the structure of the scales used to measure the constructs was, in fact, invariant across countries. In addition, the findings provided some evidence for the assumption that the relationships between the motivational variables and performance on the reading literacy test are consistent across countries. Intrinsic motivation showed a significant direct effect on performance in most countries, while the effect of instrumental motivation was largely mediated by students' reported use of control strategies. A different result emerged at the country level. A multilevel analysis with performance in the reading test as the dependent variable revealed a positive effect of motivation on the individual level but a negative effect of average motivation at the country level. This pattern was driven by such countries as Korea and Brazil. In Korea, students reached relatively high scores on the reading test but reported relatively low levels of motivation whereas the opposite pattern emerged in countries like Brazil. This provides another example for the shift in meaning that can occur when variables are aggregated at different levels.

A final set of studies we would like to mention examined gender differences at different levels and in terms of different research questions (Penner, 2003; Van Langen, et al., 2006). The study by Van Langen and colleagues explored potential determinants of performance gaps between boys and girls at the levels of school and countries. Using data from the 42 countries participating in the PISA 2000 and PISA+ assessments (OECD & UNESCO Institute for Statistics, 2003), the authors performed a series of three-level analyses to predict students' mathematics, science, and reading scores from a number of student characteristics (gender, SES, immigrant background), school characteristics (mean SES, proportion of girls and immigrant students, public and private school types, school location's degree of urbanization), and country characteristics (GENDER SES, differentiation of the school system, female economic activity rate, gender empowerment index). To estimate the extent to which these factors moderate gender differences in performance, the model included cross-level interaction terms of gender (level 1) with school characteristics (level 2) and with country characteristics (level 3). Contrary to predictions, the indicators for gender equality at the country level did not interact significantly with student gender in the prediction of mathematics or science performance. The analysis of reading test scores, however, revealed a significant interaction between gender and economic activity rates of women indicating that the reading performance gap in favor of girls tends to be larger in countries with higher female economic activity rates. In addition, school location in urban areas and differentiation of the school system interacted with gender across all three assessment domains. The disadvantage of girls in mathematics and science tended to be smaller and their advantage in reading tended to be larger in rural schools and in integrated systems than in urban schools and in differentiated systems (with the integration or differentiation of a system being represented by a composite index of such factors as number of school tracks; degree of sex, socioeconomic, and immigrant segregation; and performance differences across schools). Yet, the mechanisms underlying these effects remain largely unclear.

CONCLUSION

The goal of this chapter was to describe some of the strengths and weaknesses of international large-scale assessment studies on student performance and their potential for multilevel analyses. In terms of instrumentation and implementation, the quality of these studies has improved considerably over the past 40 years, with PISA representing the current state of the art. At the same time, a number of challenges remain. These include the use of unidimensional models as the basis for instrument development and international comparisons, which could conceivably "smooth out" relevant differences between countries (Goldstein, 2004, p. 322); the possibility that language or general cultural factors may influence overall test results (Artelt & Baumert, 2004; Bonnet, 2002); the unclear psychometric equivalence of many questionnaire scales; the omission of levels (e.g., classrooms), which may bias variance estimates; and the limited potential of the studies for the identification of causal relationships due to the lack of longitudinal data (Goldstein, 2004).

Despite these limitations, the data provide unique opportunities for multilevel analyses involving individuals, schools or classrooms, as well as countries. Even though the data are readily available on the Internet (for PISA, see: http://www.pisa.oecd.org; for TIMSS and PIRLS see: http://timss.bc.edu) and the documentation of the most recent studies in technical reports is exceptional (e.g., Adams & Wu, 2002; Martin, Gregory, & Stemler, 2000; OECD, 2005), the potential of the assessments has not yet been widely used in psychology. The few studies that we described in this chapter illustrate the diverse types of questions that can be addressed with the data.

In performing the analyses and in interpreting their results, a number of methodological challenges and potential pitfalls need to be taken into account. These include changes in the meaning of variables at different levels of aggregation, problems associated with generalizing relationships from one level to another, and omission of variables at different levels. If these issues are treated appropriately, analyses of data from international assessment studies can provide valuable information on variables at different levels, on relationships among these variables, and on between-country differences in the variables and their relationships.

It is difficult to predict in which directions this line of research will develop in the future. Especially in the case of the OECD studies, this is highly dependent on the interests of policy makers. Research teams will certainly continue to work on improving the methodology, such as the measurement models underlying the tests and questionnaires. Furthermore, a possible development that has begun to emerge in the context of PISA is the introduction of technology-based assessment. This would allow for the use of new item formats and for the implementation of adaptive testing procedures. However, the costs for such an innovation are considerable and may be prohibitive for large-scale international studies. Thus far, the issue of added costs has also prevented the collection of longitudinal datasets, which would greatly improve the scope for causal analyses.

In terms of theoretical developments, it would be highly desirable to expand existing models of student performance to take into account cultural characteristics of countries, such as the extent to which societies value education or share assumptions about teaching and learning processes. This would require a more intensive participation of cross-cultural psychologists in the conceptualization and analysis of large-scale assessment studies. The challenge of developing such models is to identify relevant cultural factors and to develop hypotheses about how they may impact teaching and learning in schools. Such an enriched framework would help to provide a better understanding of student performance in international comparison.

Note

1. Diez-Roux (1998) provides an overview of additional fallacies that may occur in interpretations of multilevel analyses. In addition to the *ecological fallacy* (drawing inferences at the individual level based on group-level data), she describes an *atomistic fallacy* (drawing inferences at the group level based on individual-level data), a *psychologistic fallacy* (assuming that individual-level outcomes can be explained exclusively in terms of individiual-level characteristics), and a *sociologistic fallacy* (ignoring the role of individual-level factors in a study of groups).

REFERENCES

Adams, R., & Carstensen, C. (2002). Scaling outcomes. In R. Adams & M. Wu (Eds.), *PISA 2000 technical report* (pp. 149–162). Paris: OECD.

Adams, R., & Wu, M. (Eds.). (2002). *PISA 2000 technical report.* Paris: OECD.

Allalouf, A. (2003). Revising translated differential item functioning items as a tool for improving cross-lingual assessment. *Applied Measurement in Education, 16,* 55–73.

Artelt, C. (2005). Cross-cultural approaches to measuring motivation. *Educational Assessment, 10,* 231–255.

Artelt, C., & Baumert, J. (2004). Zur Vergleichbarkeit von Schülerleistungen bei Leseaufgaben unterschiedlichen sprachlichen Ursprungs. *Zeitschrift für Pädagogische Psychologie, 18,* 171–185.

Artelt, C., Baumert, J., Julius-McElvany, N., & Peschar, J. (2003). *Learners for life: Student approaches to learning. Results from PISA 2000.* Paris: OECD.

Bauer, D. J., & Curran, P. J. (2005). Probing interactions in fixed and multilevel regression: Inferential and graphical techniques. *Multivariate Behavioral Research, 40,* 373–400.

Bauer, D. J., Preacher, K. J., & Gill, K. M. (2006). Conceptualizing and testing random indirect effects and moderated mediation in multilevel models: New procedures and recommendations. *Psychological Methods, 11,* 142–163.

Baumert, J., Blum, W., & Neubrand, M. (2004). Drawing the lessons from PISA-2000: Long term research implications. In D. Lenzen, J. Baumert, R. Watermann, & U. Trautwein (Eds.), *PISA und die Konsequenzen für die erziehungswissenschaftliche Forschung. Zeitschrift für Erziehungswissenschaf,* (Suppl. 3-2004), 143–157.

Beaton, A. E., Martin, M. O., Mullis, I. V. S., Gonzales, E. J., Smith, T. A., & Kelly, D. L. (1996). *Science achievement in the middle school years: IEA's Third International Mathematics and Science Study.* Chestnut Hill, MA: TIMSS International Study Center, Boston College.

Beaton, A. E., Mullis, I. V. S., Martin, M. O., Gonzalez, E. J., Kelly, D. L., & Smith, T. A. (1996). *Mathematics achievement in the middle school years*. Chestnut Hill, MA: TIMSS International Study Center, Boston College.

Bishop, J. H. (1997). The effect of national standards and curriculum-based exams on achievement. *American Economic Review, 87,* 260–264.

Blair, C., Gamson, D., Thorne, S., & Baker, D. (2005). Rising mean IQ: Cognitive demand of mathematics education for young children, population exposure to formal schooling, and the neurobiology of the prefrontal cortex. *Intelligence, 33,* 93–106.

Blakely, T. A., & Woodward, A. J. (2000). Ecological effects in multi-level studies. *Journal of Epidemiology and Community Health, 54,* 367–374.

Blalock, H. M. (1984). Contextual-effects models: Theoretical and methodological issues. *Annual Review of Sociology, 10,* 353–372.

Bliese, P. D. (2000). Within-group agreement, non-independence, and reliability: Implications for data aggregation and analysis. In K. J. Klein, & S. W. Kozlowski (Eds.), *Multilevel theory, research, and methods in organizations* (pp. 349–381). San Francisco, CA: Jossey-Bass.

Bonnet, G. (2002). Reflections in a critical eye: On the pitfalls of international assessment. *Assessment in Education, 9,* 387–399.

Bonnet, G., Daems, F., De Glopper, C., Horner, S., Lappalainen, H.-P., Nardi, E. et al. (2003). *Culturally balanced assessment of reading.* Retrieved November, 2003 from http://cisad.adc.education.fr/reva/pdf/cbarfinalreport.pdf.

Bowers, J., & Drake, K. W. (2005). EDA for HLM: Visualization when probabilistic inference fails. *Political Analysis, 13,* 301–326.

Brislin, R. W. (1986). The wording and translation of research instruments. In W. J. Lonner & J. W. Berry (Eds.), *Field methods in cross-cultural research* (pp. 137–164). London: Sage.

Bronfenbrenner, U. (1979). *The ecology of human development: Experiments by nature and design.* Cambridge, MA: Harvard University Press.

Budgell, G. R., Namburty, S. R., & Douglas, A. Q. (1995). Analysis of differential item functioning in translated assessment instruments. *Applied Psychological Measurement, 19,* 309–321.

Burstein, L. (1980). The analysis of multilevel data in educational research and evaluation. *Review of Research in Education, 8,* 158–233.

Camilli, G., & Shepard, L. A. (1994). *Methods for identifying biased test items.* Thousand Oaks, CA: Sage.

Ceci, S. J. (1991). How much does schooling influence general intelligence and its cognitive components? A reassessment of the evidence. *Developmental Psychology, 27,* 703–722.

Chan, D. (1998). Functional relations among constructs in the same content domain at different levels of analysis: A typology of composition models. *Journal of Applied Psychology, 83,* 234–246.

Cronbach, L. J. (1976). *Research on classrooms and schools: Formulations of questions, design and analysis.* Stanford, CA: Stanford Evaluation Consortium.

Cronbach, L. J., & Webb, N. (1975). Between-class and within-class effects in a reported aptitude * treatment interaction: Reanalysis of a study by G. L. Anderson. *Journal of Educational Psychology, 67,* 717–724.

Dai, D. Y. (2004). How universal is the big-fish-little-pond effect? *American Psychologist, 59,* 267–276.

Diez-Roux (1998). Bringing context back into epidemiology: Variables and fallacies in multilevel analyses. *American Journal of Public Health, 88,* 216–222.

Esping-Andersen, G., & Przeworski, A. (2001). Quantitative cross-national research methods. In N. J. Smelser & P. B. Baltes (Eds.), *International encyclopedia of the social and behavioral sciences* (Vol. 18, pp. 12649–12655). Amsterdam: Elsevier.

Firebaugh, G. (1978). A rule for inferring individual-level relationships from aggregate data. *American Sociological Review, 43,* 557–572.

Fuchs, L., & Woessmann, L. (2007). What accounts for international differences in student performance? A re-examination using PISA Data. *Empirical Economics, 32,* 433–464.

Gelman, A. (2006). Multilevel (hierarchical) modeling: What it can and cannot do. *Technometrics, 48,* 432–435.

Gierl, M. J., & Khaliq, S. N. (2001). Identifying sources of differential item and bundle functioning on translated achievement tests: A confirmatory analysis. *Journal of Educational Measurement, 38,* 164–187.

Goldstein, H. (2004). International comparisons of student attainment: Some issues arising from the PISA study. *Assessment in Education, 11,* 319–330.

Grisay, A. (2002). Translation and cultural appropriateness of the test and survey material. In R. Adams & M. Wu (Eds.), *PISA 2000 technical report* (pp. 57–70). Paris: OECD.

Grisay, A. (2003). Translation procedures in OECD/PISA 2000 international assessment. *Language Testing, 20,* 225–240.

Hanushek, E. A. (2003). The failure of input-based schooling policies. *Economic Journal, 113,* 64–98.

Hanushek, E. A., & Woessmann, L. (2005). Does educational tracking affect performance and inequality? Differences-in-differences evidence across countries. *Economic Journal, 116,* 63–76.

Harkness, J. A. (2003). Questionnaire translation. In J. A. Harkness, F. J. R. Van de Vijver, & P. P. Mohler (Eds.), *Cross-cultural survey methods* (pp. 35–56). New York: Wiley.

Härnqvist, K., Gustafsson, J.-E., Muthén, B. O., & Nelson, G. (1994). Hierarchical models of ability at individual and class levels. *Intelligence, 18,* 165–187.

Hofmann, D. A., & Gavin, M. B. (1998). Centering decisions in hierarchical linear models: Implications for research in organizations. *Journal of Management, 24,* 623–641.

Holland, P. W., & Wainer, H. (Eds.). (1993). *Differential item functioning.* Hillsdale, NJ: Erlbaum.

Hunt, E., & Sternberg, R. J. (2006). Sorry, wrong numbers: An analysis of a study of a correlation between skin color and IQ. *Intelligence, 34,* 131–137.

Husén, T. (Ed.). (1967). *International project for the evaluation of educational achievement (IEA). Phase 1: International study of achievement in mathematics.* Stockholm: Almqvist & Wiksell.

King, G., Keohane, R., & Verba, S. (1994). *Designing social inquiry: Scientific inference in qualitative research.* Princeton, NJ: Princeton University Press.

King, G. (1997). *A solution to the ecological inference problem.* Princeton, NJ: Princeton University Press.

Kish, L. (1965). *Survey sampling.* New York: Wiley.

Klieme, E., & Baumert, J. (2001). Identifying national cultures of mathematics education: Analysis of cognitive demands and differential item functioning in TIMSS. *European Journal of Psychology of Education, 16*, 385–402.

Kozlowski, S. W., & Klein, K. J. (2000). A multilevel approach to theory and research in organizations: Contextual, temporal, and emergent processes. In K. J. Klein & S. W. Kozlowski (Eds.), *Multilevel theory, research, and methods in organizations: Foundations, extensions, and new directions* (pp. 3–90). San Francisco: Jossey-Bass.

Krawchuk, S., & Rust, K. (2002). Sample design. In R. Adams & M. Wu (Eds.), *PISA 2000 technical report* (pp. 39–-56). Paris: OECD.

Krull, J. L., & MacKinnon, D. P. (2001). Multilevel modeling of individual and group level mediated effects. *Multivariate Behavioral Research, 36*, 249–277.

Lohr, S. L. (1999). *Sampling: Design and analysis.* Pacific Grove, CA: Duxbury Press.

Lynn, R., & Mikk, J. (2007). National differences in intelligence and educational attainment. *Intelligence, 35*, 115–121.

Lynn, R., & Vanhanen, T. (2002). *IQ and the wealth of nations.* Westport, CT: Praeger.

Marks, G. N. (2006). Are between- and within-school differences in student performance largely due to socio-economic background? Evidence from 30 countries. *Educational Research, 48*, 21–40.

Marks, G. N., Cresswell, J., & Ainley, J. (2006). Explaining socioeconomic inequalities in student achievement: The role of home and school factors. *Educational Research and Evaluation, 12*, 105–128.

Marsh, H. W., & Hau, K.-T. (2003). Big-fish-little-pond effect on academic self-concept. A cross-cultural (26-country) test of the negative effects of academically selective schools. *American Psychologist, 58*, 364–376.

Marsh, H. W., & Hau, K.-T. (2004). Explaining paradoxical relations between academic self-concepts and achievement: Cross-cultural generalizability of the internal/external frame of reference predictions across 26 countries. *Journal of Educational Psychology, 96*, 56–67.

Marsh, H. W., & Parker, J. (1984). Determinants of student self-concept: Is it better to be a relatively large fish in a small pond even if you don't learn to swim as well? *Journal of Personality and Social Psychology, 47*, 213–231.

Marsh, H. W., & Yeung, A. S. (2001). An extension of the internal/external frame of reference model: A response to Bong (1998). *Multivariate Behavioral Research, 36*, 389–420.

Martin, M. O., Gregory, K. D., & Stemler, S. E. (2000). *TIMSS 1999 technical report.* Chestnut Hill, MA: TIMSS & PIRLS

Martin, M. O., Mullis, I. V. S., Gonzalez, E. J., & Chrostowski, S. J. (2004). *TIMSS 2003 international science report: Findings from IEA's Trends in International Mathematics and Science Study at the fourth and eighth grades.* Chestnut Hill, MA: TIMSS & PIRLS International Study Center, Boston College.

Mehta, P. D., & Neale, M. C. (2005). People are variables too: Multilevel structural equations modeling. *Psychological Methods, 10*, 259–284.

Moerbeek, M. (2004). The consequence of ignoring a level of nesting in multilevel analysis. *Multivariate Behavioral Research, 39*, 129–149.

Mullis, I. V. S., Martin, M. O., Beaton, A. E., Gonzales, E. J., Kelly, D. L., & Smith, T. A. (1998). *Mathematics and science achievement in the final year of secondary school: IEA's Third International Mathematics and Science Study (TIMSS)*. Chestnut Hill, MA: TIMSS International Study Center, Boston College.

Mullis, I. V. S., Martin, M. O., Gonzalez, E. ., & Chrostowski, S. J. (2004). *TIMSS 2003 international mathematics report. Findings from IEA's Trends in International Mathematics and Science Study at the Fourth and Eighth Grades*. Chestnut Hill, MA: TIMSS & PIRLS International Study Center, Boston College.

Muthén, B. O. (1991). Multilevel factor analysis of class and student achievement components. *Journal of Educational Measurement, 28,* 338–354.

Muthén, B. O. (1994). Multilevel covariance structure analysis. *Sociological Methods & Research, 22,* 376–398.

Muthén, B. O., & Satorra, A. (1995). Complex sample data in structural equation modeling. *Sociological Methodology, 25,* 267–316.

OECD. (1999). *Measuring student knowledge and skills: A new framework for assessment.* Paris: OECD.

OECD. (2001). *Knowledge and skills for life: First results from the OECD Programme for International Student Assessment (PISA) 2000.* Paris: OECD.

OECD. (2003). *The PISA 2003 assessment framework—Mathematics, reading, science and problem solving knowledge and skills.* Paris: OECD.

OECD. (2004). *Learning for tomorrow's world: First results from PISA 2003.* Paris: OECD.

OECD. (2005). *PISA 2003 technical report.* Paris: OECD.

OECD. (2006). *Education at a glance: Education indicators 2006.* Paris: OEDC.

OECD & UNESCO Institute for Statistics (UIS). (2003). *Literacy skills for the world of tomorrow: Further results from PISA 2000.* Paris: OECD.

Opdenakker, M.-C., & Van Damme, J. (2000). The importance of identifying levels in multilevel analysis: An illustration of effects of ignoring the top or intermediate levels in school effectiveness research. *School Effectiveness and School Improvement, 11,* 103–130.

Ostroff, C. (1993). Comparing correlations based on individual-level and aggregated data. *Journal of Applied Psychology, 78,* 569–582.

Penner, A. M. (2003). International gender x item difficulty interactions in mathematics and science achievement tests. *Journal of Educational Psychology, 95,* 650–655.

Plucker, J. A., Robinson, N. M., Greenspon, T. S., Feldhusen, J. F., McCoach, D. B., & Subotnik, R. F. (2004). It's not how the pond makes you feel, but rather how high you can jump. *American Psychologist, 59,* 268–271.

Postlethwaite, T. N. (1999). *International studies of educational achievement: Methodological issues.* Hong Kong: Comparative Education Research Centre.

Prais, S. J. (2003). Cautions on OECD's recent educational survey (PISA). *Oxford Review of Education, 29,* 139–163.

Raudenbush, S. W., & Bryk, A. S. (2002). *Hierarchical linear models* (2nd ed.). Thousand Oaks, CA: Sage.

Robinson, W. S. (1950). Ecological correlations and the behavior of individuals. *American Sociological Review, 15,* 351–357.

Segall, M. H., Lonner, W. J., & Berry, J. W. (1998). Cross-cultural psychology as a scholarly discipline: On the flowering of culture in behavioral research. *American Psychologist, 53,* 1101–1110.

Shen, C., & Pedulla, J. J. (2000). The relationship between students' achievement and their self-perception of competence and rigour of mathematics and science: A cross-national analysis. *Assessment in Education, 7*, 237–253.

Sireci, S. G. (1997). Problems and issues in linking assessments across languages. *Educational Measurement: Issues and Practice, 16*, 12–19.

Skaalvik, E. M., & Skaalvik, S. (2002). Internal and external frames of reference for academic self-concept. *Educational Psychologist, 37*, 233–244.

Skrondal, A., & Rabe-Hesketh, S. (2004). *Generalized latent variable modeling: Multilevel, longitudinal, and structural equation models.* Boca Raton, FL: Chapman & Hall/CRC.

Snijders, T. A. B., & Bosker, R. J. (1999). *Multilevel analysis: An introduction to basic and advanced multilevel modeling.* London: Sage.

Stanat, P., & Christensen, G. (2006). *Where immigrant students succeed—A comparative review of performance and engagement in PISA 2003.* Paris: OECD.

Stanat, P., & Lüdtke, O. (2007). Internationale Schulleistungsvergleiche [International comparisons of student performance]. In G. Trommsdorff & H.-J. Kornadt (Eds.), *Enzyklopädie der Psychologie: Kulturvergleichende Psychologie: Vol. 2. Kulturelle Determinanten des Erlebens und Verhaltens* (pp. 279–347). Göttingen, Germany: Hogrefe.

Stevenson, H. W., & Nerison-Low, R. (1997). *To sum it up: Case studies of education in Germany, Japan, and the United States.* University of Michigan: Center for Human Growth and Development.

Sue, S. (1999). Science, ethnicity, and bias: Where have we gone wrong? *American Psychologist, 54*, 1070–1077.

Teddlie, C., & Reynolds, D. (2000). *The international handbook of school effectiveness research.* London: Falmer.

Van de Vijver, F. J. R., & Hambleton, R. K. (1996). Translating tests: Some practical guidelines. *European Psychologist, 1*, 89–99.

Van de Vijver, F. J. R., & Tanzer, N. K. (1997). Bias and equivalence in cross-cultural assessment: An overview. *European Review of Applied Psychology, 47*, 263–279.

Van den Noortgate, W., Opdenakker, M.-C., & Onghena, P. (2005). The effects of ignoring a level in multilevel analysis. *School Effectiveness and School Improvement, 16*, 281–30.

Van Langen, A., Bosker, R., & Dekkers, H. (2006). Exploring cross-national differences in gender gaps in education. *Educational Research and Evaluation, 12*, 155–177.

Woessmann, L. (2001). Why students in some countries do better. International evidence in the importance of education policy. *Education Matters, 1*, 67–74.

Woessmann, L. (2003). Schooling resources, educational institutions and student performance: The international evidence. *Oxford Bulletin of Economics and Statistics, 65*, 117–170.

Woessmann, L., & West, M. (2006). Class-size effects in school systems around the world: Evidence from between-grade variation in TIMSS. *European Economic Review, 50*, 695–736.

Wu, M. (2002). Test design and test development. In R. Adams & M. Wu (Eds.), *PISA 2000 technical report* (pp. 21–31). Paris: OECD.

13

Multilevel Structure Analysis for Family-Related Constructs

Kostas Mylonas, Vassilis Pavlopoulos, and James Georgas

This chapter is based on a project which studied similarities and differences in families across cultures (Georgas, Berry, Van de Vijver, Kagitcibasi, & Poortinga, 2006). The goal of the project was to study family networks, family roles, and psychological variables in different ecological and socio-political systems across 30 countries. The present chapter focuses on the issue of structural equivalence of the above measures at the individual and country level. Structural equivalence implies that the same psychological constructs are measured cross-culturally (Van de Vijver & Leung, 1997); cross-level equivalence implies that the same constructs can serve to explain differences at each of the two levels without committing an ecological fallacy (Hox, 2002). The need to compare variables at different levels of aggregation is an important aspect of multilevel analysis in cross-cultural research (Van de Vijver & Poortinga, 2002).

The purpose of the present chapter is to explore structural equivalence of the scales employed in the 30-country family study and to compare the underlying constructs at the individual and country levels of aggregation; these scales involve family constructs, such as family hierarchy, family values and roles, and presumably related variables, such as values and personality.

Family systems and family change have been studied during the past two centuries by family sociology, cultural anthropology, psychology, education, psychiatry, economics, and historical demography, among other disciplines. Theories of family change have centered on the effects of social changes, such as economic development, education, political systems, and more recently, the global influence of television, of communication through telephones, e-mail, and the Internet. Changes in family types during the past two centuries, as a result of industrialization and urbanization, have been described as transitions from extended types of family systems to the nuclear family, and more recently, to the one-parent family.

For some family researchers, these social changes are considered to lead to an inevitable convergence of family systems across the globe. Extended family in non-Western societies is thought to give way to the nuclear family and ultimately the one-person family of Western societies in North America and Northern Europe. However, other studies have shown that the extended family did not become extinct in modern cities; rather, it has changed into a "modified extended family system," in which contact and psychological bonds of nuclear family members with kin are maintained (see also Georgas et al., 2006, for detailed discussion).

The theoretical approach of the overall project was derived from cross-cultural and indigenous psychology. The formulation of research hypotheses was guided by the ecocultural framework of Berry (1976, 1979) and the model of family change of Kagitcibasi (1990, 1996). The cross-cultural analyses were based on data from variables at four hierarchically related sets of variables: Country-level ecological and sociopolitical variables; family roles; family networks; and an array of psychological variables, including emotional bonds with members of the nuclear family and kin, personality traits, self-construal, family values, and personal values (Figure 13.1). The main analyses for this project were directed toward determining similarities and differences in mean scores at country level (Georgas et al., 2006). In addition, the findings were interpreted not only across all countries, but also for clusters of countries, or "cultural zones," based on ecological and sociopolitical variables. The indigenous approach was reflected

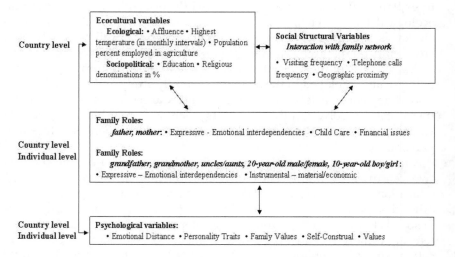

FIGURE 13.1 Overview of the levels of analyses and the variables employed based on the Ecocultural Framework. (Adapted from Georgas, Berry, Van de Vijver, Kagitcibasi, & Poortinga, 2006)

in a qualitative analysis of the relationships between cultural, family, and psychological variables in "family portraits" written by authors from each of the 30 countries. The quantitative analyses reported in this chapter are based on data from 27 of these 30 countries.

Indigenous patterns of family functions may or may not be the same across countries, which raises the issue about the similarity or dissimilarity of the underlying structure and functions across cultures. That is, to what extent can we describe the similarities and differences in the underlying psychological structure of families across cultures in terms of common variables? Such a procedure would require testing of the equivalence of central family constructs across countries (Van de Vijver & Leung, 1997). One central family construct is family values; it is of obvious importance to compare family values across countries with respect to their degree of acceptance or rejection. To be able to compare the respective constructs in a meaningful way requires at least an acceptable degree of certainty that they are invariant across the countries involved in the comparison. If such equivalence is not shown, then the family values under consideration may have a different functional meaning for some of the countries involved than they do for other countries. Several other constructs of interest (such as the ones in the four hierarchically related sets of variables as shown in Figure 13.1) can and should be explored with the same rationale of cross-level comparison, since family is well established as an important contextual agent in shaping individual behavior. This is evident in theoretical conceptualizations such as the ecological framework (Bronfenbrenner, 1979) or the ecological-social model (Georgas, 1993).

Cross-cultural studies in which individual-level family-related constructs are studied have to deal with equivalence issues in two ways. The first addresses the individual-level equivalence of the scales: Do scales measure the same psychological constructs in each culture examined? Identity of constructs is a prerequisite for comparing scores of individuals from different countries. This equivalence would be challenged if, say, obedience to the parents would be unidimensional in one culture and domain specific in another culture (e.g., parents are more focused on obedience in some domains than in others). Such a finding would imply that the global concept of obedience cannot be used to describe the behavior of children in all cultures of the study. The second type of equivalence that is relevant in cross-cultural family studies involves the comparability of constructs at individual and cultural level: Can the same constructs be used to describe individual- and culture-level constructs? Again, identity of factors is a prerequisite to make meaningful comparisons of constructs at individual and cultural level. If obedience would be unidimensional at individual level and multidimensional at cultural level, we would need to use different concepts to describe differences at the two levels. The global concept of obedience could then not be used to describe country-level differences. Analyses of individual-level and cross-level equivalence do not necessarily yield the same results. For example, an instrument that shows the same factor structure in all cultures of the study may show a different factor structure at country level.

A number of cross-cultural studies have addressed psychological aspects of family functioning at the individual level. Examples include family values in terms of acculturation effects across generations (Georgas, Berry, Shaw, Christakopoulou, & Mylonas, 1996) and family values across Europe (Georgas, Mylonas, Gari, & Panagiotopoulou, 2004). Other examples are studies of family functions and structure along with roles of family members (Georgas et al., 2001); of socialization and social skills formation through the family (Keller, Zach, & Abels, 2005); of parenting style in relation to individualism and mental health within Arab nations (Dwairy & Achoui, 2006); of perceived parental rearing (Deković et al., 2006), to name a few. Although there have been various examples of studies that test individual-level equivalence, there is little to be found on the cross-level testing of equivalence. The latter is what the present chapter focuses on. The paucity of studies dealing with cross-level equivalence could be due to the fact that the methodological and statistical tools required to fully test such multilevel hypotheses have only recently been developed. Another reason may have to do with difficulties in defining the appropriate context. Ideally, all individuals sharing a context should be subject to the same contextual conditions (Teachman & Crowder, 2002). If culture can be conceptualized as an abstract, higher level context, the definition of family may vary across cultures. This conceptual problem may challenge even the use of the concept of family in a cross-cultural context.

In the country-level analysis where the country indicators are estimated from individual-level information, the population characteristics are considered to be the basic information pool when testing for equivalence of structures across countries. Intervening factors (mediating or moderating variables) may regulate the relationships between the constructs. The role of such intervening factors which lie in between the country-population level characteristics and the individual-level manifest behaviors should necessarily be tested in a multilevel model. A cross-cultural study of the family requires the collection of data at three levels: individual, family, and culture. The higher levels, family and culture, could involve both intrinsic and derived variables. An example of an intrinsic family variable would be size and income; derived variables could be scores on family-related constructs, such as perceived hierarchy and family, which are aggregated from individual-level scores. Analogously, intrinsic and derived culture-level variables could be studied. Derived variables could be aggregated individual and family scores. The study of these complex multilevel structures requires a full understanding of the meaning of variables at each level. If we assume isomorphism between individual and cultural levels (see the introduction chapter of this volume), we can analyze how the functional ways of the family are projected on the population level, and the other way round. This requires a simultaneous analysis of the individual-level and the culture-level structure.

The present chapter addresses the question of identity of meaning of family and presumably related constructs at the individual and cultural level. Six main types of constructs are addressed: family values, emotional distance with members of the family and nonfamily community members, personal values, family roles for nine family positions/persons, personality traits, and self-construal. These sets are separately presented in the next sections in respect of their characteristics and assessment procedures; their structures are then presented—separately for each scale, and for subscales when applicable—both at the individual level and the country level. A comparison is presented between the structures found at individual and country level to test for the multilevel equivalence of the constructs.

METHOD

Participants

To test for factor equivalence of family functions at the two levels of analysis, the individual level and the country level, we employed the data available from the psychological study of families across cultures (Georgas et al., 2006). Data on the family and psychological variables were gathered from the 30 countries as follows: Algeria (N = 107), Brazil (N = 159), Bulgaria (N = 195), Canada (N = 215), Chile (N = 207), Cyprus (N = 132), France (N = 97), Georgia (N = 200), Germany (N = 153), Ghana (N = 70), Greece (N = 350), Hong Kong (N = 423), India (N = 220), Indonesia (N = 239), Iran (N = 189), Japan (N = 185), Mexico (N = 227), Nigeria (N = 337), Pakistan (N = 450), Saudi Arabia (N = 198), South Korea (N = 199), Spain (N = 111), the Netherlands (N=165), Turkey (N = 211), United Kingdom (N = 115), Ukraine (N = 65), and the United States (N = 263). The South African, Botswana, and Mongolian data were excluded for technical reasons. The total number of cases in the study was 5,482. All participants were university students aged 19 to 24; 39.5% of the overall sample were males and 60.5% were females.

Instruments

The psychological and structural family measures employed were: Family Roles, developed by Georgas, Giotsa, Mylonas, and Bafiti for the 30-nation project; Emotional Distance (Georgas et al., 2001); Personality

Traits (Williams, Satterwhite, & Saiz, 1998); Self-Construal (Singelis, 1994); Family Values (Georgas, 1989, 1991); and Values (Schwartz, 1992, 1994). Short forms of the measures for Personality Traits, Self-Construal, and Values were employed since the use of the full versions of the questionnaires would have been too lengthy for participants to respond to in a single session.

The Family Roles items were constructed in cooperation with each local research team, which generated its own suggestions for the addition, adaptation, or elimination of roles. The items and instructions of each questionnaire were translated from English into the target language by an indigenous member of each research team. They were then back translated into English and compared with the original English version for equivalence in connotation. Problematic items, in terms of equivalence of meaning were discussed with the project leader (third author) and rephrased until linguistic equivalence was satisfactory. Items were adapted when a close translation proved to be problematic (Van de Vijver & Leung, 1997).

Data collection was carried out by the local research teams. The questionnaires were administered to university students and were completed in the classroom in all countries. The time required ranged from one to two hours.

Family Values

This questionnaire (Georgas, 1999) consists of 18 questions and its theoretical structure refers to the traditional family values of agricultural societies. There are two dimensions, the *Hierarchical roles of father and mother* dimension and the *Relationships within the family and with kin* dimension. Responses were collected on a 7-point Likert scale from (7) *strongly agree* (traditional end) to (1) *strongly disagree*. Item examples of the *Hierarchical roles of father and mother* are "Father should handle the money in the house," "Mother's place is at home"; examples of the *Relationships within the family and with kin* are "Children should obey parents," and "Parents should teach behavior to children."

Emotional Distance

This questionnaire (Georgas et al., 2001) is based on Bogardus's (1925) concepts of social distance and personal space, and refers to bonds with relatives (father, mother, siblings, spouse, etc.) and members of the immediate community (friends, neighbors, fellow students, etc.). Respondents rated the perceived emotional distance for each of these social categories as emotionally distant or close. The items were scored on a 7-point scale from *very far* (1) to *very close* (7) in the form of concentric circles (the closer the circle assigned to a person to the centre, the stronger the bond).

Values

We employed the Schwartz Values scale (Schwartz, 1994) using a short form (21 items out of the original 56); the respondents used a 7-point Likert scale from *very important* (7) to *not important at all* (1) to rate value types regarding the *Hierarchy, Mastery, Embeddedness, Intellectual Autonomy, Affective Autonomy,* and *Harmony* dimensions. Examples of items for this scale are "family security," "social order," "creativity," and "wealth." Items were scored on the extent to which they are seen as guiding principles in the respondents' lives. Because of communication problems with certain research teams, *Egalitarian Commitment* was not included in all participating countries. Thus, it was decided to proceed with six scales, instead of seven, rather than not employing the questionnaire at all.

Family Roles

The items asked to which extent members of the family undertake various family roles. The family positions were: father, mother, grandfather, grandmother, uncle/aunt, 20-year-old male, 20-year-old female, 10-year-old boy, and 10-year-old girl (Georgas et al., 2006). These family positions were seen as representative of: (1) nuclear family members, namely mother, father, and children (the latter at two age levels; the approximate age of participants, 20 years old, and preadolescents, 10-year-olds); (2) three-generation family members (grandmother, grandfather); and (3) collateral relatives (aunts/uncles). It should be noted that these positions are not considered to be entirely satisfactory since they do not represent all the different types of kinship relationships in extended families throughout the world. For example, the distinction between maternal and paternal aunts and uncles, or between matrilineal and patrilineal grandparents, is not included. The questionnaire was devised by Georgas, Giotsa, Mylonas, and Bafiti on the basis of family literature and questionnaires from countries throughout the world, and the 22 items of the scale were modified in the respective countries by the indigenous members of the project. The respondents answered on a 6-point Likert scale from *almost always* (6) to *never* (1) to items such as "Father protects the family," "Grandmother plays with children," and "20-year-old daughter takes siblings to school." Of the 22 items, 11 were assigned to all family positions; these referred to emotional support, maintenance of a pleasant environment, sense of unity and family relations, conveyance of traditions and religion, financial contribution, and everyday tasks such as housework or shopping. Nine family roles were related to parents, grandparents, and uncles/aunts (not to children) since they referred to adult responsibilities (e.g., daily care and support to grandparents and children). Finally, two roles were not assigned to father and mother because they referred to situations where parents are not present.

Personality Traits

The Personality Traits scale (Williams et al., 1998) was employed in a short version (30 questions out of the 300). The items were in the form of adjectives, such as "moody," "shy," "responsible," and "adventurous." The short version was constructed so as to contain markers of the five-factor personality structure: *Extraversion, Agreeableness, Conscientiousness, Emotional Stability,* and *Openness to Experience.* Items were rated by the respondents on a 7-point Likert scale from *not like me at all* (1) to *very much like me* (7).

Self-Construal

Singelis's Self-Construal scale (Singelis, 1994) was employed using 18 questions out of the 31. The *Independent Self* dimension is assessed by nine items (e.g., "I act the same way no matter who I am with") and the other nine refer to the *Interdependent Self* dimension (e.g., "I feel good when I cooperate with others"). Responses were given on a 7-point Likert scale from *strongly agree* (7) to *strongly disagree* (1).

Statistical Analyses

The aim of the statistical analyses of the family data is to describe the factor structure of all six scales employed in this study at the individual level and at the country level. Van de Vijver and Poortinga (2002) adapted a method to examine cross-level equivalence, using exploratory factor analysis, from a method, in the context of confirmatory factor analysis, proposed by Muthén (1994). The method is particularly useful for comparing data from multiple countries.

In a previous analysis of the family data (Van de Vijver, Mylonas, Pavlopoulos, & Georgas, 2006), the focus was on individual-level factor equivalence across cultures: Do scales have the same psychological meaning in each country involved? The main strategy was to compare the factor structure obtained in each country to a pooled ("average") factor structure. The latter is based on an analysis of the pooled dataset; more specifically, an exploratory factor analysis is conducted on the average covariance matrix of the countries, weighted by sample size. The factor structure found in such an analysis provides information about the pooled individual-level structure. The question of structural equivalence at the individual level (i.e., the question of whether the same factors are found in each country) is addressed by examining the similarity of the factor structure found in each country to the pooled individual-level factors. More specifically, the pooled-within and the between-groups correlation matrices for the set of countries involved in the analysis are calculated and then factor analyzed. A target rotation follows for the two solutions (i.e., the factors found in a country are rotated toward the factors of the global solution). The similarity of the factors of the two solutions is evaluated by means of Tucker's ϕ (Tucker, 1951). If this coefficient is larger than .90, this is taken to mean that factor equivalence exists across countries and that the overall pooled structure can be described through the target-rotated solution. Such a method can be used for all factor solutions based on similar correlation matrices, for any given number of factors or even unifactorial solutions (one principal component).

The current chapter and analysis focus on the multilevel aspect of the family data. Country-level factor structures may or may not be similar to the factors found in the individual-level analyses. This question can be addressed in different ways. A first approach would be to compare the country-level factors to the factors that are found in each country; the individual-level factors in each country separately would then be compared to the country-level factors on a one-to-one basis. A second approach, which is adopted here, addresses the question to what extent the factors of the pooled solution, which represents the global individual-level factors, are similar to the factors found at country level. Preference for the second approach is based on our findings regarding the structural equivalence at individual level (Georgas et al., 2006); we found a remarkably good similarity between the factors of the pooled individual-level solution and the factor solution in each of the separate countries (Van de Vijver et al., 2006). These findings strongly suggest that there is no need to compare the factors of each of the 27 countries separately to the country-level factor structure if we are interested in cross-level equivalence. Rather, the more parsimonious approach can be followed, in which the pooled individual-level solution is compared to the country-level solution. In operational terms, the latter is computed on the basis of the correlation matrix produced by the respondents' mean scores for each variable for each country. These means were inserted into a rectangular matrix (items×countries) and the interitem correlation matrix for each of the measures was used to calculate the factor solutions.

Poortinga and Van de Vijver (2004) have summarized the three levels of equivalence for cross-cultural comparisons as (1) structural or functional equivalence which lacks quantification compatibility; (2) metric or measurement unit equivalence, which lacks a common anchor point; and (3) scale equivalence or full score comparability. The latter is an ideal level of cross-country similarity and it implies that the same constructs are measured at both levels and that scores can be compared across individuals and levels. Having ascertained equivalence at the individual level for the various constructs in the study (Georgas et al., 2006), the current analyses mainly aimed at exploring structural equivalence of factors found at individual and country level, in order to gain a deeper insight in the construct compatibility across countries. However, it should be noted that to examine full-score equivalence, other statistical tests would be needed such as confirmatory factor analysis. Factor equivalence testing for the two levels of analysis as conducted in the present analyses can exhibit similarities or differences in meaning for family-related constructs and fully (or partially) justify the aggregation methods frequently used for country means to be compared; a secondary aim of the present analysis was to compare the outcomes to the ones present at the individual level for the same measures.

RESULTS

Family Values

The 18 items of the scale were factor analyzed. In line with theory (Georgas, 1999), two factors were extracted with substantial loadings on 14 items. This analysis was carried out on the overall pooled-within correlation matrix for the 27 countries. The resulting factor structure was then compared with the global average (the 27×14 matrix of item country means). The principal components extraction method, followed by a varimax rotation of the factors, was used in both analyses and the loadings for each of the two respective factors were then compared (after target rotating the individual-level loadings toward the country-level solution). The loadings for this multilevel factor analysis are shown in Table 13.1. The Tucker φ congruence coefficients reached values of .97 for the first and .98 for the second factor, showing factor equivalence for individual and country levels.

The analysis of the data at only the individual level (Van de Vijver et al., 2006) showed similar outcomes in respect of cross-countries equivalence. The present finding supports the existence of the same constructs at the country level. It seems that the *Hierarchical roles of father and mother within the family* (first factor) and the *Relationships within the family and with kin* (second factor) are basic family value concepts or constructs not only at individual level, but also at country level. The main conclusion of the overall analysis is that the two constructs of family values are isomorphic at the country and individual level. Thus, *Hierarchical roles of father and mother* and *Relationships within the family and with kin* are constructs that are relevant to understand individual differences as well as country differences.

A close examination of the loadings of Table 13.1 suggests some further results. The factor loadings were higher at country level than at individual level. The background of this difference may be methodological-statistical. Aggregation of scores from individual to country level tends to reduce

TABLE 13.1

Rotated Component Matrices for the Family Values Scale of the Individual- and Country-Level Factor Analysis Solutions[a]

Family Values Scale items	Individual level		Country level	
	Factor 1	Factor 2	Factor 1	Factor 2
Father is the head of family	.78	.30	.86	.44
Good relationships with relatives should be maintained	.16	.61	.24	.85
Mother's place is at home	.77	.03	.94	.03
Mother is the go-between between father & children	.74	.15	.89	.19
Parents should teach behavior to children	.12	.61	.49	.69
Father should handle money in the house	.82	.14	.90	.31
Children should take care of parents when they get old	.33	.55	.80	.49
Children should help with chores at home	−.08	.64	.04	.88
Problems are solved within the family	.18	.61	.52	.62
Children should obey parents	.35	.66	.31	.87
Family's reputation should be honored and protected	.41	.64	.61	.68
Children should respect grandparents	.09	.74	.26	.92
Mother should accept father's decisions	.76	.25	.82	.50
Father is the breadwinner	.82	.18	.91	.27

Note. Out of the 18 items in the scale, 14 are a part of the 2-factor solution.

[a]The loadings reported for the individual level structure are the ones before target rotation toward the country level solution.

the size of random error in scores. As a consequence, eigenvalues of factors and reliabilities of scales based on these factors tend to be higher for aggregated than nonaggregated scores. In addition, some of the minor discrepancies between the individual and country level are of interest. The three items that show differences (after target rotation) in absolute values of at least .30 across the two levels are "Parents should teach behavior to children," "Children should take care of parents when they get old," and "Problems are solved within the family." Each of these items shows a relatively strong loading on both factors in the country-level solution. Therefore, it seems that the two factors show somewhat less differentiation in the country-level solution. This might initially suggest (although to be tested further) that both factors measure to some extent a single underlying dimension which could be related to a focus on traditions. This "traditionality" aspect might act as a homogenizing construct (second-order factor) of family values at country level.

Emotional Distance

The individual-level analysis of the Emotional Distance scale (Georgas et al., 2001), which measures emotional distance to family members and nonkin, showed agreement of the pooled solution with the factors in all countries except Germany (Van de Vijver et al., 2006). Therefore, it was expected that the country-level analysis would also show a high level of agreement. The analysis resulted in one dimension at both individual and country levels (Table 13.2). However, a number of discrepancies appeared among the items at these two levels. The pooled individual level comprised a strong component for all items, but there was a minor loading of *spouse/date*. This difference could indicate a possible relation of the item to some other underlying construct. For the country-level solution many negative or low correlations of items were found; that is, *friends, siblings, father, grandparents, spouse/date, cousins,* and *uncles/aunts.* These differences challenged the equivalence of individual and country levels. The Tucker ϕ coefficient of .82 that we found is lower than the criterion value of 0.90 for construct equivalence. In addition, the factor loadings at the pooled

TABLE 13.2

Component Matrices for Emotional Distance of the Individual- and Country-Level Factor Analysis Solutions

Emotional distance from...	Individual level	Country level
Mother	.38	.36
Neighbors	.54	.89
Friends	.36	−.29
Siblings	.43	.27
Newspaper journalists	.49	.84
Colleagues	.57	.56
Acquaintances	.57	.54
Priest	.49	.69
Father	.38	.19
Primary school teachers	.62	.64
Prime Minister	.48	.46
Grandparents	.48	−.02
Shopkeepers	.59	.88
Writers	.44	.40
Spouse/date	.26	−.39
Fellow students	.56	.67
Members of parliament	.46	.60
Cousins	.41	−.12
High school teachers	.62	.72
Uncles/aunts	.56	.03
Newscasters	.53	.63

individual level were higher than at the country level, unlike to what we found for family values.

The main persons of interest were the members of the nuclear family (father, mother, siblings) and of the extended family (grandparents, aunts/ uncles, cousins). Other persons who represent different roles in society were of minor interest. However, the initial factor structure was computed on all categories in the scale, including nonfamily members as well as all family members. It was for this reason that only the members of the nuclear and extended family were employed in the analyses of the relationships between the ecocultural variables and the family and psychological variables in the "Families across cultures" study (Georgas et al., 2006). Additionally, previous research (Georgas et al., 2001) has revealed some robust findings about emotional distance (or closeness) to relatives of the immediate family, the extended family, and nonkin members of the community. These findings suggest that there are similar patterns of emotional bonds with specific members of the nuclear family, such as mother, siblings, and father (in order of closeness) that are prevalent across countries. However, the present analyses seem to suggest that country differences in emotional distance cannot be explained in the same way as individual differences; we have to accept that the same constructs do not apply equally at both levels. A plausible reason for this would be that siblings and father are part of a different underlying construct, possibly due to specific cultural variations in the relative positions these persons hold in the nuclear family.

A final general comment is that although we specifically assumed a unifactorial structure in the analysis, the scale may not represent a unifactorial construct across countries. Further analyses of the scale, employing other methods, are required such as returning to the individual-level construct equivalence testing and searching for congruent patterns that may enhance interpretation of the factors at the country level. A possible analysis strategy to serve this aim would be to employ a "hit" matrix of all possible Tucker's ϕ coefficients among all factor solutions across countries; such an analysis has been applied with promising results to a set of family values by Georgas et al. (2004) in a comparison of 33 European countries. One might also test for possible second-order factors or multifactorial solutions or possible smaller clusters of countries for which the country-level structure might prove to be identical. Such a procedure takes advantage of the number of factor equivalence instances in a "hit" matrix computed, again, at the individual level on a country-by-country basis (Georgas & Mylonas, 2006). Through other multivariate methods (such as multidimensional scaling) this matrix may reveal clusters of countries for which cross-level structural equivalence could be studied separately (a similar method for country clustering has been proposed by Georgas & Berry, 1995).

Values

Factor analysis and multilevel comparisons were conducted for a short form of the Values scale (Schwartz, 1994). Testing all value items in a single factor analysis model would not be appropriate, because it was not our intention to represent the whole value domain of Schwartz's model. Therefore, the procedure followed was a separate component analysis of each of the six subscales. We note that the prerequisite for factor analysis to include at least 10 items in the model, as proposed by Kline (1993), was not met; still, the solutions can provide an estimate of the degree of construct equivalence. The procedure was to factor analyze the items of each subscale at the individual level and then compare each country-level factor analysis with the pooled average individual analysis. The outcomes of these analyses are shown in Table 13.3 along with the respective solutions for the two levels for the Embeddedness, Hierarchy, Harmony, Intellectual Autonomy, Affective Autonomy, and Mastery dimensions.

Tucker ϕ coefficients for all six dimensions indicated satisfactory equivalence between individual and country levels: Embeddedness .99; Hierarchy .99; Harmony .99; Intellectual Autonomy .98; Affective Autonomy .99; Mastery .97. The findings indicate that each of the subscales of the short form of the Schwartz Values scale was structurally equivalent at the individual and country level. Again, factor loadings were generally larger at country level. A social desirability effect possibly may have caused inflation of the loadings at the country level. Although this does not threaten the cross-level equivalence found, it points to potential interference of method factors, especially when values or similar constructs that have to do with *ethos*[1] are studied in multilevel analyses.

Family Roles

Family Roles for the nine family positions (father, mother, grandfather, grandmother, uncle/aunt, 20-year-old male, 20-year-old female, 10-year-old boy, 10-year-old girl) were factor analyzed separately for each position. Some roles occur for all nine family positions, some only for the adults, and some do not pertain to mother and father; for example, mother and father are not included for the item "When the parents are not home [family position specified here] babysits with grandchildren."

For mother and father, three types of family roles were distinguished, labeled *Expressive*, *Child Care*, and *Finances*. Examples of items are "keeps the family united," "contributes financially," and "helps children with homework," respectively. For grandfather, grandmother, uncle/aunt, 20-year-old male and female, 10-year-old boy and girl, the two factors of family roles are *Expressive* and *Instrumental*. Examples of the items which form the factors are "conveys traditions to grandchildren/nephews-nieces/siblings" and "does the shopping."

TABLE 13.3

Component Matrices for Values of the Individual- and the Country-Level Factor Analysis Solutions

Embeddedness	I	C
Family security	.55	.82
Respect for tradition	.69	.91
Honoring elders	.73	.88
Social order	.63	.84
National security	.72	.90
Reciprocation of favors	.47	.78

Hierarchy	I	C
Authority	.82	.90
Wealth	.70	.84
Social power	.82	.92

Harmony	I	C
World of beauty	.72	.82
Unity with nature	.83	.91
Protecting environment	.80	.89

Intellectual autonomy	I	C
Broad-minded	.63	.81
Creativity	.77	.59
Curious	.75	.80

Affective autonomy	I	C
Pleasure	.79	.90
Exciting life	.67	.58
Enjoying life	.79	.88

Mastery	I	C
Independent	.81	.90
Daring	.64	.36
Choosing own goals	.65	.73

Note: I = Individual-level analysis on the pooled-within countries correlation matrix; C = Country-level analysis.

Father's Roles and Mother's Roles

For the 22 *Father's Roles* the initial factor analysis at the individual level and the structural comparisons across countries (Van de Vijver et al., 2006) resulted in three dimensions. These are also found in the present results for the individual-level analysis and are presented in Table 13.4 as I-1, I-2, and I-3; the first factor refers to the Expressive Roles of the father, the second to Child Care, and the third to Financial Roles. All three factors in the solution were found to be correlated (an oblique rotation was applied). Although the selection of the family roles was not based on a particular theory, two of the extracted factors in the factor analyses of the family roles resemble Parsons's (1943, 1949) expressive and instrumental roles, the latter being a combination of Financial and Child Care Roles. They also resemble Durkheim's (1888, 1892/1921) description of the last two stages of family change, in which the paternal family is reduced to the conjugal or nuclear family and in which the relationships between parents and children change from a material or economic basis to a psychological basis in which "personal motives" are dominant. The two factors are also similar to Kagitcibasi's (1990, 1996) emotional interdependencies and material/economic interdependencies roles.

The same factors were found at the individual level of analysis for Mother's Roles, although the order of the factors was different, with Expressive Roles still the first factor (I-1), Financial Roles the second factor (I-2), and Child Care the third factor (I-3). Each of the three factors at the individual level showed the same patterning of high and low loadings as found in the analysis of Father's Roles, with one remarkable exception (see Table 13.4). The item dealing with housework had a loading of .68 on the second individual-level factor in the analysis of the roles of the father, but the loading was only .21 in the analysis of the roles of the mother (first factor). The mean of the mothers across all 5,482 participants was 5.47 ($SD = .99$) on a 7-point scale, compared to a mean of 2.61 ($SD = 1.49$) for the fathers. It is very clear that mothers do most of the housework in all countries studied. The three factors showed agreement indices between father and mother of .98, .97, and .87, respectively. The somewhat lower ϕ value of the third factor can be explained by the differential loadings of the item about housework in the two individual-level analyses or as a consequence of the limited variability of the scores of the mothers.

Country-level factor solutions were also computed for Father's Roles and Mother's Roles. Loadings for both solutions are reported in Table 13.4. An inspection of the first factor for Father's Roles reveals "Protective and regulatory" roles a father might undertake within a family. The second resembles the individual-level "Child care" factor, but covers also financial support and conveyance of tradition to children along with more general managing of finances. The third factor reflects father's role in contributing financially along with emotional support and protection of the emotional

TABLE 13.4

Rotated Component Matrices for Father's Roles and for Mother's Roles in the Family of the Individual- and Country-Level Factor Analysis Solutions[a]

Father / Mother …	Father						Mother					
	I-1	I-2	I-3	C-1	C-2	C-3	I-1	I-2	I-3	C-1	C-2	C-3
Provides emotional support to children	.74	.15	-.04	.06	.15	.81	.68	-.01	-.06	.90	.11	-.11
Provides emotional support to grandparents	.76	-.07	-.18	.23	-.24	.79	.58	.01	.09	.67	.07	-.32
Provides emotional support to wife	.74	.06	-.03	-.09	.17	.89	.66	-.05	.02	.83	-.01	-.02
Keeps the family united	.77	-.06	.15	.41	.06	.67	.79	.04	.07	.92	-.21	.08
Keeps a pleasant environment	.76	.04	.07	.45	.13	.54	.76	.01	.00	.89	-.18	.09
Conveys traditions to children	.56	.28	-.04	.49	.48	.08	.46	-.15	-.38	.74	.45	-.25
Conveys religion to children	.54	.01	.12	.66	.19	.29	.58	-.25	-.13	.80	-.33	.03
Preserves family relations	.70	.01	.11	.54	.06	.51	.68	-.09	-.14	.90	-.12	-.06
Supports grandparents	.59	-.13	.16	.28	-.12	.72	.58	.15	.07	.73	.09	-.06
Takes care of grandparents	.45	.06	-.02	.71	-.33	.25	.43	-.02	.00	.44	-.66	.17
Protects the family	.59	-.14	.35	.43	-.08	.65	.61	.24	.14	.44	-.64	.35
Resolves disputes	.33	-.08	.44	.60	.27	.31	.36	.26	-.05	.62	-.09	.21
Does housework	-.02	.68	-.15	-.92	.05	.13	.21	.11	-.13	.15	.00	.54
Does the shopping	-.07	.21	.60	.56	.14	.12	-.17	.66	-.13	-.46	.48	.55
Takes children to school	-.01	.54	.31	.32	.65	.06	-.23	.14	-.78	-.08	.80	.31
Plays with children	.31	.56	.09	-.09	.81	-.08	.18	.04	-.67	.45	.63	.12
Helps children with homework	.14	.62	.20	-.11	.88	.01	.11	.03	-.72	.46	.57	.17
Teaches manners to children	.43	.12	.39	.35	.54	.31	.53	.06	-.27	.90	.10	.14
Contributes financially	.09	-.13	.68	-.40	.21	.88	.02	.68	-.01	.03	.45	.67
Manages finances	-.04	-.05	.81	.55	.45	.07	.04	.76	.06	-.26	-.08	.89
Gives pocket money to children	.05	.08	.68	.43	.43	.23	.14	.56	-.09	.04	-.01	.73
Supports career of children	.16	.09	.59	.00	.79	.21	.32	.36	-.16	.59	.41	.22

Note: I = Individual-level analysis on the pooled-within countries correlation matrix (three-factor solution); C = Country-level analysis (three-factor solution).

[a] Pattern matrices are reported (oblique rotation solutions). The loadings reported for the individual-level structure are the ones before target rotation toward the country-level solution.

climate within the family. This third factor was named "Expressive/earner roles." At face value, there is clear evidence of nonequivalence across the two levels of analysis; when we rotated the loadings of the pooled individual-level solution toward the country-level solution using Procrustean rotation methods (Van de Vijver & Leung, 1997), the Tucker φ coefficients reached values of .64, .86 and .82 for the "Protective-regulatory roles," the "Child care" and the financial-supportive "Expressive/earner roles" factor, respectively. The main discrepancy in the structures was found for the "Protective and regulatory roles" factor for which congruence with the country-level factor was very low (.64). The inequivalence was caused mainly by the items on emotionally driven "protection" namely *father takes care of grandparents,...conveys tradition to children,...conveys religion to children,* and*...takes children to school* (with a mean absolute difference between individual-level and country-level solution of .52). Both factors, at individual as well as country level, seem to involve financial and emotional roles of the father in the family. This confounding might also reflect the need for an oblique rotation of the factor, rather than an orthogonal solution. The main conclusion for these findings is that although at the individual level of analysis differences can be examined under the three factors resembling Parsonian theory, a description of country differences requires some alternative formulation of constructs that can accommodate the shifts in meaning as observed for the three factors identified in father's roles.

For Mother's Roles, the first factor at the country level is the "Expressive roles" factor and it closely resembles the corresponding individual-level factor. The second factor, in addition to the child care items forming the individual-level "Child care" factor, also involves financial aspects, such as financial support of children's career and general financial contribution. It could be named "Caregiver/financial contribution" to describe more closely the specific loading of mother's roles on the factor. The third factor seems to depict mother's "Regulatory roles," including shopping and housekeeping along with financial contribution and managing finances and pocket-money for children. Like in the case of Father's Roles, for two out of the three factors, factor equivalence between the two levels of analysis was not perfect. The Tucker φ coefficient for the individual-level Expressive factor reached .98, but for the Child Care factor it was just .79, and for the Financial Role factor a borderline value of .88 was found.

Although equivalence levels were generally higher than for Father's roles, the agreement was not perfect. Therefore, we decided to search for the items responsible for the discrepancies in the factor structures of the two levels of analysis. Although we had applied Procrustean rotation of the mother's roles individual-level loadings to the country level loadings, we still could not attribute inequivalence to shifts in loadings of single items. Therefore, another index for each item was computed, namely a measure of item discrepancy calculated as the square root of the mean squared difference of the target-rotated loadings with the country-level loadings. The index measures the overall fit of the item by combining discrepancies in loadings across all items of a factor. The highest values were found for the Caregiver/financial contribution factor that appeared second in the country level solution. Some of the items with high discrepancy indices were *mother does housework...does the shopping,...contributes financially,...takes care of grandparents,* and...*supports career of children,* along with *emotional support* to both children and grandparents. By comparing the country-level factor of Caregiver/financial contribution to the individual-level loadings on the target-rotated factors, a shift in the meaning of mother's roles became more apparent. Specifically, the country-level factor emphasized the "between-generations" role of mothers, taking care of and supporting the elderly, as well as supporting children in their career, conveying religion to them, and generally protecting the family also by contributing financially. Most of these items appeared in the first target-rotated factor for the individual-level loadings as well, but there the emphasis was mainly on the emotional aspect translated into emotional support to children, husband, and the elderly, and into protecting the family by preserving relations, keeping the environment pleasant, and the family united.

In summary, the same sets of three factors can be used to describe the role of the father and the mother in all 27 countries when the individual level of analysis is of interest. However, discrepancies, especially for Father's Roles, do not allow for using the same constructs for explanation at the country level. This discrepancy was mainly due to the father's Protective and regulatory roles, the mother's Caregiver/financial contribution roles, and for both father and mother the possible interaction of financial and protective roles. This interaction is not entirely absent from the individual-level factor solution but it surfaces more clearly in the country-level structures. A possible explanation might be that financial issues and functions are understood, utilized, and interconnected in a different way within each country's aggregate scores than they do at the individual level of nonaggregated scores. Financial issues such as wealth, money management, unemployment, profit and saving, are possibly conceived in a different way across countries, being a function of the prevailing economic conditions (Furnham, 1988), a difference which does not always appear in traditional cross-cultural comparisons (Furnham & Lewis, 1986) at the individual factor analysis level.

Grandparents and Uncles/Aunts

Factor analyses conducted at the individual and then at the country level for the roles of the Grandfather, the Grandmother, and Uncles/Aunts generally revealed a two-factorial structure differentiating between Expressive and Instrumental Roles. Procedures similar to those used for analyzing Father's and Mother's Roles were employed for Grandfathers, Grandmothers, and Uncles/Aunts roles in the family. The roles analyzed are the same as for father and mother, except that in the case of grandparents the role functions are directed toward grandchildren and their parents, and in the case of uncles and aunts toward nephews/nieces and their parents. Excellent cross-level structural equivalence was found for these positions in the family (Table 13.5). The respective factors for grandfathers (at both individual and country levels) were an "Expressive functions" first factor and an "Everyday help" second factor (clearly following the instrumental dimension). Tucker φ coefficients (after target rotation of the individual level loadings) for these two factors reached .96 and .94, respectively. For Grandmother's Roles, factors were the same and also nearly identical in meaning. Tucker φ coefficients for these two factors reached .95 and .94, respectively. Finally, for the Uncles' and Aunts' Roles, the factors were again the same, but they appeared in reversed order. Tucke φ r coefficients for these two factors reached .90 and .95, respectively.

An interesting note is that in the individual-level of analysis for grandfather's and uncles/aunts roles, "taking care of the grandchildren/nephews" and "playing with grandchildren/nephews" items showed loadings of about the same size on both factors, but this is not the case for the country-level solutions. This difference may imply a possible minor shift in the factor meanings for the grandfather and uncles/aunts family positions. For grandfathers, the "playing with grandchildren" and "taking care of grandchildren" items remain at the country-level structure in the "Expressive functions" factor only and do not load on the "everyday help" factor. The same holds for uncles and aunts, but only for the "playing with nephews/nieces" item which still shows up as an expressive behavior of uncles/aunts at the country level; the "taking care of nephews/nieces" item loads at the country level only on the "Everyday help" factor. It might be argued that the respondents at the individual level of analysis sense the multiple utility of these roles and register it in their scores but when it comes to the country level, the aggregated scores feature the strongest related construct (mostly "Expressive functions"). On the other hand, for grandmother's roles, both items load on both factors at the country level as well as at the individual level, splitting the two ways in which grandmothers are functioning within the family. In this case, the multiple utility of these two roles remains active at the country level as well, possibly because grandmothers' qualities of practical and at the same time emotional help within the family as caregivers and affectionate partners in play have remained strong traits over the centuries. Still, this minor shift in meaning did not threaten cross-level equivalence for any of the three family positions.

TABLE 13.5

Rotated Component Matrices for Grandfather's Roles, for Grandmother's Roles, and for Uncle's–Aunt's Roles in the Family of the Individual- and the Country-Level Factor Analysis Solutions[a]

Grandfather/Grandmother/ Uncle-Aunt...	Grandfather				Grandmother				Uncle–Aunt			
	I-1	I-2	C-1	C-2	I-1	I-2	C-1	C-2	I-1	I-2	C-1	C-2
Provides emotional support to grandchildren	.73	.01	.89	.01	.75	-.02	.87	.00	.00	-.74	.12	.84
Provides emotional support to parents	.76	-.06	.86	-.02	.74	-.05	.83	-.01	-.12	-.78	-.22	1.02
Keeps the family united	.84	-.06	.92	-.34	.82	-.07	.87	-.32	-.01	-.79	.24	.65
Keeps a pleasant environment	.83	-.02	.90	-.07	.81	-.02	.84	-.03	-.04	-.84	.08	.87
Conveys traditions to grandchildren	.78	-.04	.90	.00	.76	-.01	.86	.20	.01	-.72	.22	.79
Conveys religion to grandchildren	.74	-.08	.92	-.27	.73	-.12	.85	-.09	.08	-.62	.42	.52
Preserves family relations	.80	-.02	.91	-.15	.78	-.03	.81	.03	.00	-.78	-.07	.91
Supports grandchildren	.64	.14	.55	.24	.62	.16	.40	.35	.09	-.69	-.12	.88
Takes care of grandchildren	.30	.43	.55	.26	.36	.39	.42	.39	.44	-.31	.74	.08
Protects the family	.59	.26	.81	.01	.57	.23	.67	-.10	.33	-.49	.43	.52
Resolves disputes	.42	.34	.86	-.07	.39	.33	.81	-.05	.57	-.15	.83	.07
Does housework	-.11	.61	-.32	.72	.07	.57	-.16	.76	.60	-.04	.13	.43
Does the shopping	-.07	.69	-.12	.69	-.13	.69	-.54	.60	.65	.02	-.04	.23
Takes grandchildren to school	-.08	.73	.16	.75	-.13	.71	-.27	.78	.75	.12	.94	-.08
Plays with grandchildren	.43	.35	.52	.21	.39	.38	.40	.45	.40	-.35	.18	.64
Helps grandchildren with homework	.03	.68	.35	.72	.02	.66	.17	.82	.72	-.02	.92	.04
Teaches manners to grandchildren	.67	.15	.90	-.19	.68	.11	.89	-.03	.34	-.48	.53	.53
Contributes financially	.03	.74	.29	.82	.00	.72	.01	.87	.80	.07	.87	.03
Manages finances	-.03	.73	.50	.47	-.04	.70	.33	.51	.83	.16	.81	.02
Gives pocket money to grandchildren	.13	.60	-.14	.76	.12	.61	-.28	.73	.64	-.08	.55	-.02
Supports career of grandchildren	.28	.49	.42	.29	.28	.46	.26	.23	.54	-.20	.54	.22
Babysits grandchildren	.30	.47	.69	.34	.36	.39	.55	.46	.54	-.20	.79	.14
Helps parents with their work	.14	.57	.61	.50	.09	.59	.35	.69	.64	-.03	.93	-.20

Note: I = Individual-level analysis on the pooled-within countries correlation matrix (2 factor solution); C = Country-level analysis (2 factor solution). For Uncles and Aunts, grandchildren is replaced by nephews/nieces in the respective items

[a] Pattern matrices are reported (oblique rotation solutions). The loadings reported for the individual-level structure are the ones before target rotation toward the country-level solution.

Siblings

Factor analyses of the roles of the siblings at the individual level (son of 10, daughter of 10, son of 20, and daughter of 20 years of age) also found the same two-factorial structure. For these analyses, data were available for 14 roles describing the nature of the relationships with grandparents and parents and also with siblings. The first factor (Table 13.6) for all positions of the pooled individual-level solutions clearly refers to "Emotional climate." The same factor is replicated at the country level in all cases (Tucker ϕ indices after target rotation of the individual-level loadings reached .98, .97, .92, and .96, for 10-year-old sons, 10-year-old daughters, 20-year-old sons, and 20-year-old daughters, respectively).

The second factor also appears to be the same in all four individual-level analyses and refers to housework, shopping, taking siblings to school, playing with siblings, baby-sitting siblings, helping parents with their work, and contributing financially. These activities form a list of obligations offspring up to 20 years of age should meet. When analyzed at the country level though, the factor is different for 10-year-old sons and daughters (after target rotation of the individual-level loadings, Tucker ϕ = .76). The country-level factor mainly focuses on children's cooperation with parents in attending to their siblings. This holds for both the 10-year-old son and the 10-year-old daughter (Tucker ϕ = .78). When it comes to 20-year-old offspring, the pattern still changes for the country-level solutions (Tucker ϕ = .74), but there is a gender difference. The role of the 20-year-old daughter still involves sibling attendance and cooperation with parents, but it also involves housekeeping and financial contribution. On the other hand, the 20-year-old son's role involves tradition conveyance to siblings and playing with them, and it also involves housework. Tucker ϕ for this second factor in the country-level structure reached a value of only .12. A close look showed that this second factor for the 20-year-old son is bipolar, with negative loadings for financial contribution and shopping items. The target-rotated loadings of the corresponding individual-level factor also form a bipolar factor; shopping, financial contribution, babysitting, and taking siblings to school have positive signs, whereas keeping the family united, keeping a pleasant environment, and supporting grandparents emotionally have negative signs. A large part of the cross-level inequivalence might be due to this bipolarity in the dimensions, especially since many positively signed items at the individual level have negative signs at the country level and vice versa.

Overall, for all four family positions, it was evident that no single item was causing inequivalence (due to possible method or item bias), but that a number of items were contributing to the discrepancies between the two levels. For the 10-year-old offspring these items were the same for both sons and daughters. Specifically, contributing financially, conveying traditions, playing with siblings, and doing the shopping seem to differ-

TABLE 13.6

Rotated Component Matrices for Offspring's Roles (10-year-olds and 20-year-olds) of the Individual- and Country-Level Factor Analysis Solutions[a]

He/she...	10-year-old son				10-year-old daughter				20-year-old son				20-year-daughter			
	I-1	I-2	C-1	C-2	I-1	I-2	C-1	C-2	I-1	I-2	C-1	C-2	I-1	I-2	C-1	C-2
Provides emotional support to grandparents	.69	-.13	.69	.18	.69	-.12	.71	.12	.66	-.11	.69	-.14	.62	-.07	.82	-.11
Provides emotional support to siblings	.74	-.08	.78	.07	.74	-.08	.80	.04	.70	-.02	.69	.23	.70	-.04	.77	.08
Keeps the family united	.79	-.08	.86	.01	.79	-.08	.87	.00	.82	-.08	.81	-.13	.80	-.09	.89	-.17
Keeps a pleasant environment	.79	-.07	.89	-.03	.79	-.07	.89	.01	.79	-.02	.85	-.25	.79	-.04	.95	-.18
Conveys traditions to siblings	.60	.15	.58	-.59	.61	.12	.55	-.54	.58	.14	.34	.58	.59	.12	.43	.17
Conveys religion to siblings	.54	.22	.63	.08	.55	.19	.61	.15	.53	.19	.87	-.15	.61	.10	.79	.19
Preserves family relations	.66	.10	.72	-.01	.65	.10	.74	-.06	.66	.09	.83	-.22	.71	.02	.92	-.22
Does housework	.12	.57	.04	.31	.18	.57	.14	.61	.06	.42	-.19	.75	.29	.44	.63	.42
Does the shopping	.03	.61	.17	.25	.04	.60	.25	.05	-.04	.63	.03	-.49	-.09	.61	-.36	-.28
Takes siblings to school	.00	.62	.01	.80	.01	.61	.10	.67	-.01	.70	.76	.33	.06	.65	.26	.78
Plays with siblings	.30	.12	.05	.55	.31	.11	.06	.56	.27	.38	.59	.55	.36	.28	.52	.48
Contributes financially	-.10	.64	.18	.26	-.10	.61	.13	.30	-.08	.65	.46	-.53	-.10	.68	-.16	.40
Babysits siblings	.04	.66	.03	.83	.04	.67	.04	.84	.12	.59	.71	.35	.26	.47	.81	.17
Helps parents with their work	-.01	.68	-.08	.74	-.02	.68	-.13	.75	-.03	.70	.68	.04	.00	.70	.19	.74

Note: I = Individual-level analysis on the pooled-within countries correlation matrix (2 factor solution); C = Country-level analysis (2 factor solution).
[a]Pattern matrices are reported (oblique rotation solutions). The loadings reported for the individual-level structure are the ones before target rotation toward the country-level solution.

entiate the structure of the two levels in the analysis. For the 20-year-old daughter just two items are creating discrepancies, namely "babysits siblings" and "does the shopping," but for the 20-year-old son, nine out of the 14 items in the scale showed high root mean squared difference indices resulting in the very low levels of cross-level equivalence. These items are (starting with the item with the highest discrepancy index) "contributes financially," "does the shopping," "conveys traditions to siblings," "helps parents with their work," "does housework," "takes siblings to school," "provides emotional support to siblings," "babysits siblings," and "plays with siblings."

Personality Traits

Five factor analyses were carried out separately, one for each of the five personality dimensions of the Williams et al.scale (1998). Each personality dimension was measured by six items (three positively keyed, three negatively keyed). The results (Table 13.7) indicate a high level of structural equivalence across the two levels of analysis for three scales. Tucker φ coefficients reached values of .97 for Agreeableness, .98 for Conscientiousness, and .97 for Openness. However, for the Extraversion and the Emotional Stability personality traits, congruence coefficients were lower (.87 and .89, respectively). A similar comparison of the five dimensions of personality was reported by Rossier, Dahourou, and McCrae (2005). They found fairly acceptable levels of cross-level equivalence for most dimensions comparing factors derived from Swiss and Burkinabé data, and from French, American, Zimbabwean, and South African data. However, for the Extraversion dimension, some of the comparisons did not reach congruence levels of .90 and the same was true to a larger extent for the Openness factor. Other smaller discrepancies were present for Agreeableness and Conscientiousness but not for Neuroticism. In the present multilevel analysis (short questionnaire forms and unifactorial structure testing) the levels of factor equivalence reached are similar.

The multilevel inequivalence found in the present analysis for the Extraversion dimension seems to be mainly produced by one item ("quiet") which has a close to zero loading for the country-level solution. Thus, at the country level "quiet" does not seem to correlate with the other five facets of this dimension, although it does so in the pooled individual-level solution. A common reason for such a finding is small item variance, which seems to be illustrated here in the case of "quiet" at the aggregated country level (the variance was only .29). The small variance resulted in low correlations of this item with the other five (outgoing, sociable, active, withdrawn, and shy) in the Extraversion scale. The substantive interpretation of this finding is that at country-level, "quiet" may be a less pronounced and more positively evaluated expression of introversion than "withdrawn" and "shy."

TABLE 13.7

Component Matrices for the Five Personality Traits of the Individual- and Country-Level Factor Analysis Solutions

	Agreeableness		Conscientiousness			Extraversion			Emotional stability			Openness	
	I	C		I	C		I	C		I	C		I	C
Understanding	.66	.89	Organized	.71	.89	Outgoing	.61	.36	Stable	.60	.88	Imaginative	.66	.81
Sympathetic	.61	.89	Reliable	.53	.75	Sociable	.69	.83	Optimistic	.57	.88	Adventurous	.70	.72
Considerate	.63	.91	Responsible	.68	.82	Active	.58	.89	Calm	.49	.73	Spontaneous	.66	.62
(Quarrelsome)	.41	.17	(Careless)	.64	.82	(Withdrawn)	.60	.78	(Moody)	.48	.36	(Rigid)	.09	.38
(Deceitful)	.53	.40	(Lazy)	.66	.81	(Shy)	.65	.57	(Irritable)	.63	.42	(Inhibited)	.30	.34
(Rude)	.64	.83	(Disorderly)	.66	.39	(Quiet)	.61	-.03	(Anxious)	.60	.16	(Conservative)	.29	.36

Note: I = Individual-level analysis on the pooled-within countries correlation matrix; C = Country-level analysis. For parenthesized items, the scores were reversed for the analysis

Although factorial agreement for the Agreeableness dimension is very high, "quarrelsome" has a much higher loading at individual level than at country level. It might be the case that "quarrelsome" is not as negatively evaluated at the country level as the items "rude" and "deceitful." The latter two items contain a moral aspect; this is not the case for "quarrelsome" which can be related to mood or temperament. Emotional Stability showed a borderline value of cross-level equivalence, which is also mainly due to a single item, namely "anxious." Again, "anxious" may be a less negatively evaluated expression of emotional instability at the country level than "moody" and "irritable," thus making it a less adequate indicator of the Emotional Stability dimension at country level.

Comparing individual-level and country-level loadings, another finding is that for half of the items, the loadings are higher at the country-level solution than at the individual-level solution, and for the other half of the items the opposite is found. This difference could be a product of low country means along with low variability at the country level. Such a state of affairs can be consequence of social desirability and aggregation of scores. The Emotional Stability dimension shows a difference between the individual- and culture-level factors in that the loadings of the positively formulated country-level items, which represent the desirable end of the continuum, have on average higher loadings than the negatively formulated items. Thus, the two ends of a continuum reflecting a bipolar factor may be accentuated at the country level due to social desirability. This was also the case in respect of the differences found for the first father's roles factor mentioned earlier.

Self-Construal

The 18 items are given in Table 13.8 in an abbreviated form. In two separate analyses (one for the Independent and one for the Interdependent Self), we computed the unifactorial solutions for each level (individual and country levels) as described before. The individual-level equivalence analyses for the Self-Construal scale, reported by Van de Vijver et al. (2006), provided strong evidence for the poor replicability of the factors across the 27 countries. The first factor "Independent Self" was not found in many countries. The current analysis, addressing the cross-level equivalence, also revealed unsatisfactory results. The Tucker ϕ coefficient of the independence factor reached a value of only .85. The lack of cross-level equivalence is probably a by-product of the lack of equivalence at the individual level.

One item is again behind the structural inequivalence, namely the item "I try to do what is best for me, regardless of how that might affect others" ("do the best for me" in Table 13.8). What is most striking is the inversion of the item's loading in the country-level solution. For the aggregate scores we would generally encounter low variances and this might affect com-

TABLE 13.8

Component Matrices for the Independent and Interdependent Self-Construal Dimensions for the Individual- and the Country-Level Factor Analysis Solutions

Independent self			Interdependent self		
	I	C		I	C
Enjoy being unique	.52	.79	Respect modest people	.58	.85
Act as independent person	.52	.80	Sacrifice self interest	.59	.75
Direct and forthright	.55	.73	Cooperate	.67	.89
Comfortable when praised	.45	.59	Relationships are important	.48	.67
Speaking up not a problem	.51	.37	Happiness depends on others	.57	.86
Act the same way	.56	.23	Stay in the group	.46	.34
Do the best for me	.23	−.55	Respect group decisions	.73	.91
Take care of myself	.51	.84	Maintain harmony	.75	.91
Act the same way	.53	.61	Go along with others	.36	.24

Note: I = Individual-level analysis on the pooled-within countries correlation matrix; C = Country-level analysis.

munalities for this factor. A methodological explanation of the cross-level inequivalence might be the social desirability of the various items. The specific item ("do the best for me") shows a negative loading at the country level and is the only one with this characteristic. Perhaps the behavior expressed is undesirable because it goes against the interest of others whereas all other items emphasize the expression of independence without harming others. This difference in valence of the item may have triggered social desirability effects for the other items in the Independent self dimension. Georgas et al. (2006) have pointed out that for this set of data "It is a recurrent theme in our findings that interpersonal aspects…behave more in line with expectations than intrapersonal aspects" (pp. 213–214). This is once again the case in the present analysis, with the Interdependent Self dimension being structurally equivalent at both individual and country levels (Tucker φ reached a value of .96).

A similar approach to the cross-level equivalence of independent and interdependent self was adopted by Van de Vijver and Watkins (2006). Using a different assessment method, the Adult Sources of Self-Esteem Inventory (Fleming & Elovson, 1988), the authors found very high levels of multilevel equivalence. In addition to this, they found imperfect equivalence in the structural equivalence at the individual level; the two factors were not retrieved in all 19 countries. They pointed out the need for assessing the degree of individual-level and country-level factor structures for other measures of self-construal. An interesting point is that Van de Vijver and Watkins found the independence factor to be made up of several skills that are desirable. Even the social and interpersonal skills load on the independence factor at the country level, such as the skill to convince others of one's ideas. The same notion of desirable skills could underlie the independence factor of the present study. Thus, in the present analysis we can support cross-level structural equivalence for the interdependent self, but not for the independent self dimension, being unable to support the etic character of this self-construal dimension.

CONCLUSION

It is clear that the overall research project had many more aims beyond testing for multilevel structural equivalence for the family functions and characteristics studied. Additionally, the present analyses did not address metric or full-score equivalence but remained limited to structural equivalence. As stated earlier in the Method section, other statistical models such as confirmatory factor analysis models or hierarchical linear models would be necessary to test for metric equivalence across the individual and country levels. Still, the question of structural equivalence is of extreme importance when one wants to ensure that the same concepts can be used to describe individual- and country-level constructs related to family functioning. The outcomes of a study are easier to interpret, if identity of the meanings found for the individual level (in a comparison of the factors found in all countries of the study) has been demonstrated for the country level as well. An important prerequisite for addressing this question is a sufficiently large number of samples so that an analysis at country level is warranted. In the case of the present analyses, the large number of countries involved in the study was helpful for the testing of equivalence.

The first series of analyses supports cross-level invariance for the Family Values scale. It seems that the two underlying factors, Hierarchical roles and Relationships within the family, have a strong etic character. For the six values dimensions as measured by the short version of the Schwartz Value scale (for each of which we specified a unifactorial structure), a strong etic character was also supported. Structural equivalence across levels was partly supported for Emotional distance, possibly indicating a nonunifactorial structure. Family roles were also partly shown to be equivalent in meaning at the two levels with grandfather's, grandmother's, uncles/aunts' and the Expressive role of mother being clearly equivalent at both levels. The "Emotional climate" factor for the offspring's roles also reached multilevel factor equivalence. For personality traits structural equivalence across levels was supported to a large extent, with small discrepancies. Equivalence was present for only one of the two dimensions in self-construal; the interdependent self appeared to have the same meaning in both individual and country levels.

Overall, it seems that values are quite clearly "transcending" the individual level and form a feature of cultures. Of course, a next question would refer to the nature of this link between the two levels; for example, might similarities in culture structures produce the construct identities at the individual level? For Emotional distance we cannot draw conclusions with such certainty on their "projection" across levels, although we can be more optimistic of cross-level equivalence when only family members will take part in the analysis (Georgas et al., 2006, reported individual-level equivalence when only family members were considered). We found support for the cross-level equivalence in factor meaning for the Expressive roles of the mother (although the factor structure was not completely identical for both factors) and the Emotional and Instrumental family roles of the "extended" family members. This equivalence may be related to the function of the modified version of the extended family observed in many contemporary cultures. In this scheme immediate proximity has been abandoned; that is, the nuclear family is no longer living in the same house with grandparents, grandmothers, uncles, aunts, and uncles/aunts, but the functional relationships of these members within the main core of the nuclear family is being maintained. The strong multilevel equivalence found possibly emphasizes the vitality of the mother's, grandparents', and uncles/aunts' roles in the family, even though living arrangements have changed over time.

A second conclusion refers to factors which, although highly equivalent at the individual level, did not reach the desired degree of equivalence when tested at the level of countries. This refers to father's family roles, two of the dimensions for mother's family roles, the second factor for offspring's family roles, and the emotional distance scale when ratings for nonfamily members are included. Starting with the last one, it is rather obvious in retrospect that equivalence for emotional distance was hindered by the fact that the analysis assumed a unifactorial structure. Recalculation of the factor structure, keeping only the family members in the model and individual-level analysis is needed before more extensive multilevel analysis can be conducted. Such an attempt would also test for another alternative but relevant explanation of the inequivalence observed, namely that low scores for nonfamily members may lead to overrepresentation of small differences.

Initially, we could not think of any apparent reason for the discrepancies (sometimes large) in some family roles. Additionally, the near-perfect equivalence found for members of the "extended" family, computed with the same items for all the different family positions, emphasizes the discrepancies that were found between individual- and culture-level analyses for father's and mother's roles. However, by exploring each item's "contribution" to the inequivalence, we found that even at the individual level of analysis, the two factors for father's and mother's roles involve both financial and emotional roles. This "interaction" is more apparent at the country-level structure and is possibly leading to inequivalence, especially if we accept that financial issues may be perceived in different ways across cultures. In addition to this, social desirability effects may also alter the items' behavior at the country level, and one might also argue that the current results should be replicated by using more samples from the same or even more countries. Cross-level deviances might be more easily attributed to structure inequivalence if the possibility of method factors can be eliminated.

Our findings, as presented in this chapter, may further guide researchers in selecting appropriate family-related variables in order to form and subsequently test specific hypotheses. Our own further aim in using the data set of the 27 countries is to reexamine equivalence and factor structures, but based on a pairwise comparison of countries. We expect to find in the 27 countries clusters of more homogeneous countries, which should be less prone to aggregation fallacies. It is to be expected that within-clusters tests for equivalence between individual-level and country-level factor structures should show fewer discrepancies than tests based on the entire set of countries. However, it is also possible that discrepancies persist in a homogeneous subset of countries, in which case there is all the more reason to look for variables that can explain these discrepancies.

With the present analyses of the "Families across cultures" data, multilevel analysis has been demonstrated to be a powerful and very useful technique in studying family variables and their correlates. Although structural equivalence was not always supported, it appeared that even small shifts in meaning can be detected, given the method's sensitivity. It takes strong, well-established constructs, firm theorizing and proper sampling and assessment techniques to be able to assume a priori that data meet acceptable levels of multilevel equivalence. The method is stringent but fair with the data; moreover, the method is necessary not only when addressing family issues cross-culturally but in any cross-cultural study that attempts a comparative description of countries. Caution should be exercised though, since this statistical method's fairness is also a function of the researcher's control of method factors and statistical artifacts, which may inflate error and, consequently, lead to inequivalence.

Note

1. The approximate meaning of the Greek word *ethos* ("ἦθος"/`iθos/) is "moral standards." *Ethos*, also in its Greek sense, does not only refer to values but beyond that represents all "must-demands" one accepts or defies through one's everyday behavior. "Right" or "wrong" is then translated into norms

that should guide human behavior (Bechtel, 1988). Greek dictionaries define "ἦθος " as the entirety of human psychological traits. In this sense, *ethos is* the mirror of the characteristics of a society or "community."

REFERENCES

Bechtel, W. (1988). *Philosophy of science: An overview for cognitive science.* Hillsdale, NJ: Lawrence Erlbaum.

Berry, J. W. (1976). *Human ecology and cognitive style: Comparative studies in cultural and psychological adaptation.* New York: Sage/Halsted.

Berry J. W. (1979). A cultural ecology of social behavior. In L. Berkowitz (Ed.), *Advances in experimental social psychology* (Vol. 12, pp. 177–206). New York: Academic Press.

Bogardus, E. S. (1925). Measuring social distance. *Journal of Applied Psychology, 9,* 299–308.

Bronfenbrenner, U. (1979). *The ecology of human development.* Cambridge, MA: Harvard University Press.

Deković, M., ten Have, M., Vollebergh, W. A. M., Pels, T., Oosterwegel, A., Wissink, I. B. et al. (2006). The cross-cultural equivalence of Parental Rearing measure: EMBU-C. *European Journal of Psychological Assessment, 22,* 85–91.

Durkheim, E. (1888). Introduction à la sociologie de la famille. *Annales de la Faculté des Lettres de Bordeaux, 10.*

Durkheim, E. (1921). La famille conjugale. *Revue Philosophique de la France et de l'Etranger, 90,* 1–14. (Original work published 1892)

Dwairy, M., & Achoui, M. (2006). Introduction to three cross-regional research studies on parenting styles, individuation and mental health in Arab societies. *Journal of Cross-Cultural Psychology, 37,* 221–229.

Fleming, J., & Elovson, A. (1988). *The adult sources of self-esteem inventory.* Northridge CA: State University of California at Northridge.

Furnham, A. (1988). *Lay theories: Everyday understanding of problems in the social sciences.* Oxford: Pergamon.

Furnham, A., & Lewis, A. (1986). *The economic mind: The social psychology of economic behaviour.* Hove, UK: Wheatsheaf.

Georgas, J. (1989). Changing family values in Greece: From collectivist to individualist. *Journal of Cross-Cultural Psychology, 20,* 80–91.

Georgas, J. (1991). Intrafamily acculturation of values in Greece. *Journal of Cross-Cultural Psychology, 22,* 445–457.

Georgas, J. (1993). An ecological-social model for indigenous psychology: The example of Greece. In U. Kim & J. W. Berry (Eds.), *Indigenous psychologies: Theory, method and experience in cultural context* (pp. 56–78). Beverly Hills, CA: Sage.

Georgas, J. (1999). Family as a context variable in cross-cultural psychology. In J. Adamopoulos & Y. Kashima (Eds.), *Social psychology and cultural context* (pp. 163–175). Beverly Hills, CA: Sage.

Georgas, J., & Berry, J. W. (1995). An ecocultural taxonomy for cross-cultural psychology. *Cross-Cultural Research, 29,* 121–157.

Georgas, J., Berry, J. W., Shaw, A., Christakopoulou, S., & Mylonas, K. (1996). Acculturation of Greek family values. *Journal of Cross-Cultural Psychology, 27,* 329–338.

Georgas, J., Berry, J. W., Van de Vijver, F. J. R., Kagitcibasi, C., & Poortinga, Y. H. (2006). *Families across cultures: A 30-nation psychological study.* New York: Cambridge University Press.

Georgas, J., & Mylonas, K. (2006). Cultures are like all other cultures, like some other cultures, like no other culture. In U. Kim, K. S. Yang, & K. K. Hwang (Eds.), *Indigenous and cultural psychology: Understanding people in context* (pp. 197–221). New York: Springer.

Georgas, J., Mylonas, K., Bafiti, T., Poortinga, Y. H., Kagitcibasi, C., Berry, J. W. et al. (2001). Functional relationships in the nuclear and the extended family: A 16 culture study. *International Journal of Psychology, 36,* 289–300.

Georgas, J., Mylonas, K., Gari, A., & Panagiotopoulou, P. (2004). Families and values in Europe. In W. Arts & L. Halman (Eds.), *European values at the end of the millennium* (pp. 167–204). Leiden, the Netherlands: Brill.

Hox, J. (2002). *Multilevel analysis: Techniques and applications.* Mahwah, NJ: Lawrence Erlbaum.

Kagitcibasi, C. (1990). Family and socialization in cross-cultural perspective: A model of change. In J. Berman (Ed.), *Cross-cultural perspectives: Nebraska symposium on motivation, 1989* (pp. 135–200). Lincoln, NE: Nebraska University Press.

Kagitcibasi, C. (1996). *Family and human development across cultures: A view from the other side.* Hillsdale, NJ: Lawrence Erlbaum.

Keller, H., Zach, U., & Abels, M. (2005). The German family: Families in Germany. In J. L. Roopnarine & U. P. Gielen (Eds.), *Families in global perspective* (pp. 242–258). Boston: Allyn & Bacon.

Kline, P. (1993). *The handbook of psychological testing.* London: Routledge.

Muthén, B. O. (1994). Multilevel covariance structure analysis. *Sociological Methods and Research, 22,* 376–398.

Parsons, T. (1943). The kinship system of the contemporary United States. *American Anthropologist, 45,* 22–38.

Parsons, T. (1949). The social structure of the family. In R. N. Anshen (Ed.), *The family: Its functions and destiny* (pp. 33–58). New York: Harper.

Poortinga, Y. H., & Van de Vijver, F. J. R. (2004). Culture and cognition: Performance differences and invariant structures. In R. J. Sternberg & E. Grigorenko (Eds.), *Culture and competence: Context of life success* (pp. 139–162). Washington, D.C.: American Psychological Association.

Rossier, J., Dahourou, D., & McCrae, R. R. (2005). Structural and mean-level analyses of the five-factor model and locus of control. *Journal of Cross-Cultural Psychology, 36,* 227–246.

Schwartz, S. H. (1992). Universals in the content and structure of values: Theoretical advances and empirical tests in twenty countries. In M. P. Zanna (Ed.), *Advances in experimental social psychology* (Vol. 25, pp. 1–65). San Diego, CA: Academic Press.

Schwartz, S. H. (1994). Beyond individualism-collectivism: New cultural dimensions of values. In U. Kim, H. C. Triandis, C. Kagitcibasi, S.-C. Choi, & G. Yoon (Eds.), *Individualism and collectivism; Theory, method and applications* (pp. 85–119). Thousand Oaks, CA: Sage.

Singelis, T. M. (1994). The measurement of independent and interdependent self-construals. *Personality and Social Psychology Bulletin, 20,* 580–591.

Teachman, J., & Crowder, K. (2002). Multilevel models in family research: Some conceptual and methodological issues. *Journal of Marriage and the Family, 64,* 280–294.

Tucker, L. R. (1951). *A method for synthesis of factor analysis studies* (Personnel Research Section Report No. 984). Washington, D.C.: Department of the Army.

Van de Vijver, F. J. R., & Leung, K. (1997). *Methods and data analysis for cross-cultural research.* Newbury Park, CA: Sage.

Van de Vijver, F. J. R., Mylonas, K., Pavlopoulos, V., & Georgas, J. (2006). Results: Cross-cultural analyses of the family. In J. Georgas, J. W. Berry, F. J. R. Van de Vijver, C. Kagitcibasi, & Y. H. Poortinga (2006). *Families across cultures: A 30-nation psychological study* (pp. 126–185). New York: Cambridge University Press.

Van de Vijver, F. J. R., & Poortinga, Y. H. (2002). Structural equivalence in multi-level research. *Journal of Cross-Cultural Psychology, 33,* 141–156.

Van de Vijver, F. J. R., & Watkins, D. (2006). Assessing similarity of meaning at the individual and country level: An investigation of a measure of independent and interdependent self. *European Journal of Psychological Assessment, 22,* 69–77.

Williams, J. E., Satterwhite, R. C., & Saiz, J. L. (1998). *The importance of psychological traits: A cross-cultural study.* New York: Plenum.

14

Acculturation

Bernhard Nauck

Acculturation is by nature a multilevel issue; it typically involves at least the current state of social groups and individual change. The current chapter concentrates on two topics. First, I discuss current conceptual developments in acculturation research from a multilevel perspective. In the second part, I review selected empirical studies to assess their contribution to multilevel analysis of acculturation phenomena.

CONCEPTUAL ISSUES

Acculturation as a Multilevel Phenomenon

The most widely accepted approach to acculturation in cross-cultural psychology is that of Berry (1980, 1997, 2002). He developed the idea of acculturation strategies as specific types of individual adaptation to culturally new social environments. This notion typically applies to immigrants in a culturally distinct receiving society. Acculturation in this sense has two characteristics: First, it presupposes the accomplishment of an individual process of enculturation, namely the learning of the knowledge and beliefs of the social group in the society of origin. This primary socialization process is part of the adaptation of human individuals to their environment. Second, acculturation is invariably confounded with the process of individual development (Schönpflug, 1997).

This narrower understanding of acculturation as an individual adaptation process (psychological acculturation) has always been embedded in a wider framework of group-related process (Graves, 1967). According to Berry (1997),

This distinction between levels is important for two reasons: first, in order to examine the systematic relationships between these two sets of variables; and second, because not all individuals participate to the same extent in the general acculturation being experienced by their group. (p. 7)

Earlier definitions of acculturation already encompassed individual- and group-level processes:

Acculturation comprehends those phenomena which result when groups of individuals having different cultures come into continuous first-hand contact with subsequent changes in the original culture patterns of either or both groups. (Redfield, Linton, & Herskovits, 1936, p. 149)

The lack of distinction between acculturation as individual adaptation and as change in the group culture has resulted in numerous misunderstandings, but has seldom inspired explanatory attempts to relate social change systematically to individual adaptation and vice versa; the seminal work of Berry is a case in point.

Basically, Berry's model of acculturation and adaptation consists of two components, namely a typology of acculturation strategies, and a coping model for acculturative stress. He argues that there are two fundamental dimensions of acculturation: maintenance of the culture of origin and maintenance of relations with other groups. Both dimensions are salient in the case of immigrants and their response to the social majority in the receiving society. The two dimensions result in two basic questions (Berry, 1980): "Is it considered to be of value to maintain cultural identity and characteristics?" and "Is it considered to be of value to maintain relations with other groups?" If the responses to these two dimensions are dichotomized, then four acculturation strategies can be distinguished:

1. Integration reflects the desire to maintain key features of the culture of origin, while also learning and adapting to relevant aspects of the receiving society. If this is achieved, it results in a double integration into two possibly distinct social contexts.
2. Assimilation relinquishes the culture of origin for the sake of learning and adopting the culture of the dominant population of the receiving society.
3. Separation maintains features of the culture of origin while rejecting contacts with members of the dominant population of the receiving society; thus it results in social segmentation (Esser, 2000).

4. Marginalization characterizes individuals who reject both their culture of origin and the culture of the dominant population of the receiving society and results in anomie or individualism (Bourhis, Moïse, Perreault, & Senécal, 1997).

This two-dimensional typology is congruent with the sociological terminology of inclusion in or exclusion from sociocultural contexts (Esser, 2004). This typology is of great value, as it overcomes one-dimensional models, which claim that assimilation is the inevitable result of culture contact and just a matter of time. Contrary to, among others, the race-relations-cycle of Park (1950; Park & Burgess, 1921), a two-dimensional typology opens up a scope for other individual choices and possibly stable different social outcomes.

So far the research program on acculturation strategies has focused on the individual consequences of the various choices. Several correlational studies have been conducted with aboriginal populations, immigrants, refugees, and sojourners (Ataca & Berry, 2002; Aycan & Berry, 1996; Berry, Kim, Minde, & Mok, 1987; Kim & Berry, 1985, 1986; Sabatier & Berry, 1994; Sam & Berry, 1995). The various effects of acculturation strategies have been largely interpreted in a framework of stress and coping (Lazarus & Folkman, 1984). This has led to the model depicted in Figure 14.1.

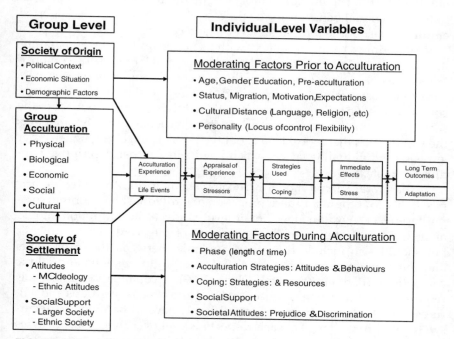

FIGURE 14.1 A framework of acculturation research. (Berry, 1997, p. 15)

Obviously, this model is conceptualized as a multilevel model. It contains explicitly the "individual level" and the "group level." Implicitly the group level is differentiated further into a societal level ("society of origin" and "society of settlement") and a group level ("group acculturation") in both of which the acculturating individual is embedded:

> It is contended that any study that ignores any of these broad classes of variables will be incomplete, and will be unable to comprehend individuals who are experiencing acculturation. (Berry, 1997, p. 15)

Although this model is meant to list and order relevant groups of variables and makes theoretical propositions only implicitly, it is to some extent misleading and deficient from a multilevel analysis perspective (the same applies to a similar model proposed by Ward, Bochner, & Furnham, 2001, p. 44). The model is misleading, because it places the society of origin and the receiving society at the same level. It is an open question, at least initially, whether the latter will be a "society of settlement," and this may influence the result of the acculturation process. The society of origin does not exercise any direct effect on the action alternatives of the individual, as it exists (contrary to the possibly existing minority group) only in the heads of the immigrants. It is brought along as imported culture obtained in the enculturation process. For the purpose of the explanation of individual behavior in the process of acculturation this imported culture is part of the individual level. The receiving society "is there" in space and time as a social context, with its opportunities and constraints, its spatial provisions, institutional regulations, and its structural composition of the population. One part of this structural composition is the existence/nonexistence of minority groups in varying size and institutional completeness. These are embedded in the receiving society, but not in the society of origin. The main reason for this deficiency in Berry's model is the absence of a theoretical idea about the possible effects of higher-order levels on individual behavior, which results in a rather descriptive handling of context effects.

Furthermore, Berry's model is incomplete as it does not provide any possibility to account for the aggregation of individual behavior into composite effects. A full-fledged, multilevel study of acculturation should analyze not only the individual outcomes of the acculturation process, but should also include the group dynamics between the immigrants and the population majority, involving intergroup relations and ethnic competition (Banton, 1967, 1983; Olzak, 1992). A combination of levels is required if acculturation is conceptualized as a change of groups and cultures. Societal, group, and individual levels have to be modeled recursively to capture change at each respective level over time. This includes not only long-term individual adaptation, but also its aggregated effect on the group composition of the ethnic minority and the receiving society.

This, in turn, leads to changes in opportunity structures and (sometimes) at a later stage in institutional regulations. The main reason for this deficit or incompleteness is the absence of a theoretical idea about the possible effects of individual behavior on collective results.

Multilevel Models of Acculturation

Social Theory

A basic model taking both types of multilevel effects into account can be specified as a special case of the micro–macro link in social theory (Coleman, 1990). For example, most psychological studies of acculturation only take into account individual perceptions of social contexts (e.g., perceived discrimination, social support, and peer group acceptance). Especially, if these are the perceptions of the acculturating individuals, the analysis remains at the individual level and no multilevel effects can be estimated. The latter effects would presuppose (at least) the existence of factual discrimination, social support, or peer group interaction, independent of whether it is individually perceived or not, and irrespective of the question of whether individual perceptions are a good proxy for its measurement. A multidisciplinary analysis of acculturation processes is needed to link the perceived characteristics of the environment to the factual environment.

As a first step, the basic model (presented in Figure 14.2) can be restricted to two levels and one cycle of interdependency. The basic principle of this methodology is the explanation of collective results as the indirect result of individual action. The social situation in the receiving society influences the immigrants' acculturation strategy. The preferred strategy will lead to a certain level of adaptation. The aggregated level of adaptation of

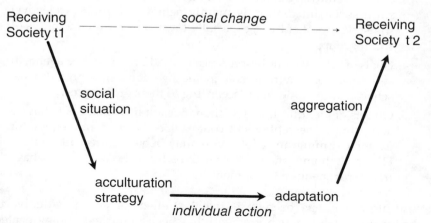

FIGURE 14.2   Acculturation in multilevel analysis.

a specific immigrant group becomes a factor on its own that influences the receiving society. So, the model estimates that characteristics of the receiving society lead to action among immigrants which can influence the receiving society. Examples include ethnic segmentation of a society, the emergence of ethnic communities or ethnically plural institutional settings, high rates of alienated second-generation immigrants, and fading away of minority languages. The minimum requirement for a complete explanation would consist of explicit assumptions about (1) the effect of societal conditions on individual choices (e.g., a specific acculturation strategy); (2) the behavioral consequences of these choices (e.g., specific strategic outcomes); and (3) the aggregation of these outcomes to changes in the social structure (e.g., interethnic conflicts, collective upward mobility of ethnic groups, an increased cohesion of the immigrant family, or ethnic school segregation). From a multilevel analysis perspective, the most challenging part of such explanations is to specify the mechanisms through which the behavior of the individual is influenced by the social context at hand (Alpheis, 1988) and how individual behavior aggregates to higher level results.

According to Nauck (1999) social contexts operate in their influence on individual behavior as:

1. Opportunity structures and constraints affecting the realization of individual action preferences, providing, for example, job offers, marriage partners, situations for practicing a language within or outside the ethnic minority;

2. Social control within the social network, which may increase the indirect costs of choices through sanctioning behavior that conforms to or is deviant from group values;

3. Places of cultural transmission for traditions and routine solutions, since social integration is mainly achieved through (selective) transmission of culture, especially toward incoming members of social groups;

4. Goals of selective migration, since individuals are active agents in selecting their environments including spouses, neighborhoods, schools, and ethnic clubs, according to their preferences;

5. Objects of identification, which may result in a choice of behavior according to perceptions of context-specific appropriateness; for example, immigrant adolescents may behave differently within ethnically homogeneous peer groups from the way they behave in heterogeneous environments.

Acculturation has been extensively studied as an individual-level phenomenon, while much less work has been published on aggregated phenomena. We know more about changes in individual behavior after acculturation than about changes in contexts as a consequence of the behavior of the acculturating groups. One prominent example of (unintended) aggregate consequences of individual action is the "tipping" theory of neighborhood segregation (Schelling, 1971, 1972). The theory is based on the assumption of randomly distributed "subjective tipping points" in neighborhood populations:

> Tipping is said to occur when some recognizable minority group in a neighborhood reaches a size that motivates the other residents to begin leaving. The term implies that subsequent entrants who take the place of those who leave are predominantly of the minority and that the process ultimately changes the composition of the neighborhood. (Schelling, 1972, p. 157)

Dynamic Modeling

Another, more elaborate model of ethnic segmentation (Esser, 1985) is based on the dynamic modeling of choices of three groups of agents: namely, the population majority (especially in its role as providing opportunities in the labor market), the immigrants (especially in their role as labor migrants), and those "left behind" (especially in their role as potential chain migrants).

The dynamic modeling approach is based on three assumptions about the interdependence of the economic and social cost–benefits structure for the members of these three groups and how each of these structures changes during the immigration process. The first interdependence assumption refers to the increasing social costs of those left behind as emigration from the area increases, which leads to an increased incentive for "social" migration instead of labor migration. The second refers to the decreasing opportunities on the labor market and the increasing social costs of in-migration for the population majority, as the proportion of social immigrants increases. The third refers to changing incentives for the various acculturation strategies within the immigrant minority as it grows larger and more ethnic institutions become available. Again, the changes in acculturation opportunities at the societal level are modeled as unintended consequences of the aggregation of individual choices and the dynamics resulting from their interdependence.

The basic multilevel model presented in Figure 14.2 can be extended in two ways; more than two levels and more than one cycle of macro–micro links may be introduced. Most of the explanatory attempts use more than two levels. As mentioned, Berry introduces explicitly an intermediate group level between the "immigrant minority" and the "population majority." Hence, explicit assumptions have to be introduced concerning the interdependent social situation of the social groups, how this affects individual choices of the members of both groups, and how the outcomes change the composition of both groups. The resulting changes, in turn, induce changes at the societal level. In empirical studies even more levels are used, be it sometimes only implicitly; extra levels can be found in studies in which acculturation in specific organizations (workplaces, schools), social groups (families, kinship systems), or ecological settings (neighborhoods) is analyzed (see the second part of the chapter). When more levels are introduced, multilevel explanations become more complex, as each level adds new causal relationships. So far, explicit attempts at complete multilevel propositions are absent in acculturation research.

There have also been studies that addressed more than one cycle of societal change during the process of acculturation. In these studies so-called genetic explanations can be applied (Hempel & Oppenheim, 1948): "The task of genetic explanations is to set out the sequence of major events through which some earlier system has been transformed into a later one" (Nagel, 1974, p. 25). In principle, genetic explanations can be extended indefinitely "at both ends." Thus, one can ask why a specific acculturation situation came about, or which further consequences are to be expected. The early race-relations cycle is a prominent example for this kind of theorizing, as is the distinction between the acculturation of first-, second-, and third-generation immigrants. There are explicit assumptions about differences in the social situation of immigrants, their children, and grandchildren, as expressed, for example, in the ethnic revival hypothesis (Gans, 1979; Hansen, 1938). Other assumptions concern systematic differences between generations in the cost–benefit structure of investments in language maintenance and opportunities for language learning (Alba, Logan, Lutz & Stults, 2002; Espenshade & Fu, 1997; Lopez, 1999; Portes & Hao, 1998; Portes & Schauffler, 1994).

Again, completeness is only achieved if the triad of multilevel explanations is explicitly stated for each cycle, which never has been the case. The research program based on Berry's acculturation strategies has concentrated almost entirely on consequences of each of the four strategies for individual adaptation, especially with regard to the individual experience and acculturative stress, as well as related changes over time. Empirical analyses in various contexts and ethnic groups have provided strong empirical evidence that integration as an acculturation strategy is accompanied with the least acculturative stress and with the highest well-being of the immigrant minority member.

Psychological adaptation has been distinguished from sociocultural adaptation and economic adaptation (Berry, 1997). Here adaptation becomes equivalent to the major dimensions of assimilation research, where personal attributes, such as "cognitive assimilation" (learning of instrumental skills and knowledge for effective behavior in the receiving society) and "identificative assimilation" (internalization of the normative culture and feelings of being part of the society) are distinguished from relational attributes, such as "social assimilation" (interethnic contacts) and "structural assimilation" (placement in the educational and labor sector and on the housing market) (Alpheis, 1988; Gordon, 1964). Empirical evidence about the causal relations between these dimensions exists for immigrant workers, with cognitive assimilation being the initial step and the determinant of both structural and social assimilation. Identification with the receiving society becomes likely, only if such assimilation is achieved and acculturative stress is largely absent (Esser, 1981, 1982; Hill, 1984).

Human Capital Theories

There is not much research on which contextual and personal conditions influence the choice of an acculturation strategy. For the relational dimensions of adaptation the choice obviously is not unconditional, but depends on opportunities in the labor and housing market as well as on the willingness of the majority population to interact. This is exemplified in the notion of social distance (Bogardus, 1933; Park, 1924). In migration research, human capital theories have provided a powerful approach. From this perspective, acculturation is seen as an investment in the human capital of the immigrant (Borjas, 1994; Kalter & Granato, 2002; Nee & Sanders, 2002). Three different kinds of capitals are distinguished, namely economic, human, and social capital, which, in principle, can be transformed from one into the other. They differ in the necessary investment of time, both in their accumulation and their maintenance.

Economic capital is the stock of money, goods or land that an actor may invest in the pursuit of his action goals. Human capital, unlike economic capital, is the added value when a laborer acquires knowledge, skills, and other assets useful to improve her or his position in the labor market. Unlike the highly exchangeable economic capital, human capital is embedded in the laborers themselves and usually measured by education, training, and experience (Lin, 2001). The concept of human capital has been extended by Bourdieu (1986) in a way that is significant for the understanding of migrant minorities, namely by introducing the concept of cultural capital. This form of capital refers additionally to the reproduction of the dominant culture and values in the next generation, resulting in a specific "habitus." Acquiring a habitus requires long training and internalization; this typically does not happen during a (late) acculturation process. As receiving societies and occupations vary much with regard to social control via the habitus, cultural capital investments of immigrants on the labor market vary extensively in their returns. Social capital is an investment in social relations and is thus not embedded in individuals, but in their social relations. Its transfer to others is quite limited (Coleman, 1988, 1990). The significance of this concept for the understanding of immigrant minorities is obvious, as migration initially is accompanied by destruction of social networks. The reorganization of social networks is time-intensive and may put immigrants at a disadvantaged position even for generations.

This capital investment explanation also covers the notion of cultural distance (Berry, 1997; Triandis, 1997). The larger the cultural distance between the culture of origin and the receiving society, the higher are the investment costs. Also, the notion of capital investment systematically relates acculturation investments (for example, in learning and maintaining the ethnic language and in building and maintaining social relationships) to the respective opportunity structures and to individual resources. Moreover, acculturation may imply not only individual costs, such as learning efforts and acculturative stress, but also the maintenance of the culture of origin and of social relationships to the country of origin. In this sense it may not be beneficial under all circumstances. Nauck (2001a, in press) has made a first attempt to relate individual resources and opportunities directly to acculturation strategies for immigrants in Europe. This study disregards economic capital, because these immigrants typically do not vary much in economic resources, as was the case in classical immigrant societies.

The relationships of cultural and social capital with the various acculturation strategies distinguished by Berry are schematically indicated in Table 14.1. The underlying assumption is that the investment balance of the various strategies differs according to individual resources, consisting of the extant social and cultural capital of the immigrant and the opportunity structures inside and outside the minority group.

Marginalization is the most likely mode of acculturation in the absence of noteworthy social and cultural capital and of opportunities; it is usually not a result of intentional choice, but of a lack of alternatives due to absence of resources and opportunities.

Segregation requires social capital within the minority or in the society of origin, but not necessarily cultural capital within the receiving soci-

TABLE 14.1

Opportunities, Social and Cultural Capital in the Process of Acculturation

Input	Output			
	Integration	Assimilation	Segregation	Marginalization
Cultural capital	+	+	−	−
Social capital	+	−	+	−
Opportunities inside/outside minority	+/+	−/+	+/−	−/−

Note. The signs in the cells indicate the investment balance. For example, the positive sign in the first cell states that cultural capital is required for a successful integration strategy.

ety. This acculturation strategy provides strong incentives for immigrants with low cultural capital, so that an optimal placement within the migrant minority becomes the preferred (or only) choice. It presupposes an institutionally relatively complete minority (Breton, 1965), but not necessarily a lack of opportunities in the receiving society.

Assimilation is based on investment in cultural capital, but it does not require necessarily social capital. Assimilation addresses an optimal placement within the majority part of the receiving society and assumes that adequate opportunity structures are available. Investments in strong relationships within the minority do not improve this strategy and a full set of minority institutions is not beneficial.

Integration is the acculturation strategy most likely leading to favorable outcomes, but it also comes with the highest required levels of investments and contextual preconditions. Integration aims at optimal placement within both social contexts and thus requires cultural capital for both, as well as the maintenance of two separate social networks. Even if the scarcity in personal resources, such as limited time and learning abilities, is disregarded, this option only remains stable if the benefits justify the intense investments. Such may be the case for cosmopolitan intellectuals, cross-nationally operating family enterprises or business networks, and members of ethnic colonies having a high level of interchange with the society of origin or other ethnic colonies.

The model in Table 14.1 does not only explain the typically homogeneous composition of friendship networks of immigrants (Esser, 1990). It also makes plausible why assimilation is such a dominant choice in the long run (Alba, 2003; Portes & Rumbaut, 2001), despite the frequently mentioned intentions to integrate made by immigrants shortly after arrival. The extra costs of additional investments in either social or cultural capital often exceed the resources of the individual. Segregation is most likely in the combination of a high social capital and a low cultural capital.

To some extent, the capital investment model challenges the conclusions drawn from empirical findings about the adaptation correlates of the four acculturation strategies. As these findings are typically based on cross-sectional data, the causal structure between adaptation and acculturation strategy remains unclear. Thus, it may well be the case that the positive outcomes of the integration strategy with regard to coping are a selection effect, as the most resourceful immigrants and those in the most favorable social contexts are most likely to choose this option and to maintain it.

Interactive Acculturation Model

The capital investment approach relates the intermediate level of opportunities within and outside the minority to individual behavior. The complementary approach of the interactive acculturation model (Bourhis et al., 1997) brings the societal level into focus by distinguishing several policy regimes of migration and the social integration of immigrants. These authors relate what they call political ideologies to the acculturation orientations of the population majority and the immigrant minority. Four different clusters of regimes are arranged on a continuum.

First, the *pluralism regime* upholds that the state has no mandate in defining or regulating the private values of its citizens. Consequently, the state is only willing to support the private activities of its indigenous minority groups financially and socially, as well as those of first- and second-generation immigrant communities. It is considered of value for the receiving society that minorities maintain key features of their cultural and linguistic distinctiveness while adopting the public values of the society. Second, the *civic regime* is based on the principle of nonintervention in the private values of particular groups, but it respects the right of minorities for self-organization and of maintaining their cultural distinctiveness. Third, the *assimilation regime* expects immigrants and minorities to abandon their own cultural distinctiveness for the sake of cultural homogeneity of the (nation-)state and for the avoidance of ethnic segmentation and inequality. Finally, the *ethnicist regime* is based on the principle that the receiving society sets standards of inclusion typically based on ascriptive attributes, such as ethnicity or religion. In its radical version this regime denies inclusion indefinitely.

This typology allows for arranging different societies, or the same societies at different historical periods, on a theoretically meaningful macrolevel, thus overcoming the most common theoretical deficit of cross-societal comparisons of acculturation research. Unfortunately, it is lacking suggestions for a valid measurement of the policy regimes. The advantage of the model is that it provides a complete explanation at least for the macro- and mesolevel, relating the policy regimes to the intermediate level of the minority and majority. The model specifies conditions under which intergroup relationships become consensual, problematic, or conflictual as a result of collectively favored acculturation strategies. It is assumed that intergroup relationships will be consensual when minority and majority pursue the same acculturation strategy. Problematic relational outcomes emerge when the majority and the minority experience both partial agreement and partial disagreement, whereas conflictual relationships are most likely when both parties pursue opposing strategies. The nature of these relationships should have subsequent effects on the microlevel of individual acculturation choices.

Although the model claims to be dynamic, in the sense that it allows for the analysis of intergroup dynamics, mechanisms are hardly specified on how the individual acculturation strategies aggregate to collective results under the respective policy regimes. Furthermore, it is still an open empirical question whether immigration policies at the societal level are the most influential regimes for individual acculturation. It has repeatedly been argued that social welfare regimes are more important, but empirical research hardly exists.

Welfare Regimes

Following the typology of Esping-Andersen (1990), three different types of welfare regimes can be distinguished; namely the *liberal* (e.g., Anglo-Saxon countries), the *corporate-conservative* (e.g., Central Europe), and the *social-democratic* regime (e.g., Scandinavia). It seems likely that these regimes have implications for acculturation. As the liberal regime is entirely based on individual resources, it provides strong incentives for the self-organization of welfare production and insurance against life risks. Hence, it promotes ethnic segmentation. On the other hand, this regime is relatively open for immigrants and for status mobility based on individual achievements. The corporate-conservative regime includes the entire population in its corporate welfare state institutions, which are typically set up to serve the mainstream population. As a consequence, these institutions are a major mechanism for assimilation. The social-democratic regime combines corporate welfare institutions with extensive income redistribution. Although similarly restrictive on the inclusion of immigrants as the corporate-conservative regime, this regime tends to provide as many opportunities for assimilation, but results in less ethnic inequality.

Although typologies of different types of regimes may be convincing at first glance, the related assumptions about their relative impact on acculturation are difficult to test empirically. The usual case studies on immigration or social policy cannot overcome this issue. Accordingly, their contribution to political advocacy often exceeds their analytical power. In principle, an empirical test should be based on a multiple stratified sampling for hierarchical modeling. This would require a sufficient number of societies for statistical analysis at the highest level, together with sufficient numbers of cases at the intermediate or the individual level.

Summarizing acculturation research on conceptual issues, it is clear that most advancement has been made in the conceptualization of the individual level. Concepts about domains of acculturation as well as the process of adaptation are suited for explanatory purposes. However, the specification of mechanisms in multilevel context affecting acculturation behavior is still in the initial stages. The same holds for the specification of the mechanisms and the dynamics of acculturation behavior aggregated over individuals on intergroup relations.

EMPIRICAL RESULTS

A discussion of empirical results of multilevel acculturation studies is hampered by both conceptual and methodological problems. The discussion on the latter can be brief: there is a limited use of statistical techniques of multilevel analysis. A first conceptual issue involves the premature state of multilevel theories of acculturation, as described in the previous section. Therefore, this overview of empirical analyses will primarily identify the various social contexts which have been taken into consideration in the analysis of acculturation processes and its outcomes. Another conceptual problem is that these contexts are not necessarily hierarchically structured, as presumed in classical ecological approaches (Bronfenbrenner, 1979) and in most statistical models of multilevel analysis. Immigrants are simultaneously embedded in various, rather independent same-level social contexts, such as kinship, neighborhood, workplace, or ethnic community. One of the challenging but rarely tackled questions has to do with whether the effect of these different contexts on acculturation is complementary (i.e., whether those contexts reinforce each other in their effects on acculturation), substitutive (i.e., whether these contexts may replace each other in their effects on acculturation), or competitive (i.e., whether these contexts have antagonistic effects on acculturation).

Only few empirical analyses have used techniques that go beyond including measures that theoretically are related to two different levels; that is, individual level and contextual measures. In most cases information about these levels is gained from the same source, namely the acculturating individual. This need not be a problem, as long as it is clear for each variable whether the individual is the informant about his or her social ecology or also the level used to analyze the data; in the latter case contextual variables are incorrectly used at individual level. Differences between levels often are not explicitly introduced or even mentioned, and only in rare cases is the term *multilevel analysis* used. In terms of modern multilevel analysis (Hox, 2002), most empirical analyses are to be classified as applications of classical linear regression models, with the exception of a few applications of Boyd and Iversen's (1979) elementary multilevel model (Alpheis, 1988; Esser, 1982). More recent developments of hierarchical linear modeling have not yet found their way into acculturation research. Thus, most empirical analyses rely on information from one source, typically individual respondents, and from one point in time (for an exception, see Silbereisen, Lantermann, & Schmitt-Rodermund, 1999). This limits the analytical potential and makes the empirical analysis of aggregation effects almost impossible.

The following analysis concentrates widely on psychological acculturation (Berry, 2002), which is to some extent synonymous with the concept of acculturation in the social sciences (Gans, 1999). Relational aspects (social relationships and structural placement of immigrants and their descendants), which are typically central for migration sociology, are mostly ignored. Instead, the analysis concentrates on the immigrant's adoption of the culture of the receiving society, its symbols, knowledge, and values, leaving open whether this is accompanied by culture maintenance or not. Needless to say, such analyses are far from being comprehensive.

The following contexts can be distinguished when acculturation studies are sorted according to the contextual level they take into consideration:

- acculturation within different receiving societies;
- interdependence of interethnic relations and acculturation;
- regional variations in acculturation;
- effects of neighborhood composition on acculturation;
- effects of network composition and peer relations on acculturation;
- effects of school on acculturation;
- effects of family structure and interaction on acculturation.

The societal level (different receiving societies) is clearly distinguished in a hierarchy from the other levels, but this is not so clear for the other categories. One may argue, for example, that families are entirely embedded in neighborhoods, but at the same time both these categories may complement or substitute for each other, or compete in their effects on individual acculturation. They then operate at the same level. However, because most of the studies consider one or at most two distinct contexts, this analytical problem occurs only in attempts to synthesize the conclusions from various studies.

Effects of the Society

One common way of studying acculturation within a multilevel perspective is to compare the acculturation and adaptation processes of individuals from identical societies of origin within different receiving societies. Numerous studies use this method to test the cross-cultural robustness of general assumptions about adaptation derived from the stress-and-coping framework. Very few studies try to account for systematic variability related to the characteristics of the receiving society. In order to detect context-specific mechanisms of adaptation, Ward and Kennedy (1993) conducted several cross-sectional studies, varying the receiving society and the immigrant group. Their major finding was that cultural distance between the society of origin and the receiving society (and intraethnic interaction) is positively correlated with adaptation problems, whereas interethnic interaction is negatively correlated. Additional analyses suggested that functionally differentiated, affluent (modern) societies provide better opportunities for adaptation than segmented, poor societies. From a multilevel perspective, this study (as well as others) is rather poor in explanatory power and empirical evidence: Beside the typical weaknesses of many cross-cultural studies, such as small convenience samples (usually students), they also fail to include independent measures of the societal context and treat these as individual properties. If, for example, cultural distance is measured by perceptions of the respective individuals, whose adaptation behavior is to be explained, it does not come as a surprise that those who report higher social distance also report more adaptation problems. In principle this is not a contextual analysis, because informant and analytical unit are identical.

Feldman and Rosenthal (1990) reported results from a comparative study on the acculturation of Chinese and Caucasian adolescents in Australia and the United States. They performed separate analyses for both countries from which they concluded that acculturation was more rapid in Australia than in the United States. However, to explain differences between the groups in both societies and with the society of origin, they did not refer to the societal level, but to differences in the immediate environment. They stated that

> in their neighborhoods and schools the Chinese-Australians constituted a tiny minority, whereas the Chinese-Americans were the most populous of all ethnic groups (including the Caucasians). In contrast to Australia, in San Francisco, where the research was conducted, it is possible to complete all daily transactions...in Chinese and with fellow Chinese nationals. Thus, Chinese parents presumably have significant support for their traditional values. (1990, p. 278)

They also stated that, compared to the society of origin, the household composition has changed from extended household to nuclear family with higher rates of female participation in the labor market, which, in turn, has reduced social control of adolescents. These explanations may be adequate because they refer to differences in opportunity structures for interethnic contacts and institutional completeness of the immigrant minority, as well as to differences in social control. Both these mechanisms of context effects are known to influence individual acculturation behavior. At the same time, neither of these effects is measured in the study.

This shortcoming was partly overcome in a study by Leung (2001) in which acculturation differences of Chinese adolescents in Australia and Canada were examined for samples with different levels of family support, thus introducing three different levels of analysis. The major finding of this study was that academic achievement was higher in Canada and for adolescents with stronger family support, while family support was also higher in Canada than in Australia. It remains unclear whether these context effects are due to selective migration (the social structure of Chinese immigrants is considerably different in Australia and in Canada), to differences in the completeness of minority institutions and resulting opportunities for social support, or to differences in the immigration regime and the related institutional structure of the receiving society.

The latter problem was tackled in a small study of Van Oudenhoven and Eisses (1998) in which the acculturation strategies of Jewish Moroccan immigrants in Israel and Islamic Moroccans in the Netherlands were related to the strategies of the majority members in the two societies. The same (Jewish) religion decreased social distance between minority and majority in Israel and less assimilation pressure was imposed on immigrants, resulting in a more frequent choice for integration in this country compared to the Netherlands where the Muslim immigrants were faced with a majority with a different (i.e., Christian) background. In a similar study, based on the interactive acculturation model of Bourhis et al. (1997), Zagefka and Brown (2002) analyzed the effects of majority–minority relations on the acculturation strategies of Turkish work migrants and German repatriates in Germany. They found higher preference for cultural maintenance (in combination with high preference for intergroup contact) in the Turkish group, but did not report whether this is linked to expectations of the majority, as both immigrant groups were combined in further analyses.

The design of neither of these two studies allows for direct empirical analysis of intergroup relations because no mechanisms were specified through which the perceptions within one group have an effect on the perceptions within the other. To decide whether there is an identification effect resulting from differences at the societal level, as the independent sampling of minority and majority members suggests, or whether a reaction to social control in the immediate social contexts plays a role, would require a research design within which both levels could be separated analytically. The minimal requirement for such a design would entail variation in neighborhood composition. An optimal design would entail a longitudinal analysis of related minority and majority members from stratified contexts. As it stands, the causal structure behind the correlational findings remains unclear.

Effects of Region

Studies on regional differences in acculturation are rather rare, although some existing studies reveal surprising results. For Germany it has been documented repeatedly that children from immigrant families are over-represented in special schools for slow learners. However, this overrepresentation varies considerably between the respective states in the country.

It seems unlikely that states in Germany differ in attracting immigrants whose children will have different learning abilities. Thus, the respective school systems apparently lead to different outcomes for immigrant children. Two context effects have been suggested. First, it has been hypothesized that composition effects of schools and classes account for the differential outcomes. The higher the proportion of foreign students in the learning environment, the fewer opportunities for acculturation are provided. As the concentration of migrants varies between states, this may explain the aggregated outcomes in school performance (Kornman & Schnattinger, 1989). The second explanation refers to selection mechanisms in the educational system. As long as slots for pupils in normal school tracks are available, these are also filled with immigrant children (Gomolla & Radtke, 2002). Differences between states in availability of slots may account for the regional variation. Empirical evidence exists for neither of these two hypotheses. Again, the appropriate explanation can only be achieved when all appropriate levels are considered explicitly.

Effects of Neighborhood

It is a common assumption in acculturation research that neighborhood composition has an effect on the individual acculturation process. High ethnic concentration and the presence of a minority institutional subculture decrease acculturative opportunities, while they increase social control on the retention of the culture of origin. At the aggregate level studies in migration sociology have repeatedly provided strong evidence for this relationship, showing that immigrants in highly concentrated quarters show higher ethnic identification, retain the language of origin and maintain intraethnic social networks. Perhaps the most convincing example for this relationship at the macrolevel is the U-curve-shape of interethnic marriages over the course of the immigration process (Kane & Stephen, 1988); pioneer migrants (who are mostly male) show a high interethnic marriage rate because of a lack of migrant women in this migration phase. The rate decreases because of increasing opportunities within the ethnic minority and its demographic completion, and increases again when higher proportions are reached of assimilated and integrated minority members. Theoretically, processes of different levels are combined in this example, namely change in the opportunity structure at the contextual level, and change in the composition of the immigrant group with regard to the state of acculturation.

The few existing German multilevel analyses on acculturation show that context effects are not very influential. Based on a research design with nested social contexts according to the proportion of immigrants at the communal, district, quarter, block, and building level, Alpheis (1990) found practically no context effects on interethnic contacts of Turks of the first and second generation, after individual-level variables, such as educational level, language skills, length of residence, and age at time of migration, had been controlled for. Individual variables explained about 17% of the variance of interethnic contacts in the first generation and 28% in the second generation, but the combined effects of all context levels explained not more than 1 percent additional variance. Similar results were found among first and second generation Yugoslav and Turkish immigrants in Germany, for the acquisition of the majority language, for subjective well-being, and for ethnic identification (Alpheis, 1988). The nested sampling design also allowed for introducing the aggregated acculturation behavior of other immigrants in the respective samples as context effects (Boyd & Iversen, 1979). Again, the context level variables explained little: "The specified models with context- and interaction-variables can explain only minor additional shares of variance beyond pure individual models. The maximum found was 5 percent of additionally explained variance" (Alpheis, 1988, p. 251). Similar results have been reported for multilevel studies on language acquisition (Dustmann, 1997; Esser, 1982) and residential choices and satisfaction (Nauck, 1988).

The conclusion of all these studies is that most of the neighborhood effects are a result of selective migration, with ethnic colonies serving as a residence for newly arriving immigrants. Those with fewer personal skills and a less stable position in the labor market will stay longer in these neighborhoods. This results in a different composition of immigrants inside and outside "ethnic colonies," but ethnic concentration seems to have no effect on cognitive or identificative assimilation (Esser, 1982). These consistent results from several independent nested sampling designs in Germany are in sharp contrast to findings from the United States and Israel, where typically strong context effects are found (Chiswick & Miller, 1992; Chiswick & Repetto, 2001; Espenshade & Fu, 1997; Linton, 2004; Portes & Rumbaut, 2001). An explanation for these systematic differences between countries in neighborhood effects is not easy. Esser (2005) has provided several hypotheses about the level of ethnic segregation and completeness of ethnic institutions (which are typically higher in the United States than in other countries studied), and about the opportunities on the housing market and the richness of the general social infrastructure (which are typically higher in central Europe). However, it is theoretically not clear whether these characteristics operate in a linear way or whether a threshold model has to be applied. Nor have any of these characteristics been measured in a way which would have allowed for cross-national comparisons.

Effects of Peer Relations

Closely related to the study of neighborhood effects on acculturation is the analysis of the effects of social networks and peer relations. Typically, the composition of networks according to ethnicity and the intensity of exposure to peer group influence are used as predictors for acculturation. Bochner (1982) has reported findings showing that assimilation is linearly related to the proportion of peers from the population majority in the social networks of adolescent immigrants and that mixed peer groups are related to openness to cultural differences. He concludes that "because of its cohesiveness, the group is able to maintain strict conformity in its members. Adolescence is also the time when most attitudes are formed, including the attitude of cultural mediation" (p. 34).

In a longitudinal study on German repatriates, Silbereisen and Schmitt-Rodermund (1999) found a mutually reinforcing process of adolescents' well-being and perceived acceptance by peers from the population majority. Phinney (2002) demonstrated that a stronger predictor for ethnic identity than language proficiency is social interaction with peers, especially for second-generation adolescents. Neto (2002), however, found that neither in-group interaction nor out-group interaction is associated with the choice for assimilation or separation as acculturation strategies by immigrant adolescents, whereas the integration mode was positively associated with in-group but not with out-group interaction. In this study there was significant variation between the immigrant minorities that were examined.

The main problem of the studies on social networks and peers is again the theoretical status of the correlational results. This may be one of the reasons for partially inconsistent empirical results, for example between ethnic groups or receiving societies. These studies also have not controlled the opportunity structure for forming networks. Moreover, it is not clear whether acculturation was the cause or the consequence of network composition. The choice of networks is to a large extent a self-selection process and only thereafter becomes a major part of the ecological niche of the acculturating individual. No empirical evidence exists so far on the extent to which this self-selection process is determined by existing opportunities, which may be shaped both by the availability of intraethnic peers and by social distance as perceived by the members of the population majority. Accordingly, the direct effect of social control on acculturation can only be assessed if at least two cycles of a two-level analysis are modeled. This would allow for the separation of the impact of acculturation on network search and effects of network exposure back onto acculturation.

Effects of Schools

The analytical problem of establishing the direction of effects was partly resolved in a study on school selection of immigrants in which the opportunity structure of available schools was related to the individual choices of immigrant families for their children according to their level of adjustment (Kristen, 2005). In this study a sequential model of school selection is suggested, which includes three stages, namely: perception of alternative schools, evaluation of these schools, and access to these schools. The study showed that already in the perception stage, the (Turkish) immigrants, especially those with low education, know about fewer school alternatives than the majority German population. This has led in turn to extreme ethnic school segregation, because all immigrant students end up in the common school of their district, whereas the native born may opt for schools outside their district with lower proportions of immigrant children. Only a few Turkish immigrant families evaluate school alternatives, whereas for the German families the ethnic composition of schools is strongly related to expected achievement outcomes. This results in alternative choices which again aggregate to stronger school segregation. Kirsten found no evidence that differential access had a substantial effect on ethnic segregation because only negligible fractions of immigrant families stated that their school of choice was denied to them. Thus, in this study school segregation was primarily the effect of unequal information access and processing rather than of social discrimination. This is an important finding because it reveals that (school-) segregation can be the result of individual (family) decisions, even if neither active identification of the minority members with their subculture (choosing schools because of the salient presence of minority students), nor active discrimination (denial of access of minority members by certain schools) operate as mechanisms at the context level.

Effects of the Family

The most frequently analyzed context of individual acculturation is the immigrant family. However, only few studies have addressed the interdependence in acculturation of spouses or siblings. A study by Ataca and Berry (2002) on immigrant couples is based on related data from husbands and wives, but these authors did not make use of information about the respective spouse or the spousal relationship as contexts for the explanation of individual acculturation. They also did not clearly separate between variables at the individual and at the couple level. Nauck (1985) and Özel and Nauck (1987) could show that the order of migration of spouses has a long-term effect on division of labor, family interaction, and individual acculturation. The pioneer migrant has a lasting lead in marital power and in contacts with members of the receiving society, and typically preserves a lead in occupational status. This makes families with female pioneer migrants sensitive to conflicts about the (re)organization of marital roles. In independent studies on various immigrant groups in Germany, Schmitt-Rodermund and Silbereisen (1999) and Nauck and Niephaus (2006) showed that unfavorable work experience and unemployment of immigrant husbands also affects the well-being of their spouses.

The vast majority of studies on families are dedicated to the effect of parents on the acculturation of their children, presupposing a unidirectional context effect of the parents on the offspring. Most empirical studies in this area do not use the full potential for multilevel analysis of the data, as they typically look at level differences between generations in the acculturation process. A better alternative would be to treat information about other family members as contexts of individual acculturation outcomes, thus analyzing families as entities of acculturation.

In a small clinical study, Pawliuk et al. (1996) compared the acculturation strategy of immigrant parents and children. They found the children to be more adjusted to the mainstream society. Children who adopted the same acculturation style as their parents scored significantly higher on social competence than those whose acculturation style differed from their parents. In addition, Gil and Vega (1996) found that acculturation stress of parents and adolescents is transmitted between generations and increases cultural conflicts in the family.

A major topic for acculturation research in the tradition of the stress-and-coping model is the effect of parental support on acculturation stress of adolescents. Family cohesion seems to be the most influential protective factor against emotional disorders of adolescent immigrants (Schmitt-Rodermund, Silbereisen & Wiesner, 1996). In line with several other studies, Liebkind and Jasinskaja-Lahti (2000) reported that

> the more our participants experienced support and understanding provided by at least one parent, the less they reported stress symptoms and behavioral problems and the higher their self-esteem, degree of life satisfaction, and sense of mastery. Experiences of maternal support seemed to be important for the girls, and experiences of paternal support seemed to be important for the boys. (p. 465)

However, in most cases the measurement of parental support is based on perceptions of the acculturating adolescent, so it is unclear whether a substantial context effect exists.

Although sometimes assumed otherwise, immigrant families seem to be more cohesive than nonmigrant families. A study on adolescents from several immigrant groups in the United States reports "a generally small amount of conflict with mothers and fathers" (Fuligni, 1998, p. 790). This repeatedly reported finding may be a consequence of the minority situation within which the intergenerational transmission of values and beliefs is not complemented by a congruent socialization process of the offspring through other agents, such as schools, mass media, or peer groups. For the majority, the transmission of culture is the result of efforts of several congruent agencies; in minorities it may become entirely the task of the family. According to Nauck (1997),

> the marked intergenerational transmission of norms leads not only to a much higher concordance in attitudes in migrant than in non-

migrant families but also to a high level of co-orientation among the family members in attitudes and values. Family members know more about each other, are more sensitive to intra-familial inactions, and are better at synchronizing their interactions. (p. 461)

Schönpflug (2001) compared the transmission of values between Turkish immigrant families in Germany and families in Turkey and found that irrespective of the societal context the intensity of transmission is moderated by parenting styles based on commitment, closeness between generations and in the marital relationship, and parents' personal resources. This pattern provides homogeneity of parental orientations, enhances the acceptability of parents as models, and provides transmission skills. Phalet and Schönpflug (2001) could test these propositions for two different immigrant groups, Moroccan and Turkish migrants, in two societal contexts, the Netherlands and Germany. They showed that intergenerational transmission is not only selective with regard to individual adaptation and intergenerational integration, but also varies with the immigrants' opportunity structure in the receiving society: In the Netherlands, with its stronger emphasis on multiculturalism, intergenerational transmission of values and of achievement goals is less intense than in the German immigrant context. Knafo and Schwartz (2001) extended these findings, comparing immigrant families and native families in Israel, and showed that intergenerational transmission of values seems to be stronger for immigrant families. These results are consistent with those obtained for Turkish families in Turkey and Germany (Nauck, 1997) as well as for other immigrant groups (Nauck, 2001a, 2001b, in press; Steinbach, 2001). These recent empirical results contradict numerous assertions expressed in traditional migration research, which focused on aggregate differences between the generations of migrants based on cohort comparisons and disregarded the intergenerational linkages in immigrant families, thus overestimating family conflicts.

Research on coping with acculturative stress and intergenerational transmission in immigrant families is mostly based on cross-sectional datasets, with or without linked records from several family members. Few longitudinal studies exist which analyze the effects of the family context on individual acculturation over time. Hänze and Lantermann (1999) observed in German repatriated families the development of family cohesion, social contacts with members of the receiving society, and family income over time, as well as the family's influence on identificative assimilation. They reported mutual reinforcement between family cohesion, social contact, and the development of identification; the material situation had no effect. Their results imply that the individual acculturation process may get into a negative repetitive cycle when neither family cohesion nor reliable social contacts exist.

Based on the same dataset, Schmitt-Rodermund and Silbereisen (1999a, 1999b, in press) studied the effect of family context on the acculturation of developmental timetables. Higher levels of conflict and permissiveness reported by parents and lower levels of monitoring and more frequent out-of-home activities corresponded with a more accelerated development toward autonomy from parental supervision, especially among newly arrived immigrant families. Higher levels of parental monitoring encouraged escape from the constraints of the newcomers' provisional homes, and thus provided opportunities to make contacts and adopt the lifestyle of adolescents from the German majority population, resulting in earlier developmental timetables. The longitudinal dataset also revealed that, contrary to the adolescents, the parental development timetables for their children remained much the same, resulting in an increasing gap. In families with conflictual relationships parents changed their developmental timetables over time toward earlier ages, whereas in families with low levels of conflicts these timetables were stable or even shifted toward later ages as a reaction to the children's behavior. This longitudinal study with linked records allowed for the first time the analysis of family context effects on individual acculturation in two directions.

Even in the relatively well-studied area of family relations, methodological deficiencies prevail. In their review of family acculturation research, Chun and Akutsu (2002) recommend multilevel analysis within a comparative longitudinal design. With regard to multilevel analysis, they stress the importance of internal dynamics of acculturation within the family context deriving from the different acculturative pace of family members, as well as external influences from social settings and institutions. With regard to longitudinal designs, not only the interplay of individual acculturation and development is seen as important, but also the rate of social change. For example, pioneer migrants face a totally different acculturative setting than members of the second or third generation who live in a minority subculture with an ethnic set of institutions. Finally, only a comparative approach can provide evidence about the interaction between context mechanisms and individual options and preferences (i.e., "culture").

CONCLUSION

In many ways, the review of Chun and Akutsu (2002) on family acculturation is symptomatic for the general state of multilevel analysis of acculturation. The majority of studies examined have been based on convenience samples, sometimes of relatively small sizes, which do not meet criteria of representativeness. The selection of immigrant groups as well as of acculturation contexts is driven predominantly by the pragmatic issue of availability, whereas theoretical considerations are introduced post hoc. Obviously, this is not a specific problem of studies with a focus on context effects, but of acculturation research in general. It seems that there is insufficient funding to realize access to larger, more carefully selected samples. In line with this, panel studies are rare exceptions, although they should be considered the backbone of empirical investigations into the process of acculturation.

More specifically, theoretical concepts and empirical methods of multilevel analysis hardly have been introduced in acculturation research; explicit reference to theoretical or methodological issues of multilevel analysis is seldom found, and adequate statistical techniques for the analysis of context effects, such as hierarchical linear modeling, are not present. Moreover, context effects are only included occasionally as part of multiple regression models, and systematic designs with independent information about levels beyond the individual are rare exceptions. Both undocumented sample biases and the absence of relevant effects from designs contribute to the sometimes inconsistent empirical results and prevent the accumulation of systematic knowledge in the field of acculturation research.

This review stands in sharp contrast to the practical implications of this research area. Ideas about context effects have long played an important role in the public discourse on immigration and acculturation and have led to a number of political and administrative measures. The busing of minority children to less segregated schools is an early example; it was based on the expectation that the composition of school classes has a positive effect on acculturation. Other examples include limits on the proportion of immigrants in a neighborhood (or society in general), and the question whether subsidies for minority organizations have an integration or a segregation effect. Even the policies of receiving nation-states on immigration and inclusion of immigrants in various institutions have unclear effects on acculturation choices and outcomes. At present, one may seriously question whether the available body of scientific knowledge is sufficient to resolve these practical questions efficiently.

Multilevel approaches to acculturation phenomena by necessity are ambitious and in many cases costly enterprises, especially if higher order levels are to be included, which is hardly avoidable in acculturation research. The interaction between social contexts, such as kinship, neighborhood, school, and workplace on the one hand and the immigrant subculture on the other hand calls for systematic variation at both levels; a lack of variation would impede the understanding of otherwise complementary, substitutive, or competitive effects of contexts on acculturation. When effects of interethnic relations or the institutional provisions of the receiving societies are part of the research focus, international comparative designs become necessary. Since acculturation of immigrant minorities is increasingly a characteristic of modern societies and a permanent practical challenge, and since the domains of individual acculturation and the process of adaptation are well conceptualized, their integration into multilevel research better serving practical needs is an urgent task for the near future.

REFERENCES

Alba, R. D. (2003). *Remaking the American mainstream: Assimilation and the new immigration.* Cambridge, MA: Harvard University Press.

Alba, R. D., Logan, J. R., Lutz, A., & Stults, B. (2002). Only English by the third generation? Mother-tongue loss and preservation among the grandchildren of contemporary immigrants. *Demography, 39,* 467–484.

Alpheis, H. (1988). *Kontextanalyse.* Wiesbaden: Deutscher Universitäts Verlag.

Alpheis, H. (1990). Erschwert die ethnische Konzentration die Eingliederung? In H. Esser & J. Friedrichs (Eds.), *Generation und Identität. Theoretische und empirische Beiträge zur Migrationssoziologie* (pp. 147–184). Opladen: Westdeutscher Verlag.

Ataca, B., & Berry, J. W. (2002). Psychological, sociocultural, and marital adaptation of Turkish immigrant couples in Canada. *International Journal of Psychology, 37,* 13–26.

Aycan, Z., & Berry, J. W. (1996). Impact of employment related experiences on immigrants' adaptation to Canada. *Canadian Journal of Behavioral Science, 28,* 240–251.

Banton, M. (1967). *Race relations.* London: Tavistock.

Banton, M. (1983). *Racial and ethnic competition.* Cambridge: Cambridge University Press.

Berry, J. W. (1980). Acculturation as varieties of adaptation. In A. M. Padilla (Ed.), *Acculturation: Theory, models, and some new findings* (pp. 9–25). Boulder, CO: Westview.

Berry, J. W. (1997). Immigration, acculturation, and adaptation. *Applied Psychology: An International Review, 46,* 5–34.

Berry, J. W. (2002). Conceptual approaches to acculturation. In K. M. Chun, P. B. Organista, & G. Marin (Eds.), *Acculturation. Advances in theory, measurement, and applied research* (pp. 17–38). Washington, D.C.: American Psychological Association.

Berry, J. W., Kim, U., Minde, T., & Mok, D. (1987). Comparative studies in acculturative stress. *International Migration Review, 21,* 491–511.

Bochner, S. (1982). The social psychology of cross-cultural relations. In S. Bochner (Ed.), *Cultures in contact. Studies in cross-cultural interaction* (pp. 5–44). Oxford: Pergamon.

Bogardus, E. S. (1933). A social distance scale. *Sociology and Social Research, 17,* 265–271.

Borjas, G. J. (1994). The economics of immigration. *Journal of Economic Literature, 32,* 1667–1717.

Bourdieu, P. (1986). The forms of capital. In J. G. Richardson (Ed.), *Handbook of theory and research for the sociology of education* (pp. 241–258). Westport, CT: Greenwood.

Bourhis, R. Y., Moise, L. C., Perreault, S., & Senecal, S. (1997). Towards an interactive acculturation model: A social psychological approach. *International Journal of Psychology, 32,* 369–386.

Boyd, L. H., & Iversen, G. R. (1979). *Contextual analysis: Concepts and statistical techniques.* Belmont, CA: Wadsworth.

Breton, R. (1965). Institutional completeness of ethnic communities and the personal relations of immigrants. *American Journal of Sociology, 70,* 193–205.

Bronfenbrenner, U. (1979). *The ecology of human development.* Cambridge, MA: Harvard University Press.

Chiswick, B. R., & Miller, P. W. (1992). Language in the immigrant labor market. In B. R. Chiswick (Ed.), *Immigration, language and ethnicity. Canada and the United States* (pp. 229–296). Washington, D.C.: AEI Press.

Chiswick, B. R., & Repetto, G. (2001). Immigrant adjustment in Israel. The determinants of literacy and fluency in Hebrew and the effect of earnings. In S. Djajic (Ed.), *International migration. Trends, policies and economic impact* (pp. 205–228). London: Routledge.

Chun, K. M., & Akutsu, P. D. (2002). Acculturation among ethnic immigrant families. In K. M. Chun, P. B. Organista, & G. Marin (Eds.), *Acculturation. Advances in theory, measurement, and applied research* (pp. 95–119). Washington, D.C.: American Psychological Association.

Coleman, J. S. (1988). Social capital in the creation of human capital. *American Journal of Sociology, 94*(Suppl. 95), S95–S120.

Coleman, J. S. (1990). *Foundations of social theory.* Cambridge, MA: Harvard University Press.

Dustmann, C. (1997). The effects of education, parental background and ethnic concentration on language. *The Quarterly Review of Economics and Finance, 37,* 245–262.

Espenshade, T. J., & Fu, H. (1997). An analysis of English-language proficiency among U.S. immigrants. *American Sociological Review, 62,* 288–305.

Esping-Andersen, G. (1990). *The three worlds of welfare capitalism.* Cambridge: Polity Press.

Esser, H. (1981). Aufenthaltsdauer und die Eingliederung von Wanderern. Zur theoretischen Interpretation soziologischer "'Variablen." *Zeitschrift für Soziologie, 10,* 76–97.

Esser, H. (1982). Sozialräumliche Bedingungen der sprachlichen Assimilation von Arbeitsmigranten. *Zeitschrift für Soziologie, 11,* 279–306.

Esser, H. (1985). Soziale Differenzierung als ungeplante Folge absichtsvollen Handelns: Der Fall der ethnischen Segmentation. *Zeitschrift für Soziologie, 14,* 435–449.

Esser, H. (1989). Die Eingliederung der zweiten Generation. Zur Erklärung "kultureller" Differenzen. *Zeitschrift für Soziologie, 18,* 426–443.

Esser, H. (1990). Interethnische Freundschaften. In H. Esser & J. Friedrichs (Eds.), *Generation und Identität. Theoretische und empirische Beiträge zur Migrationssoziologie* (pp. 185–206). Opladen: Westdeutscher Verlag.

Esser, H. (2000). *Soziologie. Spezielle Grundlagen: Vol. 2, Die Konstruktion der Gesellschaft.* Frankfurt/New York: Campus.

Esser, H. (2004). Does the "new" immigration require a "new" theory of intergenerational integration? *International Migration Review, 38*, 1126–1159.

Esser, H. (2005). *Migration, Sprache und Integration*. Berlin: Wissenschaftszentrum.

Feldman, S. S., & Rosenthal, D. A. (1990). The acculturation of autonomy expectations in Chinese high schoolers residing in two Western nations. *International Journal of Psychology, 25*, 259–281.

Fuligni, A. J. (1998). Authority, autonomy, and parent—Adolescent conflict and cohesion: A study of adolescents from Mexican, Chinese, Filipino, and European backgrounds. *Developmental Psychology, 34*, 782–792.

Gans, H. (1979). Symbolic ethnicity: The future of ethnic groups and cultures. *Racial and Ethnic Studies, 2*, 1–20.

Gans, H. J. (1999). Toward a reconciliation of "Assimilation" and "Pluralism": The interplay of acculturation and ethnic retention. In C. Hirschmann, P. Kasinitz, & J. DeWind (Eds.), *The handbook of international migration: The American experience* (pp. 161–171). New York: Russell Sage Foundation.

Gil, A. G., & Vega, W. A. (1996). Two different worlds: Acculturation stress and adaptation among Cuban and Nicaraguan families. *Journal of Social and Personal Relationships, 13*, 435–456.

Gomolla, M., & Radtke, F. O. (2002). *Institutionelle Diskriminierung. Die Herstellung ethnischer Differenz in der Schule*. Opladen: Leske & Budrich.

Gordon, M. M. (1964). *Assimilation in American life: The role of race, religion and national origins*. New York: Oxford University Press.

Graves, T. (1967). Psychological acculturation in a tri-ethnic community. *South-Western Journal of Anthropology, 23*, 337–350.

Hänze, M., & Lantermann, E. D. (1999). Familiäre, sozial und materielle Ressourcen bei Aussiedlern. In R. K. Silbereisen, E. D. Lantermann, & E. Schmitt-Rodermund (Eds.), *Aussiedler in Deutschland. Akkulturation von Persönlichkeit und Verhalten* (pp. 143–161). Opladen: Leske & Budrich.

Hansen, M. L. (1938). *The problem of the third generation immigrant*. Rock Island, IL: Augustana Historical Society.

Hempel, C. G., & Oppenheim, P. (1948). Studies in the logic of explanation. *Philosophy of Science, 15*, 137–175.

Hill, P. B. (1984). *Determinanten der Eingliederung von Arbeitsmigranten*. Königstein: Hanstein.

Hox, J. (2002). *Multilevel analysis: Techniques and applications*. Mahwah, NJ: Lawrence Erlbaum.

Kalter, F., & Granato, N. (2002). Demographic change, educational expansion, and structural assimilation of immigrants. The case of Germany. *European Sociological Review, 18*, 199–216.

Kane, T. T., & Stephen, E. H. (1988). Patterns of intermarriage of guestworker populations in the Federal Republic of Germany: 1960–1985. *Zeitschrift für Bevölkerungswissenschaft, 14*, 187–204.

Kim, U., & Berry, J. W. (1985). Acculturation attitudes of Korean immigrants in Toronto. In I. Reyes-Lagunes & Y. H. Poortinga (Eds.), *From a different perspective: Studies of behavior across cultures* (pp. 93–105). Lisse, the Netherlands: Swets & Zeitlinger.

Kim, U., & Berry, J. W. (1986). Predictors of acculturative stress among Korean immigrants in Toronto. In L. H. Ekstrand (Ed.), *Ethnic minorities and immigrants* (pp. 159–170). Lisse, the Netherlands: Swets & Zeitlinger.

Knafo, A., & Schwartz, S. H. (2001). Value socialization in families of Israeli-born and Soviet-born adolescents in Israel. *Journal of Cross-Cultural Psychology, 32,* 213–228.

Kornmann, R., & Schnattinger, C. (1989). Sonderschulüberweisungen ausländischer Kinder, Bevölkerungsstruktur und Arbeitsmarktlage-Oder: Sind Ausländerkinder in Baden-Württemberg "dümmer" als sonstwo? *Zeitschrift für Sozialisationsforschung und Erziehungssoziologie, 9,* 195–203.

Kristen, C. (2005). *School choice and ethnic school segregation: Primary school selection in Germany.* Münster: Waxmann.

Lazarus, R. S., & Folkman, S. (1984). *Stress, appraisal and coping.* New York: Springer.

Leung, C. (2001). The sociocultural and psychological adaptation of Chinese migrant adolescents in Australia and Canada. *International Journal of Psychology, 36,* 8–19.

Liebkind, K., & Jasinskaja-Lahti, I. (2000). Acculturation and psychological well-being among immigrant adolescents in Finland: A comparative study of adolescents from different cultural backgrounds. *Journal of Adolescent Research, 15,* 446–469.

Lin, N. (2001). *Social capital: A theory of social structure and action.* Cambridge: Cambridge University Press.

Linton, A. (2004). A critical mass model of bilingualism among U.S.-born Hispanics. *Social Forces, 83,* 279–314.

López, D. E. (1999). Social and linguistic aspects of assimilation today. In C. Hirschmann, P. Kasinitz, & J. DeWind (Eds.), *The handbook of international migration: The American experience* (pp. 212–222). New York: Russell Sage Foundation.

Nagel, E. (1974). *The structure of science: Problems in the logic of scientific explanation* (4th ed.). London: Routledge & Kegan Paul.

Nauck, B. (1985). "Heimliches Matriarchat" in Familien türkischer Arbeitsmigranten? Empirische Ergebnisse zu Veränderungen der Entscheidungsmacht und Aufgabenallokation. *Zeitschrift für Soziologie, 14,* 450–465.

Nauck, B. (1988). Sozial-ökologischer Kontext und außerfamiliäre Beziehungen. Ein interkultureller und interkontextueller Vergleich am Beispiel von deutschen und türkischen Familien. In J. Friedrichs (Ed.), *Soziologische Stadtforschung: Vol. 29. Sonderheft der Kölner Zeitschrift für Soziologie und Sozialpsychologie* (pp. 310–327). Opladen: Westdeutscher Verlag.

Nauck, B. (1997). Migration and intergenerational relations: Turkish families at home and abroad. In W. W. Isajiw (Ed.), *Multiculturalism in North America and Europe: Comparative perspectives on interethnic relations and social incorporation* (pp. 435–465). Toronto: Canadian Scholar's Press.

Nauck, B. (1999). Social capital and intergenerational transmission of cultural capital within a regional context. In J. Bynner, & R. K. Silbereisen (Eds.), *Adversity and challenge in life in the new Germany and in England* (pp. 212–238). London: Macmillan.

Nauck, B. (2001a). Intercultural contact and intergenerational transmission in immigrant families. *Journal of Cross-Cultural Psychology, 32,* 159–173.

Nauck, B. (2001b). Social capital, intergenerational transmission and intercultural contact in immigrant families. *Journal of Comparative Family Studies, 32,* 465–488.

Nauck, B. (in press). Intergenerational transmission, social capital and interethnic contact in immigrant families. In U. Schönpflug (Ed.), *Perspectives on cultural transmission*. Oxford: Oxford University Press.

Nauck, B., & Niephaus, Y. (2006). Intergenerative conflicts and health hazards in migrant families. *Journal of Comparative Family Studies, 37,* 275–298.

Nee, V., & Sanders, J. M. (2002). Understanding the diversity of immigrant incorporation: A forms-of-capital model. *Ethnic and Racial Studies, 24,* 386–411.

Neto, F. (2002). Acculturation strategies among adolescents from immigrant families in Portugal. *International Journal of Intercultural Relations, 26,* 17–38.

Özel, S., & Nauck, B. (1987). Kettenmigration in türkischen Familien. Ihre Herkunftsbedingungen und ihre Effekte auf die Reorganisation der familiären Interaktionsstruktur in der Aufnahmegesellschaft. *Migration, 1,* 61–94.

Olzak, S. (1992). *The dynamics of ethnic competition and conflict.* Stanford, CA: Stanford University Press.

Park, R. E. (1924). The concept of social distance. As applied to the study of racial attitudes and racial relations. *Journal of Applied Sociology, 8,* 339–344.

Park, R. E. (1950). *Race and culture.* Glencoe, IL: Free Press.

Park, R. E., & Burgess, E. W. (1921). *Introduction to the science of sociology.* Chicago: University of Chicago Press.

Pawliuk, N., Grizenko, N., Chan-Yip, A., Gantous, P., Mathew, J., & Nguyen, D. (1996). Acculturation style and psychological functioning in children of immigrants. *American Journal of Orthopsychiatry, 66,* 111–121.

Phalet, K., & Schönpflug, U. (2001a). Intergenerational transmission in Turkish immigrant families: Parental collectivism, achievement values and gender differences. *Journal of Comparative Family Studies, 32,* 489–504.

Phalet, K., & Schönpflug, U. (2001b). Intergenerational transmission of collectivism and achievement values in two acculturation contexts: The case of Turkish families in Germany and Turkish and Moroccan families in the Netherlands. *Journal of Cross-Cultural Psychology, 32,* 186–201.

Phinney, J. S. (2002). Ethnic identity and acculturation. In K. M. Chun, P. B. Organista, & G. Marin (Eds.), *Acculturation: Advances in theory, measurement, and applied research* (pp. 63–81). Washington, D.C.: American Psychological Association.

Portes, A., & Hao, L. (1998). E pluribus unum: Bilingualism and loss of language in the second generation. *Sociology of Education, 71,* 269–294.

Portes, A., & Rumbaut, R. G. (2001). *Legacies: The story of the immigrant second generation.* Berkeley: University of California Press/Russell Sage Foundation.

Portes, A., & Schauffler, R. (1994). Language and the second generation: Billingualism yesterday and today. *International Migration Review, 28,* 640–661.

Redfield, R., Linton, R., & Herskovits, M. J. (1936). Memorandum on the study of acculturation. *American Anthropologist, 38,* 149–152.

Sabatier, C., & Berry, J. W. (1994). Immigration et acculturation. In R. Y. Bourhis, & J. P. Leyens (Eds.), *Stéréotypes, discrimination et relations intergroupes* (pp. 261–291). Liège, Belgium: Mardaga.

Sam, D. L., & Berry, J. W. (1995). Acculturative stress among young immigrants in Norway. *Scandinavian Journal of Psychology, 36,* 10–24.

Schelling, T. C. (1971). Dynamic models of segregation. *Journal of Mathematical Sociology, 1,* 143–186.

Schelling, T. C. (1972). The process of residential segregation: Neighborhood tipping. In A. H. Pascal (Ed.), *Racial discrimination in economic life* (pp. 157–184). Lexington, MA: Heath.

Schmitt-Rodermund, E., & Silbereisen, R. K. (1999a). Determinants of differential acculturation of developmental timetables among adolescent immigrants to Germany. *International Journal of Psychology, 34*, 219–233.

Schmitt-Rodermund, E., & Silbereisen, R. K. (1999b). Differentielle Akkulturation von Entwicklungsorientierungen unter jugendlichen Aussiedlern. In R. K. Silbereisen, E. D. Lantermann, & E. Schmitt-Rodermund (Eds.), *Aussiedler in Deutschland. Akkulturation von Persönlichkeit und Verhalten* (pp. 185–201). Opladen: Leske & Budrich.

Schmitt-Rodermund, E., & Silbereisen, R. K. (in press). Immigrant parents' age expectations for the development of their adolescent offspring—Transmission effects and changes after immigration? In U. Schönpflug (Ed.), *Perspectives on cultural transmission.* Oxford: Oxford University Press.

Schmitt-Rodermund, E., Silbereisen, R., & Wiesner, M. (1996). Junge Aussiedler in Deutschland: Prädiktoren emotionaler Befindlichkeit nach der Immigration. *Zeitschrift für Entwicklungspsychologie und Pädagogische Psychologie, 28*, 357–379.

Schönpflug, U. (1997). Acculturation: Adaptation or development? *Applied Psychology:An International Review, 46*, 52–55.

Schönpflug, U. (2001). Intergenerational transmission of values: The role of transmission belts. *Journal of Cross-Cultural Psychology, 32*, 174–185.

Silbereisen, R. K., Lantermann, E. D., & Schmitt-Rodermund, E. (1999) (Eds.), *Aussiedler in Deutschland. Akkulturation von Persönlichkeit und Verhalten.* Opladen: Leske & Budrich.

Silbereisen, R. K., & Schmitt-Rodermund, E. (1999). Wohlbefinden der jugendlichen Aussiedler. In R. K. Silbereisen, E. D. Lantermann, & E. Schmitt-Rodermund (Eds.), *Aussiedler in Deutschland. Akkulturation von Persönlichkeit und Verhalten* (pp. 257–275). Opladen: Leske & Budrich.

Steinbach, A. (2001). Intergenerational transmission and integration of repatriate families from the Former Soviet Union in Germany. *Journal of Comparative Family Studies, 32*, 466–488.

Triandis, H. C. (1997). Where is culture in the acculturation model? *Applied Psychology:An International Review, 46*, 55–58.

Van Oudenhoven, J. P., & Eisses, A. M. (1998). Integration and assimilation of Moroccan immigrants in Israel and the Netherlands. *International Journal of Intercultural Relations, 22*, 293–307.

Ward, C., Bochner, S., & Furnham, A. (2001). *The psychology of culture shock* (2nd ed.). Hove, UK: Routledge.

Ward, C., & Kennedy, A. (1993). Where's the "culture" in cross-cultural transition? Comparative studies of sojourner adjustment. *Journal of Cross-Cultural Psychology, 24*, 221–249.

Zagefka, H., & Brown, R. (2002). The relationship between acculturation strategies, relative fit and intergroup relations: Immigrant-majority relations in Germany. *European Journal of Social Psychology, 32*, 171–188.

Part IV

Integration

15

Multilevel Models of Individuals and Cultures: Current State and Outlook

Dianne A. van Hemert, Fons J. R. van de Vijver, and Ype H. Poortinga

The chapters in this book demonstrate that many fields in the social and behavioral sciences are inherently multilevel. Studies in cross-cultural psychology almost by definition have a multilevel nature, as context–behavior relationships often involve variables at different levels of aggregation. This book illustrates how we have conceptually and statistically advanced in the field of multilevel cross-cultural research in the last decades. Cross-level relations and questions concerning similarity of concept meaning at different levels of aggregation can now be addressed in a more rigorous manner than ever before. Examples are the meaning of response styles (Smith & Fischer, this volume) and the psychological meaning of control at individual and cultural level (Yamaguchi, Okumura, Chua, Morio, & Yates, this volume). In addition, several chapters provide examples of studies in which the structure of a concept found at individual level is compared to the structure at country level (Leung & Bond, this volume; Lucas & Diener, this volume; McCrae & Terracciano, this volume; Mylonas, Pavlopoulos, & Georgas, this volume).

This final chapter attempts to integrate the various perspectives on multilevel models that have been proposed in the previous chapters. Our analysis is meant to identify strengths and weaknesses of such models and their applications. The first section provides an overview of how multilevel models are used in cross-cultural research. The second section describes conceptual and methodological limitations in the application of multilevel models. The third section explores how we can create designs in which the potential of multilevel models can be more fully realized. Conclusions are drawn in the final section.

USE OF MULTILEVEL MODELS IN CROSS-CULTURAL RESEARCH

In the first chapter we presented a taxonomy of multilevel models (reproduced here in Table 15.1). Before providing an overview of the current usage of multilevel models in cross-cultural research, we briefly recapitulate the taxonomy, which is based on two underlying dimensions. The first dimension draws a distinction between aggregated and disaggregated concepts versus nonaggregated (intrinsic) concepts. (Dis)aggregated concepts are split up depending on whether structures across levels are different or identical (also labeled as isomorphism or homology; see Adamopoulos, this volume, Fontaine, this volume, and Van de Vijver, Van Hemert, & Poortinga, this volume). The second dimension refers to how concepts and variables interact across levels. Cross-level relations constitute the core of multilevel models and it is in the study of these relations that most conceptual and methodological progress has been made in the last decades. Three types of interactions are postulated: no interaction, static interaction, and dynamic interaction. Static interaction in a multilevel analysis is similar to an interaction component in analysis of variance; for example, a tendency to display extraverted behavior may be suppressed in a culture where introversion is valued. Dynamic interaction (called reciprocal relationships by Adamopoulos, this volume) refers to feedback loops in which concepts at different levels influence each other. For example, infant–caregiver interactions in collectivistic cultural contexts put relatively much emphasis on the relatedness and interdependence of infants, which facilitates the reproduction of interaction and relationship patterns among adults and hence, the collectivistic nature of society (Keller, 2007).

Overview of Multilevel Models in Terms of Taxonomy

The first case in Table 15.1 (intrinsic concepts, no cross-level interaction) is the standard model in research examining the effect of variation in ecocultural or sociocultural conditions on behavioral variables. Even if they fall within the scope of a broad conceptual framework, these studies only address the nonrecursive influence of culture-level characteristics. The model is relatively popular in international applications of educational achievement (Stanat & Lüdtke, this volume). For example, educational achievement is described as a function of individual-level factors (e.g., intelligence and socioeconomic background), school factors (e.g., characteristics of the curriculum or school), and country differences (e.g., educational expenditure). If these studies only examine the effects of each context on performance and do not address cross-level interactions, they are illustrations of case 1. A second and classic example is the study by Segall, Campbell, and Herskovits (1966) on illusion susceptibility. They argued in their "carpentered world hypothesis" that living in an environment where geometric shapes such as rectangles, straight lines, and square corners abound will result in higher susceptibility to certain visual illusions such as the Müller–Lyer illusion than living in an environment low on carpenteredness. The hypothesis stated a causal, nonrecursive relation between an ecological feature, carpenteredness of the environment, and a psychological outcome, illusion susceptibility.

Case 2 (static interactions involving nonaggregated concepts) includes research in which cultural variables are taken as moderators of psychological outcomes (Baron & Kenny, 1986; see also Lonner & Adamopoulos, 1997). Nauck (this volume) discusses how adjustment of immigrants (an individual-level variable) is influenced both by various culture-level variables, such as policies toward immigrants, and by individual-level variables, such as personality and individual acculturation preferences (Bourhis, Moïse, Pereault, & Senécal, 1997). The culture-level variables can be linked to adjustment in various ways. The most commonly examined relations are (partial or full) mediation and moderation. With mediation, culture-level variables influence individual acculturation orientations, which in turn influence adjustment. With moderation, culture-level variables have a direct influence on adjustment as well as an indirect influence through acculturation orientations. Another instance of case 2 can be found in the literature on subjective well-being (Lucas & Diener, this volume). The relation of income and subjective well-being is weak at individual level (with correlations that are hardly ever larger than .20) but considerably stronger at country level (with correlations typically in the range of .50 to .70). Moreover, the correlation at individual level varies with the income level of the participants; it tends to be stronger among poorer groups than among richer groups.

Case 3 refers to studies in which nonaggregated culture-level variables are dynamically linked to individual-level variables. Examples are the ecocultural framework (Berry 1976; see also Figure 1.1 in Van de Vijver et al., this volume) and the framework of acculturation (Figure 1.2 in Van de Vijver et al., this volume). Both frameworks specify recursive relations between cultural and individual factors. They also share a high level of complexity and would require considerable effort to test, if testing is feasible at all. Their primary role is not to generate testable models of complex processes, but to provide conceptual guidance for designing new studies and developing new theories. These models summarize our thinking in a specific domain. Empirical studies could address the testing of specific parts of the framework. For example, ethnic vitality (the presence of institutions and support networks for immigrant groups) is an important group-level variable that has an influence on acculturation outcomes, such as adjustment. In turn, these outcome variables could have an impact on ethnic vitality in that immigrants who feel more connected to their ethnic community may also be inclined to invest more in providing support to their community. Such a study would require a longitudinal study design.

Historically, cross-cultural theories have used simple models of cross-level relations. Theories in the culture-and-personality tradition (psychological anthropology) tended to postulate complete isomorphism of culture-level structures and individual personalities (see Adamapoulos, this volume; Van de Vijver et al., this volume). These theories belong to case 7 in Table 15.1 (aggregated data, isomorphic structure, no interaction). The main difference between the original and contemporary approaches is the status of isomorphism. Modern research views isomorphism as a condition to be tested with empirical evidence. The change of isomorphism from assumption to testable condition has important implications for theory and research. The discussion in the new generation of multilevel models is not about the question of *whether or not* there is isomorphism but about the question *when* isomorphism can be expected. Our empirical database about the cross-level equivalence of psychological phenomena is still limited, and the evidence is somewhat mixed. Depending on the outcomes, evidence for case 4 (nonisomorphism) or case 7 (isomorphism) is found.

An example of case 7 is given by McCrae and Terracciano (this volume). These authors show that the Five-Factor Model of personality has an identical structure at individual and cultural level. Lucas and Diener reach the same conclusion for subjective well-being (SWB) in their chapter:

> At the individual level, SWB reflects an individual's subjective evaluation of the quality of his or her life as a whole. The research reviewed in this chapter suggests that at a national level, SWB measures may have a similar meaning—they appear to tap between-nation differences in the quality of life as a whole. (pp. 242–243)

The chapter by Mylonas et al. (this volume) contains examples of both case 4 and case 7. They report high cross-level equivalence for most family

TABLE 15.1

Taxonomy of Multilevel Models: (Non)aggregation and Interaction

Type of interaction	Intrinsic concepts and variables	Derived (disaggregated/aggregated) concepts and variables	
		Nonisomorphic relations between levels	Isomorphic relations between levels
No interaction	Case 1	Case 4	Case 7
Static	Case 2	Case 5	Case 8
Dynamic	Case 3	Case 6	Case 9

roles (case 7). A high cross-level agreement was also found for the two factors of the family values scale (Hierarchy and Relationships in the Family); yet, the small observed cross-level discrepancies were psychologically salient. Some items in the country-level solution showed secondary loadings, which suggested that the country-level solution did not show the independence of factors that was found at individual level. The authors attributed the difference to "traditionality" as a second-order factor at country level. The latter example illustrates case 4. Cross-level studies of human values as conducted by Schwartz also reflect instances of both case 4 and case 7 (see the chapter by Fontaine). Social axioms (Leung & Bond, this volume) provide another example of essentially nonisomorphic structures at individual and cultural level. The culture-level structure has two factors, labeled dynamic externality and societal cynicism, whereas the individual-level structure has five factors, among which social cynicism. The latter factor corresponds to societal cynicism at country level. Leung and Bond provide a rationale for the dissimilarity of social axioms at both levels. The core of their argument is that social axioms are embedded in different nomological networks of associated constructs at individual and cultural level. It is important to note that these authors employ different terms to describe constructs that do not show cross-level equivalence, because the constructs have a different meaning at both levels. The use of labels with a clear reference to their intrinsic level, such as the distinction between social cynicism and societal cynicism, is an effective safeguard against incorrect cross-level inferences.

Examples of cases 8 and 5 (static interactions in isomorphic and non-isomorphic structures) are reported in educational applications of multilevel models (Stanat & Lüdtke, this volume). Examples of relevant questions in these cells are: What is the influence on student performance of gender composition, average intelligence in the class, or other group characteristics that are derived from individual students? Fischer (this volume) provides examples from the organizational literature where relationships are modeled between work-related variables at individual level and various collective levels in the work organization. Smith and Fischer (this volume) present an analysis of the interaction between culture-level values and individual-level response styles. In the near future we expect to see many applications of this kind of reasoning, in which cultures are defined and measured in terms of characteristics such as individualism-collectivism, that are aggregated from the individual level. Interactions of individual scores and cultural scores are conceptually interesting, because they indicate that similar cultural antecedents do not always lead to similar outcomes. Furthermore, it is important to acknowledge that the presence or absence of these interactions is not merely a matter of armchair theorizing, but that the significance and relevance of these interactions can be tested with the help of standard multilevel statistical packages.

Dynamic interactions in aggregated models (cases 9 and 6) are not popular in cross-cultural empirical research; the present book hardly contains explicit examples. The scarcity of such studies is not surprising because dynamic interactions between (dis)aggregated concepts are hard to study in a quantitative manner. The notion that individual and cultural characteristics dynamically influence each other is more popular in cultural psychology (e.g., Adamopoulos, this volume; Miller, 1997; Shweder, 1990). However, some authors allude to dynamic interactions, and several models could be extended easily to include dynamic interactions (e.g., Oyserman & Uskul, this volume; Nauck, this volume), if data suitable for analysis with multilevel models would be available (see below).

Representations of Aggregated Individual-Level Variables

Aggregation and disaggregation models work with representations of phenomena at intrinsic and derived levels. The chapters in the present book give numerous examples of derived representations, many more of aggregated representations than of disaggregated representations. The various chapters of this book have at least three models that use aggregated representations. The first are *composition models* (Chan, 1998; see also the chapter by Fischer, this volume). These models define cultural characteristics on the basis of aggregated individual-level characteristics such as mean scores or standard deviations (Chan, 1998). For example, individual team members are used to describe the team's climate; scores of individual members are then aggregated to provide measures of the average climate or heterogeneity of the team. These models are in their early stages of development; publications that apply these models often focus on their measurement and statistical aspects. The second kind of aggregated representation is the so-called *citizen score* (Leung & Bond, 2004, this volume). The score is statistically defined as the typical level (e.g., the average score) of a psychological construct among the members of the cultural system, usually a nation. The authors use citizen scores as indicators of the psychological makeup of countries; the scores are correlated with other country-level indicators to gain insight in the nomological network of the psychological variables at country level. We are in the early stages of development of this concept, too. Future studies may address the question of how these citizen scores can yield information about cross-level interactions. The third kind of representation of aggregation is the so-called *virtual denizen* (Adamopoulos, this volume). It is the prototype of a culture, the shared elements that together constitute its core. Adamopoulos defines the concept primarily in cognitive terms, such as schemas, whereas composition models and citizen scores are couched in statistical terms. Still, the correspondence between the concepts is clear; each provides a mapping of lower level, usually psychological characteristics, at a higher level of aggregation.

The three aggregate-level representations of psychological characteristics can be viewed as the successors of old concepts such as modal personality and social representations (see introductory chapter, this volume). The latter concepts have met with criticism and were never widely accepted and applied. It is difficult to foresee whether more modern aggregate-level representations will have a similar destiny. Future studies need to elaborate these models and provide them with richer conceptual underpinnings so that they help to unravel cross-level interactions.

Interim Conclusion

Our overview of multilevel studies, though very short and primarily focused on the contents of this book, leads to several conclusions. First, we can conclude that the distribution of studies reported in the literature across the nine cells of the table is skewed. Second, domains in psychology differ in the type of questions studied. For example, establishing isomorphism across levels is an important focus in the personality domain, but it is hardly addressed in social-psychological research. Third, the literature on multilevel models seems to show certain biases. Interest in dynamic interactions is often more conceptual than empirical, which is not surprising given the considerable research efforts required to study dynamic interactions, such as the use of longitudinal designs. The other types of interaction (static and no interaction) are examined more often in empirical studies. Fourth, in recent models there is more statistical precision and more emphasis on testability. The models that are studied have not changed much over time, but techniques have become more precise. A last point we like to mention is that modern applications of multilevel models may involve more than one cell of Table 15.1. For example, cross-national comparisons of educational achievement typically address both cross-level equivalence of individual characteristics and their aggregations (case 4 and 7) and the interaction of the aggregations with other country variables, such as educational expenditure. It is exactly in such combinations of questions that multilevel models can realize their potential.

PROBLEMS IN APPLICATIONS OF MULTILEVEL MODELS

Multilevel models hold important promise for cross-cultural research. Still, problems can arise in applications of these models. In our view, two main types of problems, described below in more detail, hamper the successful exploitation of the potential of multilevel models. The first is mainly technical and involves the relatively large number of countries that is needed to conduct multilevel analysis. The second involves the poor link between conceptual and statistical advancements in the field.

Sample Size and Multilevel Models

The most important limiting factor in applying multilevel models is the sample size at the highest level; in cross-cultural research this is usually the number of cultures involved. The sample size at the level of cultures has far-reaching implications for the kind of analysis that can be conducted in cross-cultural research. It is instructive to take a closer look at the two approaches described by Selig, Card, and Little (this volume) to deal with multilevel issues. The first, multiple group mean and covariance structures (MACS; e.g., Browne & Arminger, 1995), focuses on the comparison of means across cultures or on within-culture relations between observed or latent variables across cultures. MACS can be used when the number of countries or cultures studied is relatively small. The second approach, multilevel structural equation modeling (ML SEM; e.g., Hox, 2002), can be used to address the multilevel equivalence of constructs. ML SEM presupposes a larger number of countries in the dataset. Common rules for required sample sizes in psychology do not apply to country-level analyses, as data at this level tend to be more reliable and stable than individual-level data. Nevertheless, it is clear that studies with a handful of units at the highest level (say, five or six countries) cannot meaningfully apply the sophisticated statistical machinery of multilevel modeling. Selig et al. mention a sample size of 20 countries as the minimum number.

The distinction between the more direct approach to multilevel equivalence that is used in studies involving many countries (ML SEM) and the more indirect approach necessitated by a small sample size at country level (MACS) has major implications for the analysis and interpretation of cross-cultural differences. MACS does not address the question of whether individual- and country-level differences can be described in the same way, because it does not compare latent variables across levels but across countries. ML SEM can compare variables across both levels and countries. As a consequence, ML SEM can address the issue of cross-level equivalence in an adequate manner. However, interpreting the meaning of individual and cultural differences does not only matter in studies involving many countries. There can be a shift in meaning also when in a two-country comparison individual scores on a target variable are aggregated to represent a country's standing on the target variable. Such a shift in meaning is likely to go unnoticed.

In studies with small numbers of countries only conventional methods are available to address aggregation issues. Such methods require that variables accounting for cross-cultural differences in a dependent variable have been measured at individual level; these explanatory constructs are called context variables by Poortinga and Van de Vijver (1987) because they are meant to explain contextual (cultural) variation. No conceptual restrictions are imposed on these variables. Any variable that can explain cross-cultural differences in some target variable is a potentially useful context variable. Examples include response sets and number of years of education. These variables, measured at individual level, can serve as possible candidates to explain observed cross-cultural score differences in target variables, such as personality or cognitive test scores. An analysis of covariance or regression analysis with the context variable(s) as covariate(s) can account statistically for cross-cultural differences that are not due to the target construct. Thus, context variables are confounding variables in the sense that a statistical control of these variables may reveal that cross-cultural differences in target variables become smaller or may even disappear altogether. This approach is one of the standard tools to "unpackage" culture (Bond & Van de Vijver, in press; Poortinga & Van de Vijver, 1987; Whiting, 1976).

Context variables can also refer to constructs that are located at the cultural level. Suppose that we are interested in the influence of immigration policies on acculturation outcomes of immigrant groups in two countries. Immigration policy is a country-level construct that does not show differences at the individual level within countries. A country comparison of mean scores on acculturation outcomes is inadequate to test the influence of immigration policies if only a few countries are involved in the comparisons; differences in immigration policy are confounded with numerous other differences of the countries and ethnic groups. This problem is sometimes addressed by "psychologizing" the context variable, in which case attitudes toward immigration policies become the context variable. Technically speaking, the disaggregation of a culture-level to an individual-level variable ensures that the study design deals with one level only, thereby enabling a statistical evaluation of the influence of perceived immigration policies. From a conceptual point of view, however, this transformation introduces an ambiguity. Perceived immigration policies are undoubtedly influenced by actual policies, but they may also be influenced by acculturation orientations and indeed by acculturation outcomes. More successful immigrants may prefer more lenient immigration policies. It can be concluded that different approaches can be adopted to explore or validate differences at country level if relatively few countries are involved in a study. Still, the difference with a direct test of cross-level equivalence in studies involving many cultures should be acknowledged. A context-variables approach tests specific interpretations of cross-cultural differences. We find in practical applications of this approach that context variables can often explain only part of the cross-cultural differences. Hence, the cross-cultural differences are only partly understood.

Linking Statistical and Conceptual Multilevel Models

Conceptual and statistical developments in multilevel models are often loosely linked. First, complex models of environment–organism interactions, such as the ecocultural framework, lack precision and testability. As a consequence, the adequacy of such a framework is difficult to evaluate. Tests of elements of the framework tend to be seen as support for the whole framework. For example, cross-cultural differences in cognitive styles (higher scores of nomadic hunters on field independence tests and higher scores of sedentary agriculturalists on field dependence; Berry, 1976) have been interpreted as support for the ecocultural framework. However, it is virtually impossible to design a study that would provide a comprehensive test of the entire framework; advanced conceptual models are usually difficult to "translate" in empirical designs and data.

Second, advanced statistical models cannot be easily linked to conceptual models either. This relative independence of conceptual and statistical developments impedes progress in the field. For example, various techniques have become available in the last decades to test multilevel equivalence, but we do not have a theoretical rationale that indicates when equivalence should be expected. Much of the current research seems to focus on isomorphism because of its parsimony (i.e., the same concepts and theories can be applied at multiple levels), but Adamopoulos (this volume) argues that isomorphism is the exception rather than the rule in an open-system theory of multilevel structures; levels tend to show their own dynamics. As a consequence, there may be little reason to expect that constructs used to describe individual differences (e.g., personality traits) also will describe country differences in personality. If traits are influenced by different factors at individual and cultural level a lack of isomorphism will be the result. The merits of the reasons for and against isomorphism are not easy to evaluate; yet, it is clear that isomorphism cannot be treated as the default case and that isomorphism also requires an explanation.

Lucas and Diener conclude on the basis of extensive evidence that at a national level, subjective well-being measures may have a similar meaning at individual level. Nevertheless, if well-being is influenced by cultural factors, isomorphism of well-being at individual and cultural level is not self-evident. There is a long tradition of research showing cross-cultural differences in mother–child interactions starting at a very early age (Super & Harkness, 1986; Keller, 2007). Most understanding of individual functioning in cultural context makes it almost inescapable that there should be differential shaping of traits by differential systems of rewarding and sanctioning. However, we are largely unable to model the interaction of individual and cultural factors in specific cases. Our current theories and models of interaction lack the detail and specificity that is needed to expand our horizon.

In summary, the transition from statistical tests of multilevel equivalence to theory about equivalence is often problematic; the step from advanced conceptual models of relations between individual and cultural phenomena to manageable statistical designs is equally problematic. Ideally, analyses of multilevel structural equivalence are to be informed by substantive theories specifying where to expect complete or partial isomorphism and where isomorphism will be largely absent. Progress in this direction is critically dependent on data sets including samples from many cultural groups needed to make sufficiently accurate estimates of interactions between levels as well as more precise theories about cross-level interactions.

PROMISING DOMAINS OF APPLICATION OF MULTILEVEL PERSPECTIVES

Not all areas of cross-cultural research are equally troubled by the unevenness in conceptual and methodological developments that was described in the previous section. There are various lines of research in which the link between conceptual and statistical modeling can be made closer. In this section we describe a number of such promising areas in cross-cultural psychology, mainly based on studies that are discussed in the preceding chapters.

Several large-scale educational studies are mapping the nature and size of cross-national differences (cf. Stanat & Lüdtke, this volume). These studies call for the application of advanced multilevel statistical tools; in fact the statistical innovations in the field of multilevel research have been largely driven by research in education (e.g., Goldstein, 1987; Härnqvist, 1978). Level-oriented analysis techniques as implemented in HLM (Raudenbush & Bryk, 2002) and MLwin (Goldstein, 2003) can evaluate the relative size of individual, school, district, and country differences and contribute to insights in which antecedents can statistically account for the differences at supraindividual level. The possibility that researchers could deal with nested data structures (and their complex error structures) has enabled new studies which have increased our insights. At the same time, international comparisons of educational achievement are often fact-finding enterprises that focus on assessing the size of the cross-national differences rather than on the antecedents of these differences. So far much of this research is based on simple input–output models and the theoretical depth of the studies tends to be limited. Cross-cultural educational studies offer scope for further conceptual developments. The previous decades of research have generated numerous models of teaching and learning that can be extended to multilevel models. What is needed in this area is an extension of these theories into testable multilevel models. Stanat and Lüdtke provide examples of this approach in the second part of their chapter.

Social psychology and personality are other examples of promising domains. Several chapters that deal with topics from social psychology and personality show how the explicit introduction of multiple levels impacts on the conceptualization of commonly studied concepts. Yamaguchi et al. (this volume) show how control orientations can differ at individual and cultural level. Individuals can achieve control either by personal action or by relying on significant others or groups that can help to establish control. Control is a multilevel concept in this line of argument, because it combines personal and group characteristics. Oyserman and Uskul (this volume) present two partially overlapping and complementary frameworks of individualism at the individual and the societal level. The need for two representations underlines the complexities of theorizing on culture–behavior relationships in a comprehensive manner; these authors, too, point to the need of a simultaneous study of individual and cultural features in understanding a particular construct. Historically, the blind assignment of countries to either individualism or collectivism is a notorious example of inadequate dealing with multilevel issues. Hofstede (1980) recognized the importance of distinguishing between levels and limited his findings to the national level; individualism-collectivism is a country-level characteristic in his work. The subsequent distinction between individual-level and culture-level concepts of individualism by Triandis, Leung, Villareal, and Clack (1985) strengthened the notion of level. It seems only a matter of time before such multilevel analyses of individualism and collectivism will be reported in the literature.

The scope for multilevel analysis in cross-cultural research is demonstrated convincingly in the chapters that report empirical findings. As mentioned, in the chapters by Lucas and Diener (this volume) and by McCrae and Terracciano (this volume) evidence of isomorphism is found. In a multilevel analysis of social axioms Leung and Bond (this volume) report isomorphism for one dimension, but differences in the individual-level structure and the culture-level structure for other dimensions.

Industrial and organizational psychology (cf. Fischer, this volume) is a domain in psychology where further conceptual and statistical sophistication are likely to go hand in hand. There is currently a strong interest in the use of aggregated and disaggregated concepts and various models have been formulated to deal with the interrelations of concepts at various levels. As Fischer describes, enough empirical evidence has been collected in this domain to generate and test multilevel hypotheses, such as the influence of individual value homogeneity and heterogeneity on organizational culture.

Another potentially rich domain of application of multilevel models is acculturation research (Nauck, this volume). Traditionally, acculturation has been studied by different disciplines, each using a fairly strict perspective, such as demographics, sociology, and cross-cultural psychology. As Nauck's chapter shows, acculturation issues have a strong multilevel component. Psychologists are usually interested in individual-level outcomes such as knowledge of the language of the host country and mental health, while the distal data with a bearing on these outcomes are usually nonpsychological and involve cultural distance, ethnic vitality, and immigration policies. As explained before, it is possible to "psychologize" these variables by examining the perception of the cultural distance by participants. Such an approach can be sensible if only a single group of immigrants is studied who by definition all have the same standing on the antecedent variables. However, a study in which a sufficient number of immigrant groups are included to enable multilevel analysis offers a much better approach to address the influence of the antecedent variables. We expect to see a growing number of acculturation studies that use multilevel approaches such as proposed by Nauck.

Some promising areas in cross-cultural multilevel analysis reach across content domains. The study of response styles is a good example. Although response styles play a role in monocultural studies, their influence tends to be more salient but also more elusive in cross-cultural studies. Cross-cultural studies have shown that response styles can act as filters that distort the researcher's view of the underlying reality of the participant (e.g., providing incorrect self-presentations). However, this view is insufficient for the understanding of the origins of cross-cultural differences in response styles. For example, the view that social desirability leads to an incorrect self-presentation cannot explain the negative relationship between social desirability and the level of affluence of a country (Van Hemert, Van de Vijver, Poortinga, & Georgas, 2002). Smith and Fischer (this volume) show how multilevel statistical models can help us to compare the meaning of response styles at individual and cultural level. Applications of these models can facilitate understanding of the contingencies of response styles, such as which individuals and countries are likely to show more response styles and which psychological instruments are more susceptible to response styles.

Over the last decade a new research paradigm has been emerging in cross-cultural social psychology. The influence of broad cultural constructs, such as individualism-collectivism, is measured in a detailed manner in specific domains of psychological functioning, quite often among acculturating groups. In studies using priming of bicultural individuals, who are often Asian Americans, respondents are presented with elements of either an American or an Asian context in order to trigger their respective cultural frames. It is investigated to what extent priming of immigrants with symbols of either their culture of origin or their culture of settlement leads to different psychological responses or to what extent bicultural individuals can switch their cultural frames (e.g., Benet-Martinez, Leu, Lee, & Morris, 2002; Verkuyten & Pouliasi, 2002). In these studies distant cultural factors are related to proximal consequences. From the present perspective, frame-switching studies are good examples of multilevel studies, even though they have not used the statistical machinery of multilevel models. We expect that microlevel analyses, as conducted in cross-cultural developmental science and in acculturation research, will become increasingly important. It may be too much to ask for microlevel studies with such extensive data sets that multilevel statistical analysis can be applied. Nevertheless, multilevel analyses and the findings they will lead to are likely also to have an effect on conceptualizations of microlevel studies.

CONCLUSION

Further developments of multilevel models will come from three sources: conceptual developments, methodological developments, and their further integration. Most of this chapter has dealt with conceptual issues of multilevel research. A multilevel perspective can help researchers to make explicit how they see the relationships between behavior and culture, the two levels that are of primary interest in most cross-cultural research. The various forms of interaction, summarized in Table 15.1, can lead to different families of theories; they can also help researchers to express their ideas in a common language. For example, the culture-comparative and cultural tradition, which constituted a major dichotomy in the 1990s, look much less controversial if they are seen as different cases in Table 15.1, with the cultural approach emphasizing dynamic interactions and the culture-comparative approach emphasizing static interactions between levels.

Further statistical and methodological refinements of multilevel models can be expected, but the major technical problems of estimation have been solved. New developments will focus on broadening the scope of models and addressing relations between multilevel and other statistical models rather than on novel statistical techniques. Moreover, it can be expected that statistical software to deal with multilevel models becomes more widely available. In addition to dedicated software such as HLM (http://www.ssicentral.com/hlm/index.html) and MLwin (http://www.mlwin.com), programs for multilevel models are now also available in major statistical packages such as SAS (http://www.sas.com) and SPSS (http://

www.spss.com). Furthermore, there is an increase in the number of programs for structural equation modeling that have modules for dealing with multilevel structural equivalence, such as AMOS (http://www.spss.com/amos/?source=homepage&hpzone=tech), LISREL (http://www.ssi-central.com/lisrel/index.html#lisrel), and M*plus* (http://www.statmodel.com). Growing numbers of researchers will have access to the statistical software needed to compute the parameters of multilevel models.

The third locus of potential development, the further integration of conceptual and statistical models, is probably the most promising area, but it is also the most difficult one to realize. It requires a close interaction of substantive and methodological kinds of knowledge. Experiences of the past decades do not make us optimistic about this kind of development. It is uncommon that experts from both domains meet in order to join forces to deal with multilevel issues. This may be due to some extent to the focus on slightly different questions in the substantive and methodological literature. A more direct confrontation is necessary of questions in which the substantive researcher is interested and questions that can be answered by the statistician. Answering these new questions will advance our insights in level issues. For example, advanced statistical tools can be used to address the question of how cultural knowledge varies as a function of acculturation level.

The three kinds of developments may show their own dynamics. The current state of the field is still uneven. An emphasis on the development of either conceptual models or methodological models is unlikely to overcome this unevenness. It would be regrettable if the conceptual and methodological models were further developed in the independent ways that have happened in the past. It is difficult to see how we can make real achievements in this area if we focus on one kind of development only. The chapter by Yamaguchi et al. gives an interesting example of how we can proceed in the development and application of multilevel models. The chapter starts from current theory on control and extends the notion of individual control by also including collective control. Hypotheses with a clear multilevel structure are derived from this model. Multilevel approaches can then be applied to simultaneously examine individual- and group-level differences in control.

Multilevel models were already an area of much interest among our intellectual ancestors. The question of similarity of personality at individual and cultural level was already addressed in the 1930s. Compared to these early researchers, we have methodologically more sophisticated tools and we have a larger empirical database to rely on. As a consequence, the answers we provide are less speculative and more empirically based. Still, we are still relatively far from overcoming the dualism between the individual and the culture. An adequate combination of conceptual and statistical advances in multilevel models may help our understanding of the intricate relationship between individual and cultural factors.

REFERENCES

Baron, R., & Kenny, D. A. (1986). The moderator-mediator variable distinction in social psychological research: Conceptual, strategic, and statistical considerations. *Journal of Personality and Social Psychology, 51,* 1173–1182.

Benet-Martinez, V., Leu, J., Lee, F., & Morris, M. W. (2002). Negotiating biculturalism: Cultural frame switching in biculturals with oppositional versus compatible cultural identities. *Journal of Cross-Cultural Psychology, 33,* 492–516.

Berry, J. W. (1976). *Human ecology and cognitive style: Comparative studies in cultural and psychological adaptation.* New York: Sage/Halsted.

Bond, M. H., & Van de Vijver, F. J. R. (in press). Making scientific sense of cultural differences in psychological outcomes: Unpackaging the magnum mysterium. In D. Matsumoto & F. Van de Vijver (Eds.), *Cross-cultural research methods.* Oxford: Oxford University Press.

Bourhis, R. Y., Moïse, L. C., Pereault, S., & Senécal, S. (1997). Towards an interactive acculturation model: A social psychological approach. *International Journal of Psychology, 32,* 369–386.

Bronfenbrenner, U. (1979). *The ecology of human development: Experiments by nature and design.* Cambridge, MA: Harvard University Press.

Browne, M. W., & Arminger, G. (1995). Specification and estimation of mean- and covariance-structure models. In G. Arminger, C. C. Clogg, & M. E. Sobal (Eds.), *Handbook of statistical modeling for the social and behavioral sciences* (pp.185–241). New York: Plenum.

Chan, D. (1998). Functional relations among constructs in the same content domain at different levels of analysis: A typology of compositional models. *Journal of Applied Psychology, 83,* 234–246.

Goldstein, H. (1987). *Multilevel models in educational and social research.* New York: Oxford University Press.

Goldstein, H. (2003). *Multilevel statistical models* (3rd ed.). London: Arnold.

Härnqvist, K. (1978). Primary mental abilities at collective and individual levels. *Journal of Educational Psychology, 70,* 706–716.

Hofstede, G. (1980). *Culture's consequences: International differences in work-related values.* Beverly Hills, CA: Sage.

Hox, J. J. (2002). *Multilevel analysis: Techniques and applications.* Mahwah, NJ: Lawrence Erlbaum.

Jahoda, G. (1982). *Psychology and anthropology: A psychological perspective.* London: Academic Press.

Keller, H. (2007). *Cultures of infancy.* Mahwah, NJ: Erlbaum.

Leung, K., & Bond, M. H. (2004). Social axioms: A model of social beliefs in multicultural perspective. In M. P. Zanna (Ed.), *Advances in experimental social psychology* (Vol. 36, pp. 119–197). San Diego, CA: Elsevier Academic Press).

Lonner, W. J., & Adamopoulos, J. (1997). Culture as antecedent to behavior. In J. W. Berry, Y. H. Poortinga, & J, Pandey (Eds.), *Handbook of cross-cultural psychology: Vol. 1. Theory and method* (pp. 43–83). Boston, MA: Allyn & Bacon.

Miller, J. G. (1997). Theoretical issues in cultural psychology. In J. W. Berry, Y. H. Poortinga, & J. Pandey (Eds.), *Handbook of cross-cultural psychology: Vol. 1. Theory and method* (pp. 85–128). Boston: Allyn & Bacon.

Poortinga, Y. H., & Van de Vijver, F. J. R. (1987). Explaining cross-cultural differences: Bias analysis and beyond. *Journal of Cross-Cultural Psychology, 18,* 259–282.

Raudenbush, S. W., & Bryk, A. S. (2002). *Hierarchical linear models* (2nd ed.). Newbury Park, CA: Sage.

Shweder, R. A. (1990). Cultural psychology—What is it? In J. W. Stigler, R. A. Shweder, & G. Herdt (Eds.), *Cultural psychology: Essays on comparative human development* (pp. 1–43). New York: Cambridge University Press.

Segall, M. H., Campbell, D. T., & Herskovits, M. J. (1966). *The influence of culture on visual perception.* Indianapolis, IN: Bobs-Merrill.

Super, C. M., & Harkness, S. (1986). The development niche: A conceptualization at the interface of child and culture. *International Journal of Behavioural Development, 9,* 545–569.

Triandis, H. C., Leung, K., Villareal, M. J., & Clack, F. (1985). Allocentric versus idiocentric tendencies: Convergent and discriminant validation. *Journal of Research in Personality, 19,* 395–415

Van de Vijver, F. J. R., & Leung, K. (1997). *Methods and data analysis for cross-cultural research.* Newbury Park, CA: Sage.

Van Hemert, D. A., Van de Vijver, F. J. R., Poortinga, Y. H., & Georgas, J. (2002). Structural and functional equivalence of the Eysenck Personality Questionnaire within and between countries. *Personality and Individual Differences, 33,* 1229–1249.

Verkuyten, M., & Pouliasi, K. (2002). Biculturalism among older children: Cultural frame switching, attributions, self-identification, and attitudes. *Journal of Cross-Cultural Psychology, 33,* 596–609.

Whiting, B. B. (1976). The problem of the packaged variable. In K. Riegel & J. Meacham (Eds.), *The developing individual in a changing world* (Vol. 1, pp. 303–309). The Hague: Mouton.

Author Index

Subject Index